Good luck @ School
regards,
Tom Michael.

FOOT ORTHOSES

and Other Forms of Conservative Foot Care

FOOT ORTHOSES

and Other Forms of Conservative Foot Care

Thomas C. Michaud, D.C.

Newton, Massachusetts

*Additional copies of this book may be
purchased from Dr. Thomas Michaud:
Phone: (617) 969-2225
Fax: (617) 527-5927
E-mail: Tommichaud@aol.com*

Copyright © 1997
Thomas C. Michaud
517 Washington Street
Newton Massachusetts, 02158, USA

Accurate indications, adverse reactions, and dosage schedules for drugs are provided in this
book, but it is possible that they may change. The reader is urged to review the package information data of the manufacturers of the medications mentioned.

Printed in the United States of America

Library of Congress Cataloging in Publication Data

Michaud, Thomas C.
    Foot orthoses and other forms of conservative foot care / Thomas
  C. Michaud
        p.   cm.
    Includes index.
    ISBN 0-683-05974-2
    1. Foot—Abnormalities—Treatment.   2. Gait disorders—Treatment.
  3. Orthopedic apparatus.   I. Title.
    [DNLM: 1. Foot.   2. Foot Deformities—rehabilitation.   3. Gait–
  –physiology.   4. Orthotic Devices. WE 26 M622f]
  RD756.42.M5 1993
  617.5′85043—dc20
  DNLM/DLC
  for Library of Congress   92-48944
                                                   CIP

            93 94 95 96 97
          1 2 3 4 5 6 7 8 9 10

ADDENDUM

Since the initial printing of this book in 1993, several important articles have been published that deserve discussion. First and foremost is the repeated observation by McPoil and Cornwall (1,2) that the subtalar joint, contrary to the majority of previously published data, remains almost fully pronated throughout the entire midstance period. Because there is little doubt regarding the validity of their observations, the graphs and text throughout this entire book have been modified to reflect this new information.

A somewhat controversial off-shoot of this information is that some researchers have suggested that because the subtalar joint does not intersect with its neutral position prior to heel lift, orthotics should not be made from neutral position impressions. This directly conflicts with statements by Weed et al. (3) as they claim that the rearfoot post on an orthotic should place the subtalar joint in its neutral position and a four degree biplanar grind should be added to allow the subtalar joint to pronate during the contact period. As stated on pages 209-211 of this book, the technique described by Weed et al. (3) is dangerous as it does not allow for the range of subtalar pronation necessary for adequate shock absorption and it blocks the normal coupled movements of calcaneal eversion - tibial internal rotation normally occurring during the contact period. These combined actions may produce iatrogenic injury in various locations along the entire kinetic chain (particularly the knee).

This is not to say that neutral position impressions should be abandoned. On the contrary, this technique is the only method capable of capturing flexible forefoot deformities and it gives the practitioner a picture of the foot in its most stable position: the subtalar joint is maximally congruent and, perhaps more importantly, the head of the talus is firmly stabilized in a closed-packed position in the navicular acetabulum.

An extremely important concept regarding the manufacture of orthotics from neutral position impressions is that they should never hold the foot in the neutral position during stance phase. When made properly, the positive neutral model is modified by adding a specific amount of plaster to the medial arch area (laboratories typically add 1/4 inch of plaster but any amount may be added in order to allow for a specific range of midtarsal motion). By lowering the medial arch a specific amount, the practitioner controls the exact distance that the talus will adduct and plantarflex during the contact and midstance periods (i.e., because the foot is in its neutral position early in the contact period [4,5,6], the lowered arch allows the talus to pronate a precise range from the neutral position). This action is essential for adequate shock absorption and to allow for the storage and eventual return of energy associated with deflection of the midtarsal joint. Exact control of the talar head is extremely important as recent research demonstrates that of all the joints in the mid and rearfoot, the talonavicular joint undergoes the most significant changes during weight-bearing; i.e., on average, the talonavicular joint moves 9.4 degrees while the talotibial and subtalar joints move only 5.2 and 4.4 degrees respectively (7). Furthermore, O'Malley et al. (8) recently demonstrated that the talonavicular joint exhibits marked control over the subtalar and calcaneocuboid joints. This is consistent with the observation by Mann (9) that talonavicular fusion markedly limits subtalar motion due to coupling between the joints.

In addition to allowing for adequate midtarsal motion, an orthotic should also be manufactured to allow the subtalar joint to pronate a minimum of 6-8 degrees from the neutral position. This is accomplished by determining the degree of rearfoot varus by adding subtalar varum and lower leg varum and then subtracting either 6 or 8 degrees from this number (see page 211). In situations where the rearfoot angle is less than 6 degrees, the orthotic should be posted at 0 degrees and excessive pronation would be controlled by the orthotic shell. This posting technique allows the practitioner to design an orthotic in which the talonavicular and subtalar joints pronate a specific range from the neutral position present during the early contact period. Even though it is made from a neutral position impression, the orthotic does not hold the foot in this position as it blocks only excessive pronation, allowing the range necessary for midtarsal deflection and shock absorption.

An important consideration regarding the research demonstrating that the subtalar joint is pronated during heel lift is that the majority of it is based upon two-dimensional imaging techniques. While this approach allows for accurate evaluation of joint interactions during the contact and midstance periods, it is unable to capture movements occurring during the propulsive period. Fortunately, the technical difficulties associated with evaluating joint motions occurring after heel lift have been resolved with the more advanced 3-D imaging techniques. In one of the more interesting 3-D evaluations, Nigg et al. (4) demonstrated that although the subtalar joint is pronated during midstance, it manages to supinate approximately 10 degrees beyond neutral during the propulsive period. This is consistent with the windlass mechanism proposed by Hicks (10). Perhaps the most surprising observations in the study by Nigg et al. (4) is that the degree of rearfoot motion present during stance phase does not correlate with arch height (i.e. low arched individuals often pronate through small ranges while many high arched individuals are hyperpronators) and that the transfer of calcaneal eversion to internal tibial rotation increases as arch height increases. This explains why individuals with cavus feet so often present with knee and hip problems. Along this same line of research, Sommer et al. (11) demonstrated that sectioning the lateral ankle ligaments increased the transfer of calcaneal eversion to internal tibial rotation while cutting the deltoid ligament decreased the transfer of these motions.

Although the observation by Nigg et al. (4) that the subtalar joint supinates beyond neutral is consistent with another 3-D evaluation (5), it is at odds with a 3-D study demonstrating continued subtalar pronation throughout propulsion (12). More recently, Siegel et al. (13) incorporated a new method of 3-D evaluation and found that the position the rearfoot assumes during stance is dependent upon the individual's foot type: the uncompensated rearfoot varus foot type strikes with the heel inverted and pronates slightly to an aligned rearfoot-lower leg position and then supinates approximately 5 degrees during propulsion. This is in contrast to the hypermobile pronated foot that makes ground contact with the rearfoot-lower leg aligned and pronates excessively during contact and midstance. Although this foot type begins supinating during propulsion, it is unable to get to a point within 5 degrees of neutral.

The study by Siegel et al. (13) emphasizes the need for quality 3-D evaluations in which individuals are categorized by osseous alignment patterns in the lower extremity (e.g., rearfoot varus, external tibial torsion, etc.) and the ranges of motion available to specific joints (particularly the first ray, talonavicular and subtalar joints).

It should be emphasized that decisions concerning orthotic fabrication should not be based upon osseous alignment of the foot alone. This information should be coupled with a complete structural evaluation that includes assessment of bony alignment, strength, flexibility and joint ranges of motion present along the entire kinetic chain. The overprescription of orthotics based upon a limited evaluation of subtalar and forefoot alignment has led McPoil and Hunt (14) to develop a "soft tissue stress model" as a basis for evaluation and treatment of foot injuries. In this model, a management scheme is developed to identify the specific tissue being stressed, evaluate factors contributing to the injury and, if symptoms are the result of a biomechanical problem, initiate a treatment that emphasizes decreasing tissue stress. This may be accomplished by activity modification, using soft tissue techniques to enhance flexibility, modalities to accelerate healing and exercises to improve strength and endurance. Excessive pronation, when present, may be controlled via modifications in shoe gear, stock arch supports, paste-in techniques and, if necessary, a functional orthotic. The authors emphasize that "foot orthoses should be a small part of the treatment plan rather than the entire emphasis of treatment" (14).

Perhaps the most intensively studied subject concerning lower extremity biomechanics relates to the reproducibility of various measuring techniques. It has been recently demonstrated that weight-bearing measurements of foot alignment and motion are easier to perform and provide more consistent data than off-weight-bearing measurements (15). For example, various researchers have found high levels of interrater reliability for the standing subtalar joint neutral position (15), standing foot angle (16), navicular drop test (15), medial talonavicular bulge (17), static calcaneal stance position (15) and the rearfoot- lower leg angle present during single leg stance (18). (This last angle is important as it measures the maximum degree of rearfoot eversion available during walking [2].)

It should be stressed that off-weight-bearing measurements should not be abandoned as Diamond et al. (19) demonstrated that experienced practitioners were able to obtain acceptable levels of interrater reliability for determining the off-weight-bearing neutral subtalar joint position while Smith-Oricchio and Harris (18) found moderate levels of interrater reliability for that angle. More recently, Sommer and Vallentyne (16) demonstrated that qualitative measurements of the off-weight-bearing neutral subtalar position had an acceptable interrater reliability (with subtalar varum being associated with a past history of medial tibial stress syndrome) while Astrom and Arvidson (19) demonstrated that an experienced examiner is capable of taking extremely reliable off-weight-bearing measurements (i.e., ICC averaging .91).

This is not to say that all off-weight-bearing measurements are valid as several studies have demonstrated that both experienced and inexperienced practitioners are unable to accurately reproduce off-weight-bearing measurements of subtalar inversion/eversion (18,20,21). Because of this, these measurements should be avoided. (Besides, Lattanza et al. [23] conclusively demonstrated that off-weight-bearing measurements of subtalar motion do not reflect ranges available during weight-bearing.)

In defense of these measurements, Garbalosa et al. (23) found extremely high levels of interrater reliability when evaluating off-weight-bearing ranges of subtalar inversion/eversion. Unfortunately, unlike the previously mentioned studies (18, 20, 21), Garbalosa et al. (23) did not erase the lower leg and rearfoot bisection lines used between repeat measurements. Because of this, their conclusions regarding interrater reliability must be considered invalid.

The final topic to be discussed relates to the actual prevalence of the forefoot varus deformity. Depending upon the source, the percentage of the population possessing this foot type ranges from 8 to 87 percent. This disparity is important as inappropriate treatment of a neutral forefoot with a forefoot varus post may lead to iatrogenic injury of the first metatarsophalangeal joint as it could limit first ray plantarflexion during propulsion (see figure 2.20 on page 37).

As mentioned in this text, the primary reasons for the overreporting of forefoot varus deformities are the failure to identify functional forefoot varus deformities (e.g., a functionally dorsiflexed first ray is often mistakenly identified as a forefoot varus deformity) and the continued reliance on the outdated method of determining subtalar neutrality by measuring off-weight-bearing inversion/eversion ranges (24).

As already discussed, these measurements are extremely unreliable and, even if they were valid, the ideal inversion/eversion ratio of 2:1 as described by Root et al. (24) rarely occurs. For example, in a recent study evaluating subtalar inversion/eversion ratios as compared to the palpated subtalar neutral position, Astrom and Arvidson (19) found the ratio closer to 2.8 to 1. In perhaps the most detailed study evaluating the relationship between subtalar range of motion and the palpated neutral position, Bailey et al. (25) used tomograms to evaluate lines parallel to the tibial plafond and the superior aspect of the calcaneus while the subtalar joint was maintained in neutral and when maximally inverted and everted. These researchers concluded that although on average, subtalar neutrality occurred when the calcaneus was inverted 36.2 percent from the maximally everted position, individual variation allowed for a neutral subtalar position with inversion/eversion ratios ranging from 19:1 to 1:2.3. Because very few people were close to the suggested 2:1 ratio, Bailey et al. (25) concluded that the range of motion method for determining subtalar neutrality is invalid.

Putting all this aside, another reason to abandon the 2:1 movement ratio is that, as recently demonstrated by Nigg et al. (26), inversion/eversion ratios vary between men and women and change over time. In fact, the range of eversion in women was particularly sensitive to changes with age as young women (ages 20-39) averaged 17.2 degrees of eversion while the older group (ages 70-79) averaged 11.4 degrees.

Needless to say, such variation will significantly effect the ideal 2:1 movement ratio and, as such, this technique should be abandoned.

In closing, although the number of quality scientific studies related to lower extremity biomechanics is rapidly increasing, it is clear that there is still much to learn. Future studies, in addition to identifying the most accurate in-office methods for evaluating shank rotation during stance phase, will hopefully resolve the controversy surrounding various casting techniques by evaluating the differences, if any, in patient satisfaction, ability to control motion (particularly talonavicular) and return rates for orthotics made from off-, semi-, and full-weight-bearing impressions. Another important project would be to perform 3-D evaluations of various foot types to determine how articular interactions may be modified with different forms of conservative care; e.g., orthotics, strengthening exercises, shoe gear, gait modifications, etc. It would also be interesting to categorize a large number of high school or college athletes according to osseous alignment and range of motion and then follow them for several years to determine if specific alignment patterns are associated with specific injuries (i.e., Do the "classic signs and symptoms" described in this text for each foot type actually occur?). This study could also be performed with some individuals receiving prophylactic orthotic intervention in order to evaluate the efficacy of orthotics in preventing injuries. It is only by critically evaluating many of the currently accepted beliefs that improved methods of evaluation and treatment will come to light.

REFERENCES

1) McPoil T, Cornwall, MW. Relationship between neutral subtalar joint position and the pattern of rearfoot motion during walking. Foot Ankle Int 1994; 15 (3): 141-145.

2) McPoil T, Cornwall MW. Relationship between three static angles of the rearfoot and the pattern of rearfoot motion during walking. J Orthop Sports Phys Ther 1996; 23(6): 370-375.

3) Weed JH, Ratliff FD, Ross SA. Biplanar grind for rearfoot posts on functional orthoses. J Am Podiatr Assoc 1978; 69(1): 35.

4) Nigg, BM, Cole GK, Nachbauer W. Effects of arch height of the foot on angular motion of the lower extremities in running. J Biomechanics 1993; 26(8): 909-916.

5) Areblad M, Nigg BM, Ekstand, J. Olsson I, Ekstrom H. Three dimensional measurements of rearfoot motion during running. J Biomechanics 1990; 23(9): 933-940.

6) Soutas-Little RW, Beavis GC, Verstraete MC, Markus, TL. Analysis of foot motion during running using a joint coordinate system. Med Sci Sports Exercise 1987; 19(3): 285-293.

7) Kitaoka HB, Lunenberg A, Ping Luo Z, An KN. Kinematics of the normal arch of the foot and ankle under physiologic loading. Foot Ankle Int 1995; 16(8): 492-499.

8) O'Malley MJ, Deland JT, Lee KT. Selective hindfoot arthrodesis for the treatment of adult acquired flatfoot deformity: an in vitro study. Foot Ankle Int 1995; 16(7): 411-417.

9) Mann RA. Flatfoot in adults. In: Surgery of the Foot and Ankle, Ed 2. Mann RA, Coughlin M (eds.), St. Louis: Plenum, 1992: 757-784.

10) Hicks JH. The mechanics of the foot II. The plantar aponeurosis and the arch. J Anatomy 1954; 88:23-31.

11) Sommer C, Hinterman B, Nigg BM, vanderBogart A. Influence of ankle ligaments on tibial rotation: an in vitro study. Foot Ankle Int 1996; 17(2): 79-84.

12) Engsberg JR, Andrews JG. Kinematic analysis of the talocalcaneal/talocrural joint during running. Med Sci Sports Exercise 1987; 19(3): 275-284.

13) Siegal KL, Kepple TM, O'Connell PG, Gerber LH, Stanhope SJ. A technique to evaluate foot function during stance phase of gait. Foot Ankle Int 1995; 16(12) 764-770.

14) McPoil TG, Hunt GC. Evaluation and management of foot and ankle disorders: present problems and future directions. J Orthop Sports Phys Ther 1996; 21(6): 381-388.

15) Sell KE, Verity TM, Warrell TW, Pease BJ, Wigglesworth J. Two measurement techniques for assessing subtalar joint position: a reliability study. J Orthop Sports Phys Ther 1994; 19(3): 162-167.

16) Sommer HM, Vallentyne SW. Effect of foot posture on the incidence of medial tibial stress syndrome. Med Sci Sports Exercise 1995; 27(6): 800-804.

17) Jonson SR, Gross MT. Intraexaminer reliability, interexaminer reliability and normal values for nine lower extremity skeletal measures. J Orthop Sports Phys Ther 1996; 23(1): 70-71.

18) Smith-Oricchio K, Harris BA. Interrater reliability of subtalar neutral, calcaneal inversion and eversion. J Orthop Sports Phys Ther 1990; 12(1): 10-15.

19) Astrom M, Arvidson T. Alignment and joint motion in the normal foot. J Orthop Sports Phys Ther 1995; 22(5): 216-222.

20) Baumhauer JF, Alosa DM, Renstrom PA, Trevino S, Beynnon B. A prospective study of ankle injury risk factors. Am J Sports Med 1995; 23(5): 564-570.

21) Picciano AM, Rowlands MS, Worrell T. Reliability of open and closed kinetic chain subtalar joint neutral positions and navicular drop test. J Orthop Sports Phys Ther 1993; 18(4): 553-558.

22) Lattanza L, Gray G, Kanther R. Closed versus open kinematic chain measurements of subtalar joint eversion: implications for clinical practice. J Orthop Sports Phys Ther 1988: 9(9):310.

23) Garbalosa JC, McClure, MH, Catlin PA, Wooden M: The frontal plane relationship of the forefoot to the rearfoot in an asymptomatic population. J Orthop Sports Phys Ther 1994; 20: 200-206.

24) Root ML, Orien WR, Weed JM. Biomechanical Examination of the Foot, Vol. 1. Los Angeles: Clinical Biomechanics, 1971.

25) Bailey DS, Perillo JT, Foremann M. Subtalar joint neutral: a study using tomography. J Am Podiatr Med Assoc 1984; 74: 59-64.

26) Nigg BM, Fisher V, Allinger TL, Ronsky JR, Engsberg JR: Range of motion of the foot as a function of age. Foot Ankle 1992; 13: 336-343.

CONTENTS

Chapter Three   Abnormal Motion during the Gait Cycle   57

Chapter One

Structural and Functional Anatomy
of the Foot and Ankle

The human foot and ankle contain 28 bones (Fig.1.1) with 55 articulations (1) that function in synchrony to allow for a variety of activities during the different phases of gait: during early stance phase the foot dissipates ground-reactive forces associated with heel-strike and becomes a "mobile adaptor" necessary to accommodate discrepancies in terrain. During late stance, the foot becomes a "rigid lever arm" necessary to effectively transfer body weight from rearfoot to forefoot after heel lift occurs. The foot is able to accomplish these diverse activities via a series of complex and delicately balanced interactions occurring be-

tween the various articulations and their supporting soft tissues. In order to fully appreciate these complex and often confusing movement patterns, the following section will review the different planes of motion and explain how variation in axis positioning may result in uni-, bi-, or triplanar motion. This information will then be related to the primary articulations of the foot and ankle with regard to the locations of the individual axes and their available motions. Also included in this section is a description of the various osseous and ligamentous restraining mechanisms. Finally, the mechanical advantages afforded individual muscles, as

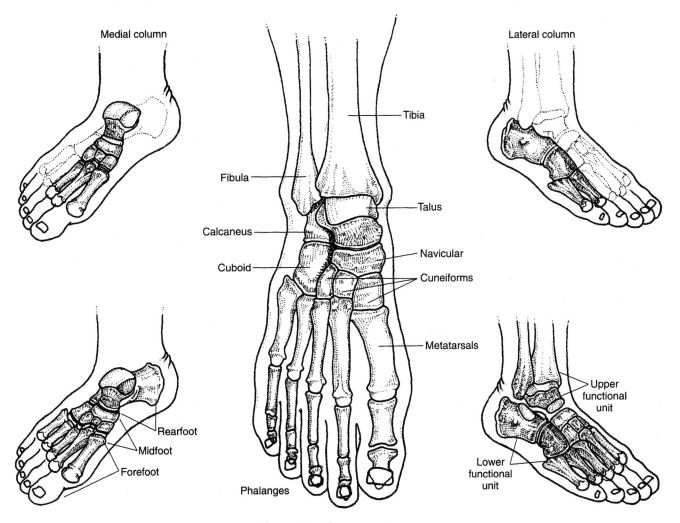

Figure 1.1. Osseous anatomy.

1

determined by their angle of approach and distance from each of the various axes, will be described in this chapter.

PLANES OF MOTION

In order to describe various movements accurately, the human body has been divided into three reference planes of motion: frontal, sagittal, and transverse. As illustrated in Figure 1.2, each of these planes is perpendicular to the other two and has a cardinal plane that bisects the body's center of gravity. (Note that there are an infinite number of corresponding planes paralleling each of the cardinal planes.) As related to most of the body, abduction/adduction occurs in the frontal plane; flexion/extension occurs in the sagittal plane; and rotation occurs in the transverse plane (Fig. 1.3).

As related to the foot and ankle, however, motions differ as inversion/eversion occurs in the frontal plane,

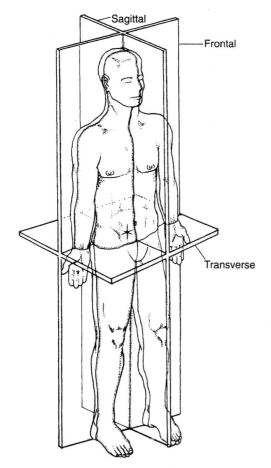

Figure 1.2. Cardinal planes of the body. The sagittal plane divides the body into equal right and left halves; the frontal plane (also referred to as the coronal plane) divides the body into asymmetrical front and back halves; the transverse plane (also known as the axial plane) divides the body into asymmetrical upper and lower halves. The cardinal planes intersect at the body's center of gravity *(x)*, which is located just anterior to the second sacral tuberosity (slightly lower in women).

dorsiflexion/plantarflexion occurs in the sagittal plane, and abduction/adduction occurs in the transverse plane (Figs. 1.4–1.6). In addition to denoting motion, it is also possible to use the reference planes to describe fixed positions (Figs. 1.7–1.9). Notice in Figures 1.4–1.9 that terms denoting motion end with the suffix "-ion," whereas static or fixed position terms end with "-us" or "-ed."

An important consideration is that motion in each of the reference planes occurs about an axis lying in the two remaining reference planes. (An axis is described as the line about which all motion takes place.) For example, transverse plane motion occurring in Figure 1.6 takes place about the frontal/sagittal axis while the sagittal plane motion in Figure 1.5 takes place about the frontal/transverse axis.

To demonstrate the relationship between the position of an axis and the potential motion available about that axis, Root et al. (2) used an analogy in which a hinge is situated in a box with each wall representing one of the reference planes. Figures 1.10–1.12 illustrate how an axis lying in two planes will allow for pure motion in the remaining plane, i.e., uniplanar motion.

Biplanar motion will result when an axis is situated in such a way that it rests in only one of the reference planes. For example, the axis in Figure 1.13, which was originally in the frontal and transverse plane, has been shifted so as to lie 45° to the transverse plane. This axis now lies in the frontal plane only, and the swing arm of its hinge describes a path allowing for biplanar motion (in this case, transverse and sagittal plane motion). Because the axis lies 45° to both planes, the amounts of transverse and sagittal plane motions are equal. If the same axis had been tilted only 10° to the transverse plane (as in Fig. 1.14), the resulting motion would still be biplanar, but then the sagittal plane component of motion would greatly exceed the transverse plane component of motion. Conversely, if the axis had been tilted 80° to the transverse plane (10° to the sagittal plane), the transverse plane component of motion would greatly exceed the sagittal plane component (Fig. 1.15). As a rule, the more parallel an axis lies to a plane, the less motion it will allow on that plane.

Triplanar motion will result when an axis deviates from all of the reference planes (Fig. 1.16). Because the axis in this illustration lies 45° to each plane, the swing arm will describe a path allowing for equal amounts of frontal, sagittal, and transverse plane motion. If the axis were to lie closer (or more parallel) to a specific plane, less motion would be possible in that plane.

Note that in all of these illustrations the swing arm moves only in one plane (i.e., the plane perpendicular to its axis of motion) and that plane may describe a path that is uniplanar, biplanar, or triplanar, depending on the spacial relationships between the axis and the reference planes. To put it another way, motion about a long axis, regardless of its position in space, will always occur in a single plane, and the terminology used to describe pathways relative to

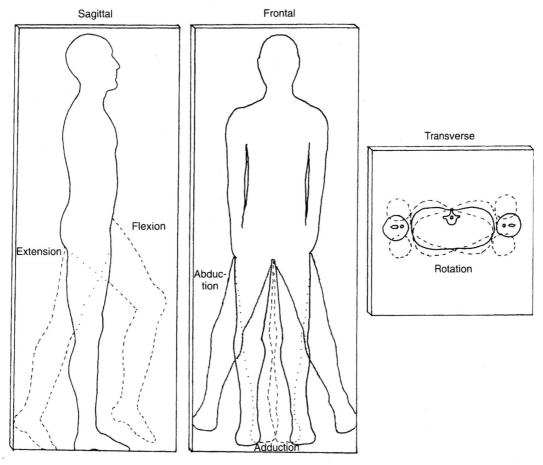

Figure 1.3. Body motions in each of the reference planes.

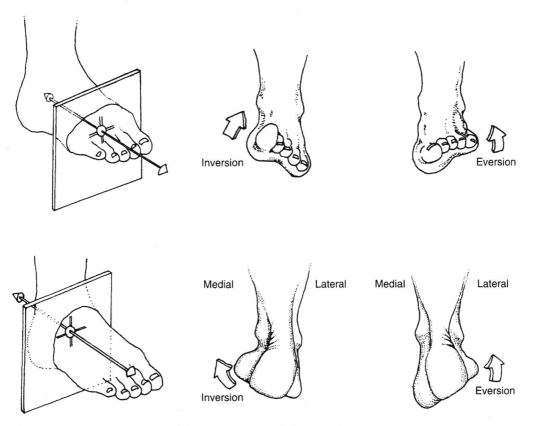

Figure 1.4. Frontal plane motions.

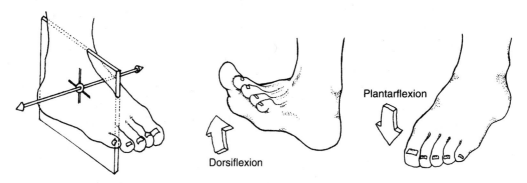

Figure 1.5.   Sagittal plane motions.

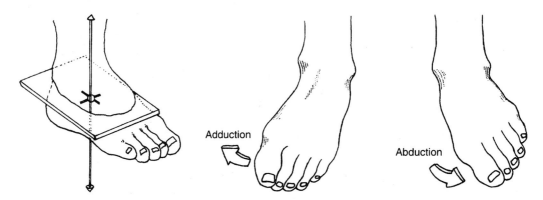

Figure 1.6.   Transverse plane motions.

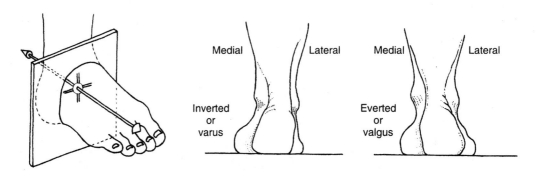

Figure 1.7.   Static frontal plane positions.

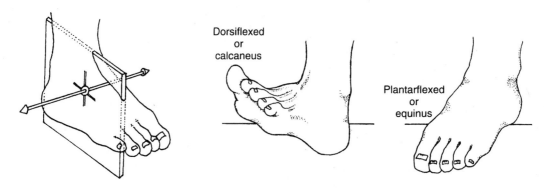

Figure 1.8.   Static sagittal plane positions.

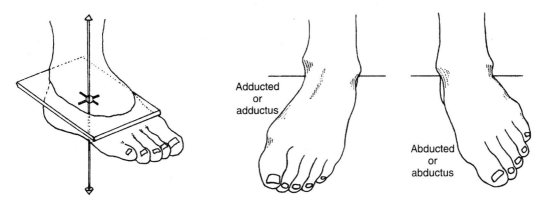

Figure 1.9.   Static transverse plane positions.

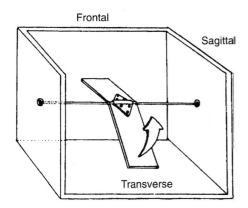

Figure 1.10.   Axis: frontal and transverse. Motion: sagittal.

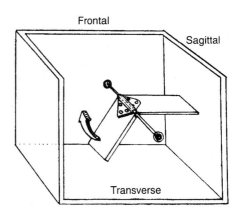

Figure 1.12.   Axis: transverse and sagittal. Motion: frontal.

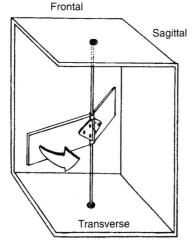

Figure 1.11.   Axis: frontal and sagittal. Motion: transverse.

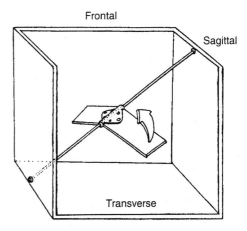

Figure 1.13.   Axis: frontal (45° to transverse). Motion: equal amounts of transverse and sagittal.

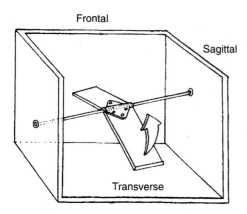

Figure 1.14. Axis: frontal (10° to transverse). Motion: primarily sagittal with some transverse.

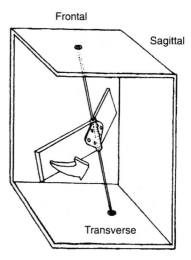

Figure 1.15. Axis: frontal (10° to sagittal). Motion: primarily transverse with some sagittal.

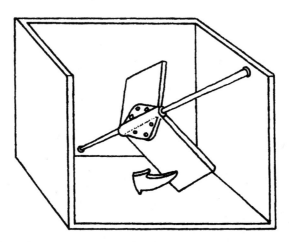

Figure 1.16. Axis: outside reference planes (45° to each plane). Motion: equal amounts of frontal, sagittal, and transverse.

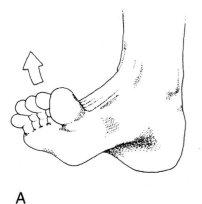

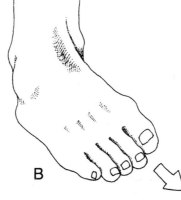

Figure 1.17. Pronation. (A) abduction, dorsiflexion, and eversion. **Supination. (B)** Adduction, plantarflexion, and inversion.

the cardinal planes must not be taken to imply that the individual components of motion can ever be segregated.

To describe triplanar motions (which are by far the most commonly seen motions in the body), the terms pronation and supination are used. Pronation refers to the combined movements of abduction, dorsiflexion, and eversion whereas supination refers to adduction, plantarflexion, and inversion (Fig. 1.17). These motions occur in the transverse, sagittal, and frontal planes, respectively.

FUNCTIONAL ANATOMY

The articulations of the foot and ankle with respect to the locations of axes and motions available will be reviewed in the following section. It is important to stress that when describing actual joint motions, rotation is an imprecise term, as it is used to describe movement about a long axis. Because most articulations move with a combination of spin, glide, and/or rock, identifying a single axis of motion is actually impossible, as its location is constantly changing as the joint moves through the available range of motion.

Ankle Joint

Also known as the talocrural joint, the ankle joint is the articulation between the talar trochlea and the distal tibia and fibula. Although the average axis of motion for this joint lies approximately 8° to the transverse plane and 20–30° to the frontal plane (3) (Fig. 1.18), numerous investigators (9–11) have demonstrated that the irregularly curved contour of the medial talus allows for a constant repositioning of the axis as the ankle is moved (Fig. 1.19). Wyller (6) likens the shift of the ankle axis to the rotation of a badly mounted wheel.

While the ankle's axis of motion may take varying inclinations between horizontal and vertical throughout the ankle's range of movement, more recent investigation demonstrates that all axes are close to the midpoint of a line connecting the tips of the malleoli (7). Because of its proximity to the transverse and frontal planes, this axis typically allows for almost pure dorsiflexion/plantarflexion (although the slight deviation from the transverse plane allows for a small but clinically significant range of talar abduction with ankle dorsiflexion [2]). It should be noted that Inman et al. (8) stated that the ankle axis may deviate by as much as 23° from the transverse plane and that the added range of talar adduction/abduction associated with this higher axis plays an important role in absorbing the rotational motions of the shank. Root et al. (2) claim that such large variation in the location of this axis is relatively uncommon and is usually found only in individuals possessing limited ranges of subtalar joint motion during the early years of skeletal growth. The authors stated that the unusually high axis results from a functional adaptation of bone as the ankle attempts to compensate for the limited subtalar joint motion by developing a supinatory/pronatory axis.

Regardless of the position of its axis of motion, plantarflexion about this axis is limited by tension created in the surrounding soft tissues (particularly the anterior talofibular ligament) and by an osseous block produced when the posterior tubercle of the talus contacts the posterior margin of the articular surface of the tibia (9) (see Fig. 1.20). Motion in the direction of dorsiflexion is limited primarily by tension in the triceps surae musculature and the posterior restraining ligaments, i.e., the posterior deltoid and the posterior talofibular ligaments (Fig. 1.21). Also, because the talus is wider anteriorly, ankle dorsiflexion may also be restricted by a bony block when the widened aspects of the talus come into contact with the distal tibia and fibula. The clinical significance of a premature osseous block will be discussed later.

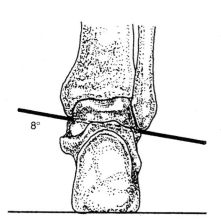

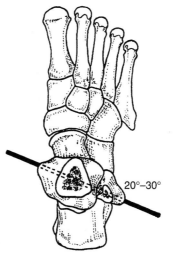

Figure 1.18. Average axis of motion for the ankle joint.

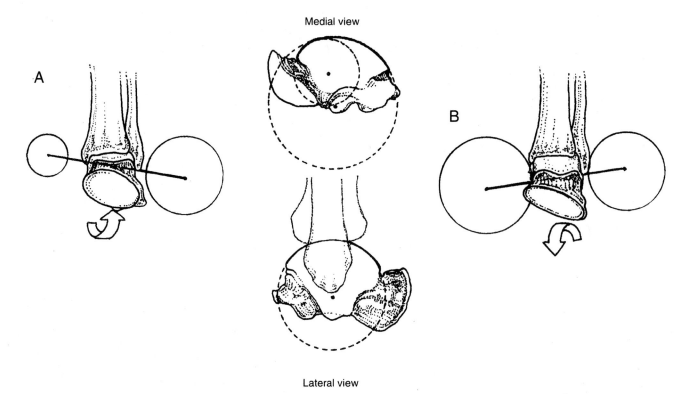

Medial view

Lateral view

Figure 1.19. Shifting of the ankle joint axis of motion. Whereas the lateral talus almost always forms a true circle, the variable radius of the medial talus *(inset)* allows for a downward and lateral projection of the axis when the ankle is dorsiflexed **(A)** and a superior and lateral projection of the axis when the ankle is plantarflexed **(B).** (Adapted from Barnett CH, Napier JH. The axis of rotation on the ankle joint in man. Its influence upon the form of the talus and the mobility of the fibula. Anatomy 1952; 86: 1–8.)

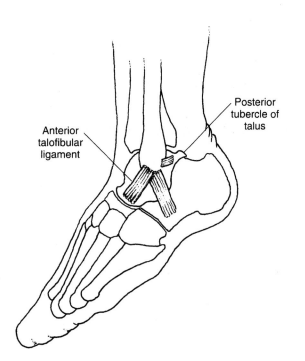

Anterior talofibular ligament

Posterior tubercle of talus

Figure 1.20. Ankle plantarflexion (lateral view of the left ankle).

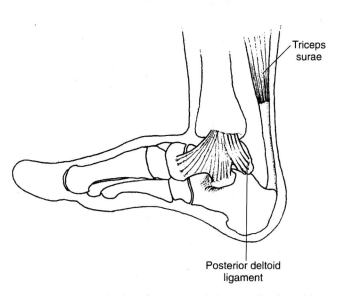

Triceps surae

Posterior deltoid ligament

Figure 1.21. Ankle dorsiflexion (medial view of right ankle).

Subtalar Joint

The subtalar joint is located between the talus and calcaneus. Though rarely mentioned, individual variation in the development of this joint may result in the formation of one, two or three separate articulations (Fig. 1.22). Bruckner (10), in his study of 32 cadaveric subtalar joints, noted that 20 specimens had two distinct articulations (with slight variation between each one) whereas the remaining 12 had 3 separate articulations. Upon being placed through their full ranges of pronation and supination, the articular surfaces of the biarticulated subtalar joints remained congruous, and movement was restricted by soft tissue-restraining mechanisms, i.e., the posterior and lateral talocalcaneal ligaments and the interosseous ligament. Although not present in his sample group, Bruckner (10) mentions the single facet configuration would be extremely mobile, as all the facets have blended into one, thereby allowing for a maximal gliding area without the stabilization afforded by the interosseous ligament.

In contrast to the more mobile single- and double-facet configurations, the subtalar joints with three articulations possessed smaller amounts of combined articular surface area and exhibited far less motion. When stressed in supination, the anterolateral articulation of the talus col-

lided with the anterolateral articulation of the calcaneus, thereby producing an osseous block that prevented further motion. When stressed in pronation, variation in the shape of the three articulations resulted in rapid joint incongruity, which limited further motion. These actions allow for a functional locking mechanism which, according to Elftman and Manter (11), is a uniquely human trait that allows for improved bipedal ambulation.

Motion in the average subtalar joint occurs about an axis that lies 42° to the transverse plane and 23° to the sagittal plane (ref. 18) (Fig. 1.23). The position of this axis allows for triplanar motion with almost equal amounts of frontal (eversion/inversion) and transverse plane motion (adduction/abduction). Although Inman and Mann (12) compared motion at the subtalar joint to that with a mitered hinge, the accuracy of this model is questioned because of a small range of translation occurring between the combined subtalar and ankle articulations (13). Because the axis lies so close to the sagittal plane, only limited amounts of dorsiflexion/plantarflexion are possible.

Just as there is much individual variation in the shape of the subtalar articulations, there is also much variation in the location of the axis of motion. Numerous investigators (14–16) have noted positional variation in the subtalar joint axis, ranging from 20° to 68.5° from the transverse plane

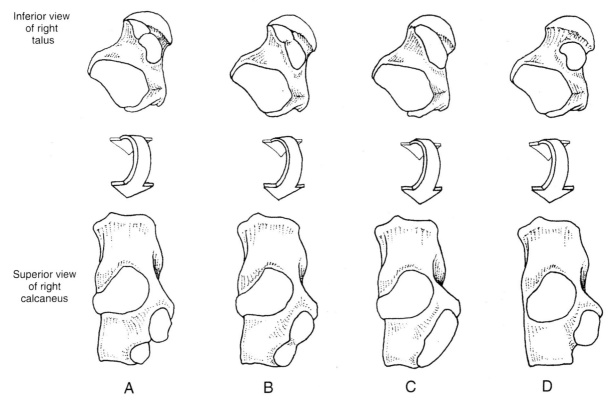

Inferior view of right talus

Superior view of right calcaneus

A   B   C   D

Figure 1.22.   Variation in subtalar joint anatomy. (A) Three-facet configuration. **(B)** Transitional two-facet configuration. **(C)** Simple two-facet configuration. **(D)** Special two-facet configuration. (Adapted from Bruckner J. Variations in the human subtalar joint. J Orthop Sports Phys Ther 1987; 8: 489–494.)

Figure 1.23.   Axis of motion for the subtalar joint.

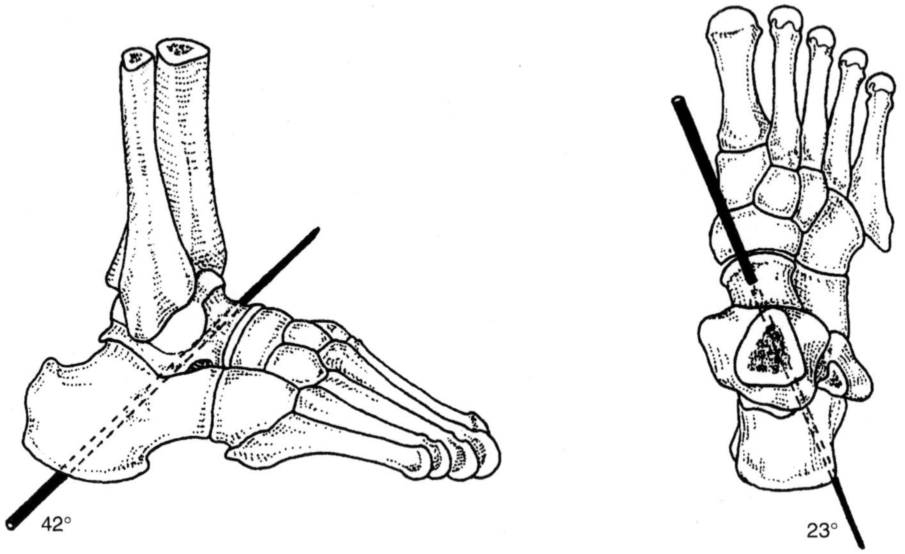

42°

23°

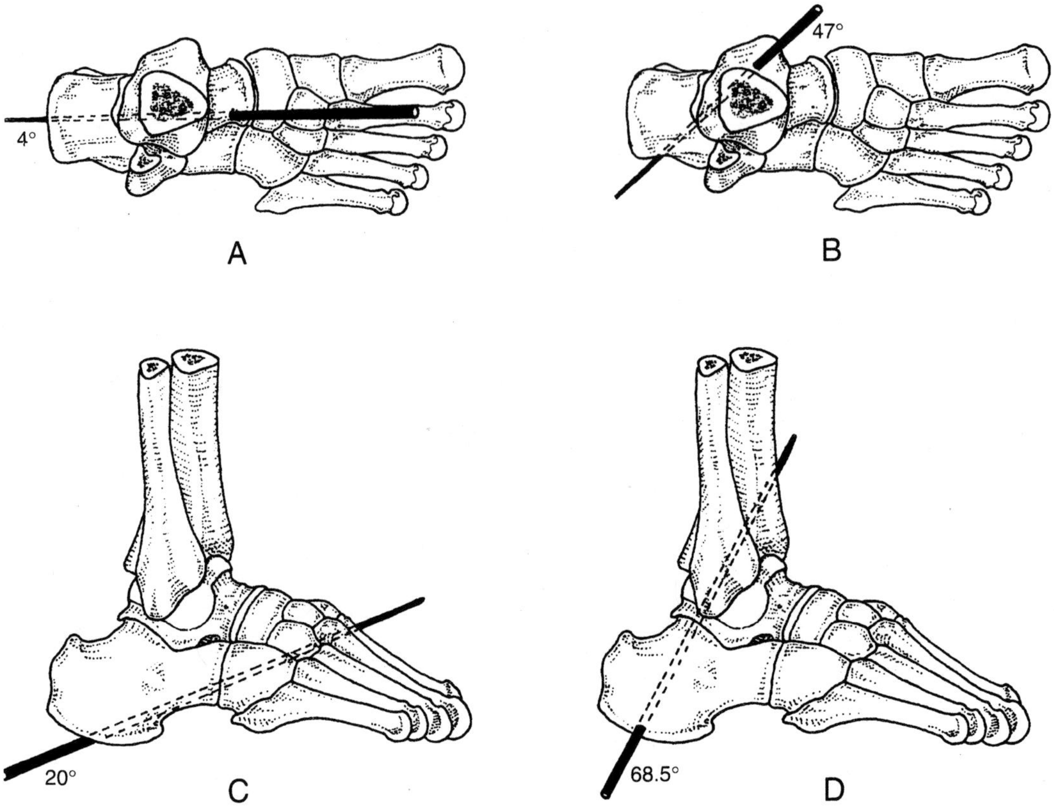

A

4°

B

47°

C

20°

D

68.5°

Figure 1.24.   Variations in positioning of the subtalar joint axis. (A) 4° from sagittal. **(B)** 47° from sagittal. **(C)** 20° from transverse. **(D)** 69° from transverse.

and 4° to 47° from the sagittal plane (Fig. 1.24). In practice, the approximate position of the subtalar joint axis can be determined by comparing the range of rearfoot inversion/eversion with the range of tibial rotation as the standing patient pronates and supinates the subtalar joint. If the axis lies 45° to the transverse plane, every 1° of rearfoot motion will produce 1° of tibial rotation. If the axis is positioned near 70° to the transverse plane, the amount of tibial rotation will greatly exceed rearfoot motion (e.g., 2° of rearfoot eversion will be accompanied by 8° of internal tibial rotation). The location of the subtalar joint axis is clinically significant as a high axis could be responsible for chronic injury to structures proximal to the subtalar joint, while a low axis could be responsible for chronic injury to structures distal to the subtalar joint.

The Midtarsal Joint

The midtarsal joint consists of the combined articulations between the talonavicular and calcaneocuboid joints. These joints function as a unit to allow for triplanar motion that occurs about two distinct axes: the oblique midtarsal joint axis and the longitudinal midtarsal joint axis (4). Although individual variation exists, the oblique midtarsal joint axis lies 52° to the transverse plane and 57° to the sagittal plane whereas the longitudinal midtarsal joint axis lies 15° to the transverse plane and 9° to the sagittal plane (14) (Fig. 1.25).

The location of the oblique midtarsal joint axis allows for large amounts of sagittal and transverse plane motion (dorsiflexion/plantarflexion and abduction/adduction, respectively) with relatively small amounts of frontal plane motion (inversion/eversion). The longitudinal midtarsal joint, because of its close proximity to the transverse and sagittal planes, allows for almost pure inversion/eversion.

The midtarsal joint is similar to a triarticulated subtalar joint in that it has an osseous locking mechanism to prevent excessive motion (17). Whereas movement in the direction of supination is resisted by soft tissue-restraining mechanisms, movement in the direction of pronation comes to an abrupt halt when the superoproximal border of the pronating cuboid comes into contact with the dorsal border of the overhanging calcaneus (Fig. 1.26). Further midtarsal pronation is prevented by tension in the various restraining ligaments (primarily the long and short plantar ligaments, the calcaneonavicular ligament, and the bifurcate ligament; see Fig. 1.27). Midtarsal pronation beyond this point is not possible without overwhelming the restraining ligaments and subluxing the calcaneocuboid joint (2). As with the subtalar joint locking mechanism, the midtarsal locking mechanism is a uniquely human trait that allows for improved bipedal ambulation (14).

First Ray

The first ray is a functional unit consisting of the medial cuneiform and the first metatarsal. First ray motion occurs about an axis that lies approximately 45° to both the frontal and sagittal planes (Fig 1.28).The location of this axis allows for relatively equal amounts of dorsiflexion/plantarflexion and inversion/eversion. Because the axis lies so close to the transverse plane, the range of adduction/abduction is clinically insignificant. Note that motion about the first ray axis in both pronation and supination is limited by soft tissue-restraining mechanisms.

Second, Third, and Fourth Rays

The second and third rays consist of the second and third metatarsals with their respective cuneiforms whereas the fourth ray is the fourth metatarsal alone. Although the exact locations of their axes have not yet been determined, Root et al. (2) postulate they lie in the transverse plane just proximal to the tarsometatarsal articulations. Because of this, motion about these axes occurs in the sagittal plane only, i.e., pure dorsiflexion/plantarflexion.

Fifth Ray

The fifth ray is the fifth metatarsal alone. This metatarsal moves about an axis that lies approximately 20° to the transverse plane and 35° to the sagittal plane (Fig.

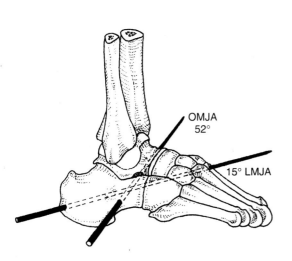

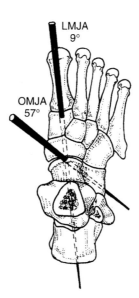

Figure 1.25. The midtarsal joint axes of motion: the oblique midtarsal joint axis (OMJA) and the longitudinal midtarsal joint axis (LMJA).

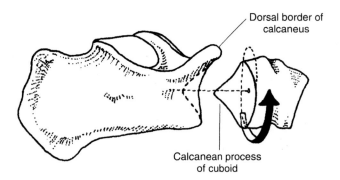

Dorsal border of
calcaneus

Calcanean process
of cuboid

**Figure 1.26. The pronating cuboid pivots about the cal-
canean process until its dorsal border contacts the overhanging calcaneus.** (Adapted from Bojsen-Moller F. Calcaneocuboid
joint and stability of the longitudinal arch of the foot at high and
low gear push-off. J Anat 1979; 129: 165–176.)

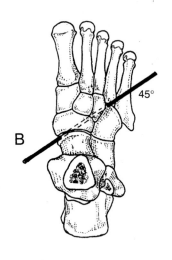

B

45°

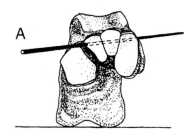

A

Figure 1.28. Axis of motion for the first ray. (A) Anterior
view (sectioned at the cuneiforms). **(B)** Dorsal view.

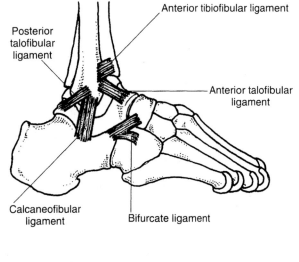

Posterior
talofibular
ligament

Anterior tibiofibular ligament

Anterior talofibular
ligament

Calcaneofibular
ligament

Bifurcate ligament

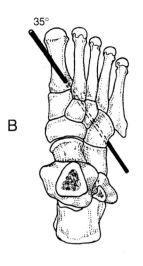

35°

B

20°

A

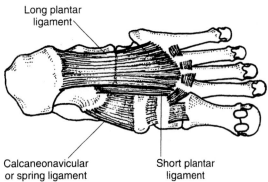

Long plantar
ligament

Calcaneonavicular
or spring ligament

Short plantar
ligament

Figure 1.27. Ligamentous anatomy of the foot and ankle.

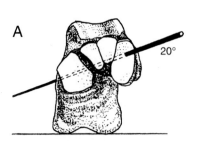

Figure 1.29. Axis of motion for the fifth ray.

1.29). The position of this axis allows for relatively large amounts of dorsiflexion/plantarflexion and inversion/eversion. Because the axis tilts 20° to the transverse plane, there is a small but clinically significant amount of abduction/adduction present. As with the first ray, motion about the fifth ray axis is also limited by tension in the restraining ligaments.

Metatarsophalangeal Joints

These joints represent the articulations between the distal first through fifth metatarsal heads and their respective proximal phalanges. Each of these joints has two distinct and separate axes that allows for pure sagittal (dorsiflexion/plan-

tarflexion) and transverse (abduction/adduction) plane motion (Fig. 1.30).

Because of the locations of these axes, frontal plane motion is not possible, and any attempt to invert or evert a normal digit may result in subluxation of the metatarsophalangeal joint (2). Furthermore, although sagittal plane motion at the metatarsophalangeal joint is extremely important for normal locomotion, the range of transverse plane motion is relatively small and of no functional significance during the gait cycle. Also, in regards to transverse plane motion of the metatarsophalangeal joints, there has been historically much controversy regarding terminology differentiating abduction and adduction. For example, the early

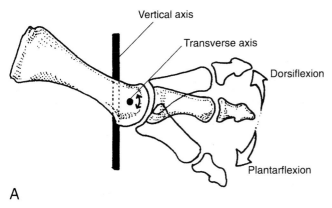

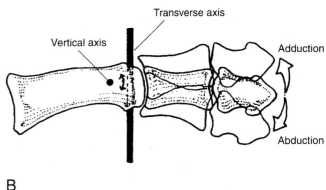

A

B

Figure 1.30.   The metatarsophalangeal joint axes. (A) Lateral view demonstrating sagittal plane motion about the transverse

axis. **(B)** Dorsal view demonstrating transverse plane motion about the vertical axis. **(Adapted from Root et al.[2].)**

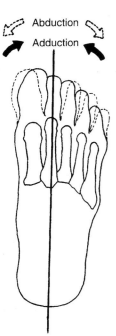

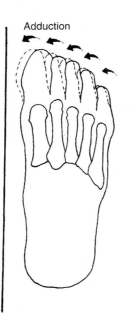

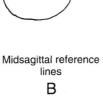

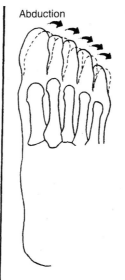

Axial reference line

A

Midsagittal reference lines

B

Figure 1.31.   Digital motions as related to an axial reference line (A) and a midsagittal line (B and C).

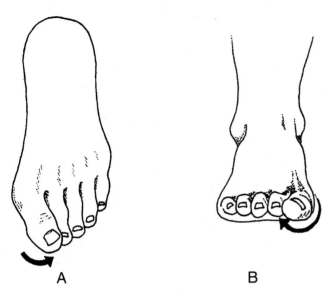

Figure 1.32. Digital positions. (A) Abducted refers to the transverse plane position while valgus **(B)** refers to the frontal plane position.

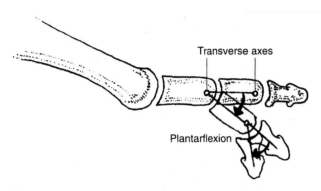

Figure 1.33. Lateral view demonstrating pure sagittal plane motion about the transverse axes of the interphalangeal joints.

anatomists responsible for naming the muscles referred to abduction at the metatarsophalangeal joint as movement of a digit away from an axial reference line projecting distally through the second metatarsal with adduction representing movement towards this axial reference line (Fig. 1.31A). Contrary to this, the more current orthopaedic and podiatric literature refers to abduction as movement of a digit away from the midsagittal plane of the body, with adduction representing movement towards the midsagittal plane (Fig. 1.31B and C). To be consistent with the more current literature, this text will refer to metatarsophalangeal joint motions as they relate to the midsagittal plane.

Another point of confusion regarding terminology concerns the use of the terms varus and valgus to describe digital positions. Whereas many authors refer to transverse plane malpositions as either varus (representing adduction) or valgus (representing abduction), this is actually incorrect

as varus and valgus refer to frontal plane positions only, e.g., hallux abductovalgus represents a deformity in which the hallux is both abducted (Fig. 1.32A) and in valgus (Fig. 1.32B).

Interphalangeal Joints

Each of the interphalangeal joints possesses a transverse axis that allows for pure sagittal plane motion (Fig. 1.33).

INTERACTION OF FORCES

Whereas the locations of the various axes are determined by the shape of the articular surfaces (4), movement about these axes is determined by the combined interactions of all forces acting on the body (with the most common forces being muscular, gravitational, inertial, frictional, and ground-reactive forces). In order to appreciate just how these forces produce or resist motion, it is important to understand that all forces possess magnitude, direction, a line of application, and a point of application (Fig. 1.34).

A force will most effectively produce motion when its line of application occurs in a plane perpendicular to the joint's surface (or its axis) and when the perpendicular distance between this line of action and the axis is greatest, i.e., when it has the longest lever arm. This is readily

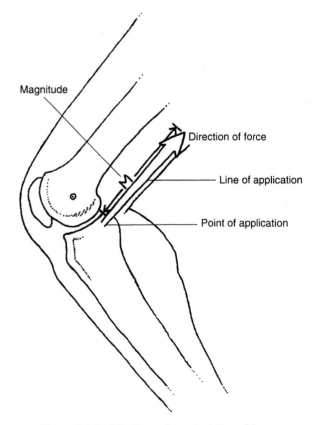

Figure 1.34. The four characteristics of force.

ment" refers to the tendency or measure of tendency to produce motion), F equals the component of force perpendicular to the lever arm, and D equals the length of the lever arm.

In this example, because the force being applied was perpendicular to the door, the length of the lever arm could be determined by measuring the distance from the axis (the hinge) to the doorknob. If these same forces were applied at different angles to the door (while remaining perpendicular to the axis), the length of their respective lever arms would significantly change (Fig. 1.36). (Remember that the length of a lever arm is the perpendicular distance between the force's line of action and the axis of motion.)

If forces F1 to F4 were equal in magnitude, F1 would have the greatest moment, followed by F2 and F3. F4, regardless of its magnitude, would be unable to move the door because its line of action passes directly through the axis. This illustration also serves to demonstrate how one force can produce two distinct actions. Notice that if you were to attempt to open the door by pulling along line F2, part of the force would go into opening the door and part of the force would go into compressing the hinge. This represents an important concept regarding the application of forces in the body: When a force is applied perpendicular to an axis (or perpendicular to a joint's surface), the force may be resolved into rotational and nonrotational components, and the nonrotational component will either compress or distract the joint surfaces. A simple example of this action occurs in the knee (Fig. 1.37).

Whereas the rotational component is obviously important as it is responsible for producing motion about an axis, the compressive component is also important, as it may be responsible for stabilizing a joint. For example, as heel lift occurs, various muscles and ligaments must work together to create the strong compressive forces necessary to stabilize the osseous structures as vertical forces reach their highest levels. Failure to generate sufficient compressive forces would allow the bony structures to shift as vertical forces peaked.

In all of the illustrations so far, forces have been applied perpendicular to the axis of motion and have been resolved into rotational and nonrotational components. However, as one might suspect, the forces in the body are not so cooperative as to align themselves perpendicularly to a joint's axis. When a force's line of action deviates from perpendicular (as it most frequently does), determining the rotational and nonrotational components requires first resolving the line of action into forces acting perpendicular to the axis and forces acting parallel to the axis. For example, Figure 1.38 illustrates the same door pictured previously in Figure 1.35, only now Force F1 is angled 30° superior to the perpendicular plane of the axis. This force can now be resolved into what is termed a normal component (Fx), which is applied perpendicular to the axis and possesses rotational and nonrotational components, and a tangential or

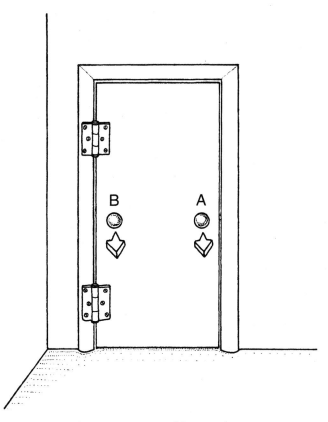

Figure 1.35.   Door hinge analogy.

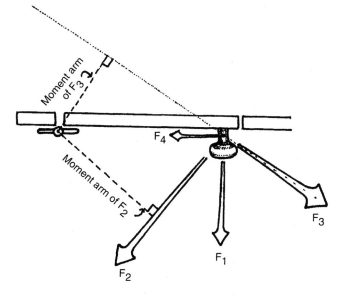

Figure 1.36.   Door hinge analogy.

demonstrated with a door hinge analogy (Fig. 1.35). If equal forces were used to open this door by pulling on doorknob A or B, the force generated at A would be much more effective than the force generated at B. The relative effect of each force could be determined by the formula $M = F \times D$, where M equals the moment of force (the term "mo-

Figure 1.37. When the knee is flexed **(A),** the semimembranosus muscle exerts a strong rotational component of force *(R)* and a small nonrotational or compressive component *(C).* Upon straightening **(B),** the length of the muscle's lever arm decreases and the nonrotational component greatly exceeds the rotational component, thereby compressing the articular surfaces.

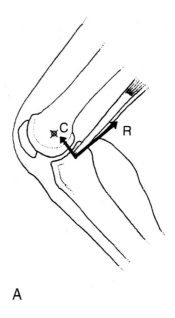

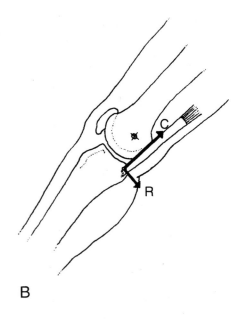

A

B

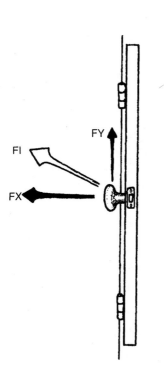

Figure 1.38.   Force: FI (line of application of force) is resolved into a normal component *(FX)* and a shearing component *(FY).*

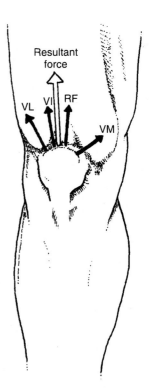

Figure 1.39.   The combined line of drive of all muscles stabilizing a joint is termed the resultant force *(open arrow).* *VM* = vastus medialis, *RF* = rectus femoris, *VI* = vastus intermedius, *VL* = vastus lateralis.

shearing component (Fy), which is applied parallel to the axis and is typically unable to produce motion without subluxing or dislocating the joint.

Fortunately, the shearing component of force present in most joints is resisted by bone/ligament-restraining mechanisms and/or the pull of antagonistic muscles. A classic example of how muscles interact to prevent shearing forces occurs in the knee as vastus medialis and lateralis create antagonistic forces to maintain the patella between the femoral condyles (Fig. 1.39). Because there is minimal bony restriction (the intercondylar groove is shallow), the antagonistic forces created by these muscles must be relatively equal, otherwise the patella may stray from its groove, damaging the articular surface.

Figure 1.40 demonstrates the various component forces present as tibialis anterior attempts to overcome inertial forces associated with the early swing phase of gait. (Note: Although inertia is not actually a force, it is typically referred to as one because of its tendency to resist motion.) Because tibialis anterior's line of action is almost perpendicular to the ankle's axis, shearing forces at the mortise are minimal and would normally be resisted by the antagonistic pull of peroneus tertius.

It is possible to determine the magnitude of each force (shearing vs. normal and rotational vs. nonrotational) by setting up an equation in which the components of force are made analogous to the legs of a right triangle. For example, if tibialis anterior were contracting with a force of 10 lbs and its insertion angled 75° to the joint's surface (15° from perpendicular), the normal component of force (which is equivalent to the adjacent leg of the formed right triangle) would equal 9.7 lbs, and the shearing component (which is equivalent to the opposite leg of the formed right triangle) would equal 2.6 lbs (see Fig 1.41)

The rotational and nonrotational components can be determined by taking the normal component (9.7 lbs), noting its angulations from the point of attachment (in this case, 65°), and then setting up a similar equation (Fig. 1.42).

The dorsiflectory force generated by contraction of tibialis anterior can now be determined by taking the rotational component (8.8 lbs) and multiplying it by the perpendicular distance between the tibialis anterior's tendon and the ankle's axis of motion. Hopefully, the resultant force will be sufficient to overcome inertial forces and initiate the dorsiflectory motions necessary for the forefoot to clear the ground during midswing.

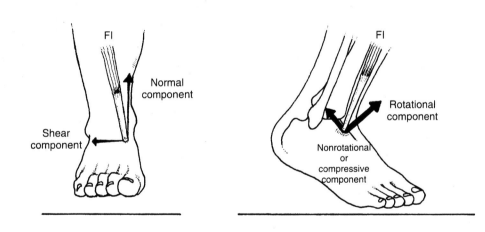

Figure 1.40. The resolution of forces associated with contraction of tibialis anterior. Note that for purposes of simplification, these actions are described only as they relate to the ankle joint, and the effect of the anterior retinaculum and the multiple articulations that the tibialis anterior tendon crosses is not considered. *FI* = line of application of force.

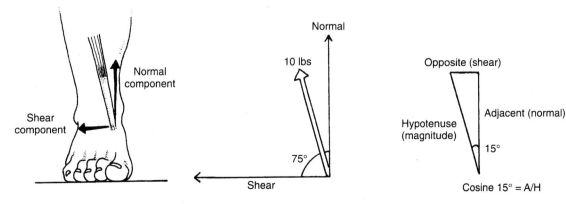

Figure 1.41. Determining relative amounts of force using the acronym "sohcahtoa." When solving biomechanical equations, the force's magnitude and line of action are referred to as the vector.

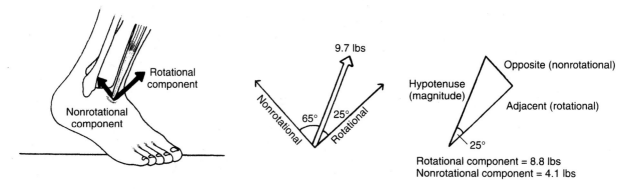

Figure 1.42.   Determining rotational and nonrotational components.

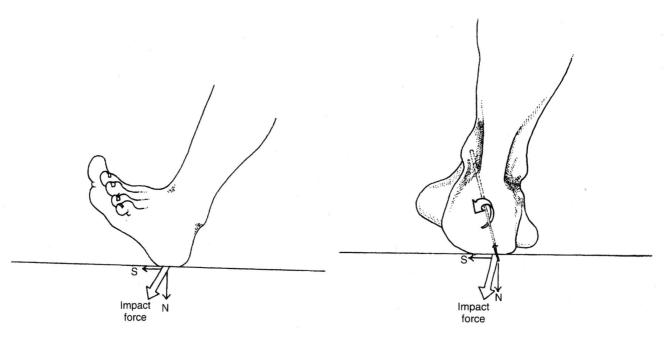

Figure 1.43.   Resolution of ground-reactive force. N = normal component, S = tangential or shearing component.

Figure 1.44.   A lateral-to-medial heel strike allows frictional forces to pronate the subtalar joint (arrow).

In this example, inertia was the only force considered. A much more significant force is encountered during the stance phase of gait: ground-reactive force. Ground-reactive force is also referred to as contact force, and it is consistent with Newton's Third Law, which states that an object will react with a force of equal magnitude and in the opposite direction to the first force. Thus, when the heel strikes the ground with a force of 200 lbs, it can also be said that the ground strikes the heel with a force of 200 lbs.

Ground-reactive forces are similar to those paralleling an axis in that they are divided into normal and shearing components. (The normal component is synonymous with vertical force.) Figure 1.43 demonstrates that when the heel strikes the ground in front of the body's center of mass, part

of the force is directed downward (and is considered the normal component), and part of the force is directed along the surface (and is referred to as the tangential, or shearing, component).

The magnitude of each component is determined by the heel's angle of approach as it strikes the ground: as this angle nears perpendicular, the normal component is greatly increased; as the angle nears horizontal, the shearing component is greatly increased. The shearing component of force (which may be applied anteriorly, posteriorly, medially, laterally, or torsionally) must be resisted by a high coefficient of friction; otherwise, the foot will remain in motion (e.g., taking a large stride on ice may result in a fall as the anterior shear forces are unrestrained and the heel continues to move forward). High coefficients of friction are responsible for the development of frictional forces that play important roles during static and kinetic activity. (The magnitude of frictional force is determined by multiplying the coefficient of friction between the two surfaces by the normal component of force.)

During static stance, frictional forces markedly reduce tension on the supporting ligaments by resisting the forward slide of the metatarsal heads. This acts to create a retrograde compressive force that maintains height of the medial longitudinal arch, thereby minimizing the need for ligamentous/muscular stabilization. Note that periods of pure static stance typically last less than 1 min and are interrupted with temporary bursts of muscle activity that serve to reposition the metatarsal heads, thereby reestablishing frictional forces.

During kinetic activity, frictional forces have the potential to generate large moments of force about the various axes, depending on their angle of application and the body's momentum. In Figure 1.43, the frictional force generated between the heel and the ground is applied perpendicular to the ankle axis and has a long lever arm to this axis (longer even than the normal component's lever arm). As a result, the frictional force creates a strong plantarflectory motion that is partially resisted by eccentric contraction of the anterior compartment musculature. Contraction of these mus-

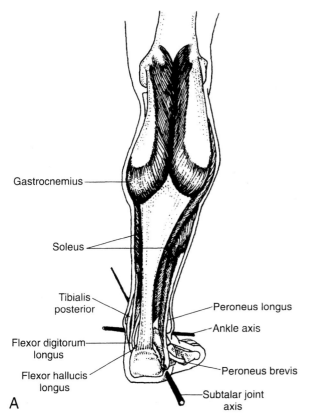

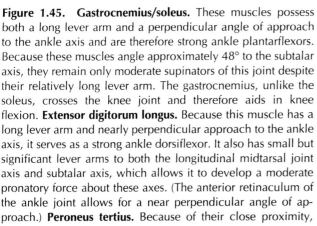

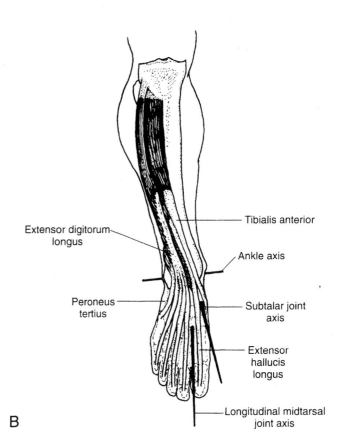

Figure 1.45. Gastrocnemius/soleus. These muscles possess both a long lever arm and a perpendicular angle of approach to the ankle axis and are therefore strong ankle plantarflexors. Because these muscles angle approximately 48° to the subtalar axis, they remain only moderate supinators of this joint despite their relatively long lever arm. The gastrocnemius, unlike the soleus, crosses the knee joint and therefore aids in knee flexion. **Extensor digitorum longus.** Because this muscle has a long lever arm and nearly perpendicular approach to the ankle axis, it serves as a strong ankle dorsiflexor. It also has small but significant lever arms to both the longitudinal midtarsal joint axis and subtalar axis, which allows it to develop a moderate pronatory force about these axes. (The anterior retinaculum of the ankle joint allows for a near perpendicular angle of approach.) **Peroneus tertius.** Because of their close proximity,

the actions of peroneus tertius and extensor digitorum longus are considered identical (although peroneus tertius has a longer lever arm for producing pronation about the longitudinal midtarsal and subtalar joint axes). **Extensor hallucis longus.** This muscle has a long lever arm and a perpendicular angle of approach to the ankle axis and is a strong dorsiflexor of this joint. In fact, Root et al. (2) noted that extensor hallucis longus is the strongest dorsiflexor of the ankle as swing phase begins. Because of its insignificant lever arm to the subtalar and longitudinal midtarsal joint axes, it is unable to produce motion about these axes and is considered a neutral dorsiflexor of the foot. **Note:** Extensor digitorum longus and extensor hallucis longus create strong compressive forces at the interphalangeal joints that act to resist clawing or hammering of the digits as they maintain extensor rigidity (see Fig. 1.46).

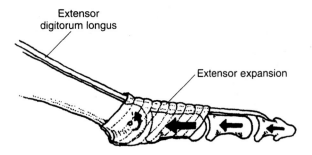

Figure 1.46.   Resolution of forces at the interphalangeal joints. Extensor digitorum longus exerts a pure compressive force at the proximal and distal interphalangeal joints with no rotational component. Extensor hallucis longus exerts primarily a compressive force with a slight dorsiflectory component. Both muscles produce dorsiflexion at the metatarsophalangeal joint.

cles (particularly tibialis anterior) serves to decrease momentum of the forefoot, thereby minimizing soft tissue damage as the plantar forefoot strikes the ground.

If the heel were striking the ground from a lateral-to-medial direction, frictional forces generated would be applied nearly perpendicular to the subtalar axis and would therefore pronate that joint (Fig. 1.44). Because the force is applied parallel to the ankle axis, it is unable to produce motion at that joint (although the normal component applied posterior to the axis or gravitational force applied anterior to the axis would produce a plantarflectory motion of the ankle). The frictional forces in this case are best resisted by tibialis posterior, which has nearly a perpendicular angle of approach and a significant lever arm for controlling motion at the subtalar joint.

The illustrations in this section have hopefully demonstrated some simple but important concepts regarding force interactions, specifically, that the muscular system works through a series of bony levers to either accelerate,

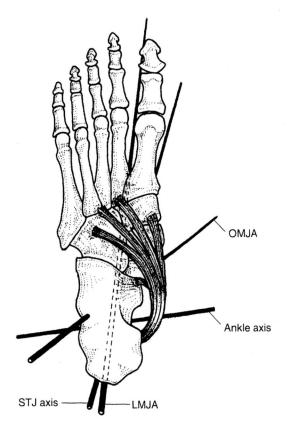

Figure 1.47.   Tibialis posterior. This muscle has a long lever arm and an almost perpendicular angle of approach to both the oblique midtarsal joint axis and subtalar axis. (The medial malleolus serves as a pulley supplying the near perpendicular approach to the subtalar axis.) Tibialis posterior also acts to create a strong posteromedial compressive force that is important in stabilizing the lesser tarsals. The posteromedial pull of tibialis posterior is balanced and reinforced by the posterolateral pull of peroneus longus. Tibialis posterior also possesses a small but significant lever arm for producing plantarflexion at the ankle joint. OMJA = oblique midtarsal joint axis, LMJA = longitudinal midtarsal joint axis, STJ axis = subtalar joint axis.

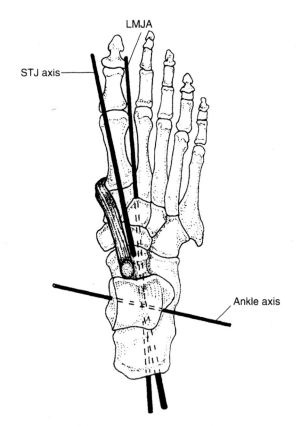

Figure 1.48.   Tibialis anterior. The tibialis anterior muscle produces a strong dorsiflectory force about the ankle and the first ray axes. It possesses a moderate lever arm for supinating the longitudinal midtarsal joint axis and a shorter lever arm for supinating the subtalar joint axis. Because its tendon frequently passes directly through the oblique midtarsal joint axis, it is unable to produce motion about this axis. STJ axis = subtalar joint axis, LMJA = longitudinal midtarsal joint axis.

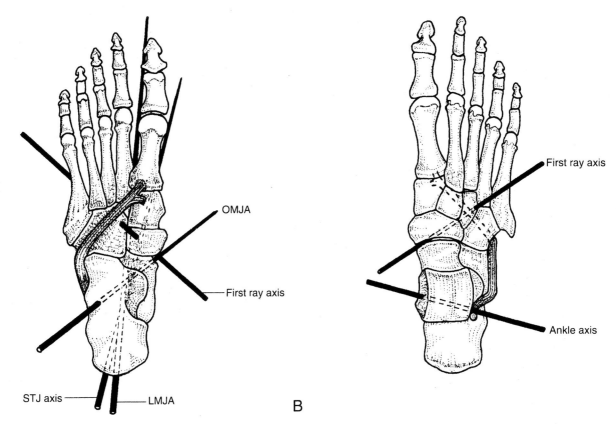

A

B

Figure 1.49.   Peroneus longus. In addition to its already discussed role of stabilizing the lesser tarsals, the peroneus longus muscle is capable of generating a powerful plantarflectory force about the first ray axis. (The peroneal groove of the cuboid acts as a pulley supplying this muscle with an improved angle of approach to the first ray axis.) Peroneus longus is also capable of producing a strong pronatory force about the longitudinal midtarsal joint axis. Because its tendon passes so close to the ankle axis, it is unable to produce significant amounts of plantarflexion at that joint. *OMJA* = oblique midtarsal joint axis, *STJA* = subtalar joint axis.

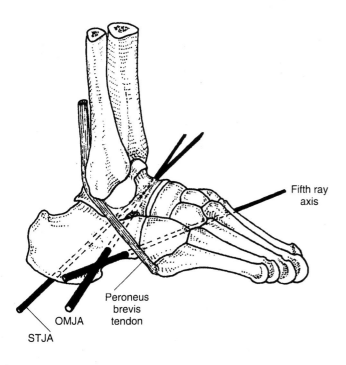

Figure 1.50.   Peroneus brevis. This muscle functions agonistically with peroneus longus to compress the tarsals. Because peroneus brevis has a longer lever arm to the subtalar axis *(STJA)*, it is a stronger pronator of this joint. Also, the peroneus brevis tendon possesses a small but significant lever arm to the oblique midtarsal joint axis *(OMJA)* and is therefore able to produce a moderate pronatory force about this axis.

decelerate, or stabilize the various articulations against a multitude of forces, primarily inertial, gravitational, and ground-reactive forces. The ability of a muscle to produce motion at a particular joint depends on the length of its lever arm (which may be increased via sesamoid bones) and the angle in which it approaches the axis (which can be improved or made more perpendicular with the help of various pulleys, i.e., the retinacular sheath, peroneal tubercle, sustentaculum tali, etc.).

Figures 1.45–1.56 demonstrate the relationship between the various muscles and axes of the foot and ankle. This information is invaluable when designing an exercise program to help stabilize damaged or hypermobile joints. (Note that Figures 1.47–1.56 have been adapted from Root

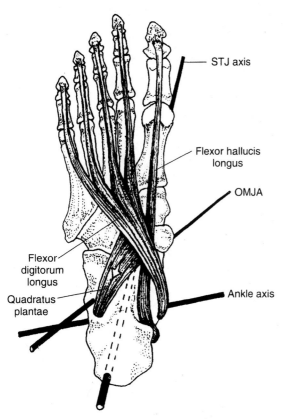

Figure 1.51.   Flexor digitorum longus. This muscle possesses a long lever arm and a nearly perpendicular angle of approach to both the ankle and oblique midtarsal joint axes. (This approach is maintained by the medial malleolus and sustentaculum tali.) As a result, flexor digitorum longus is a strong ankle plantarflexor and midtarsal joint (oblique axis) supinator. Note that the quadratus plantae muscle exerts a posterolateral pull on the flexor digitorum longus *(white arrow)* that acts to improve alignment of its tendons. If quadratus plantae were unstable, flexor digitorum longus would bowstring medially, thereby producing a shearing force at the metatarsophalangeal joints. **Flexor hallucis longus.** The tendon of flexor hallucis longus passes posterior to the ankle axis in a groove behind the talus. This groove serves as a pulley giving this muscle a longer lever arm for producing ankle joint plantarflexion. Because its tendon passes close to the subtalar axis, it is only a moderate supinator of the subtalar joint. Also, like flexor digitorum longus, it is a strong supinator of the oblique midtarsal joint axis.

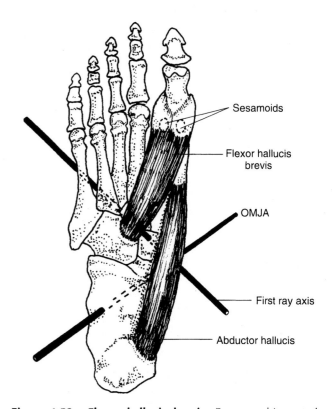

Figure 1.52.   Flexor hallucis brevis. Because this muscle originates so close to the first ray axis, it is unable to produce significant amounts of first ray plantarflexion. However, the tendons of flexor hallucis brevis contain sesamoid bones that act as pulleys to make this muscle a strong plantarflexor of the first metatarsophalangeal joint. Note that the medial and lateral attachments of these tendons produce almost pure sagittal plane motion of the first metatarsophalangeal joint with minimal transverse plane shearing of the hallux. These attachments also serve to stabilize the first metatarsophalangeal joint by creating a strong compressive force. **Abductor hallucis.** This muscle has a significant lever arm and adequate angle of approach for producing plantarflexion at the first ray and supination at the oblique midtarsal joint axes *(OMJA)*. Because abductor hallucis also has a significant lever arm to the vertical axis of the metatarsophalangeal joint, it is capable of producing a strong rotational component in the transverse plane. This abductory force is usually resolved into a pure compressive force by the antagonistic pull of adductor hallucis.

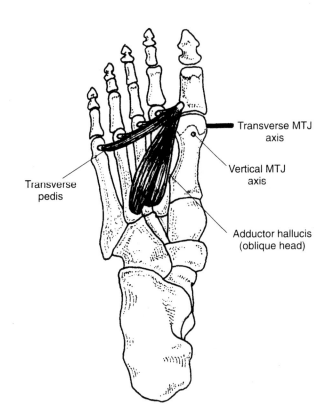

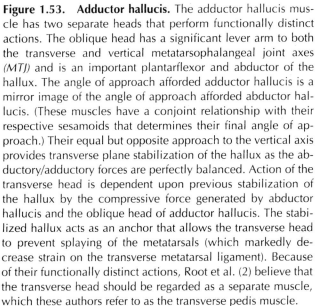

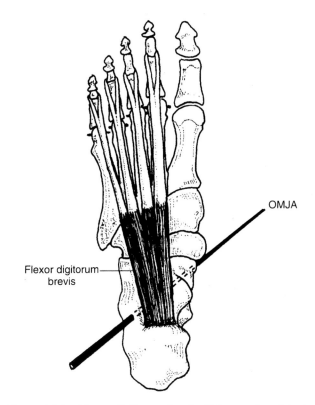

Figure 1.53.   Adductor hallucis. The adductor hallucis muscle has two separate heads that perform functionally distinct actions. The oblique head has a significant lever arm to both the transverse and vertical metatarsophalangeal joint axes *(MTJ)* and is an important plantarflexor and abductor of the hallux. The angle of approach afforded adductor hallucis is a mirror image of the angle of approach afforded abductor hallucis. (These muscles have a conjoint relationship with their respective sesamoids that determines their final angle of approach.) Their equal but opposite approach to the vertical axis provides transverse plane stabilization of the hallux as the abductory/adductory forces are perfectly balanced. Action of the transverse head is dependent upon previous stabilization of the hallux by the compressive force generated by abductor hallucis and the oblique head of adductor hallucis. The stabilized hallux acts as an anchor that allows the transverse head to prevent splaying of the metatarsals (which markedly decrease strain on the transverse metatarsal ligament). Because of their functionally distinct actions, Root et al. (2) believe that the transverse head should be regarded as a separate muscle, which these authors refer to as the transverse pedis muscle.

Figure 1.54.   Flexor digitorum brevis. This muscle originates from the medial condyle of the calcaneus and possesses both a significant angle of approach and lever arm to supinate the oblique midtarsal joint axis *(OMJA)*. Because its tendinous insertion is below the transverse metatarsophalangeal joint axis, it is an important plantarflexor of the digits. However, its effectiveness as a digital plantarflexor is dependent on the compressive force generated across the interphalangeal joints by the digital extensors (refer back to Fig. 1.46). Failure of the digital extensors to adequately compress the interphalangeal joints will allow flexor digitorum brevis to plantarflex only the intermediate phalanx, thereby predisposing to toe deformity as the plantarflexing intermediate phalanx produces retrograde dorsiflexion of the proximal phalanx.

Figure 1.55.   Lumbricales. The four lumbricale muscles originate from flexor digitorum longus, passing medial and inferior to the vertical and transverse metatarsophalangeal joint *(MTJ)* axes, respectively. Their tendons continue on to wrap around the medial shaft of the proximal phalanx, giving off a small attachment on the mediodorsal aspect of the head of the proximal phalanx. The final point of attachment for each lumbricale is on the lateral dorsal shaft of the distal phalanx. The medial passage of this tendon around the vertical metatarsophalangeal joint axis allows for a mild adductory moment, although its primary action is to rigidly extend the distal and intermediate phalanges (the tendon passes dorsal to the transverse axes) while creating a simultaneous compressive force at these joints. Because its tendon passes inferior to the transverse metatarsophalangeal joint axis, it is also able to plantarflex the proximal phalanx.

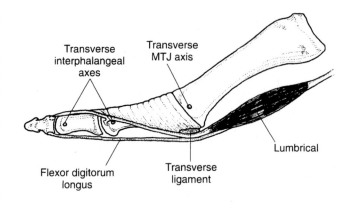

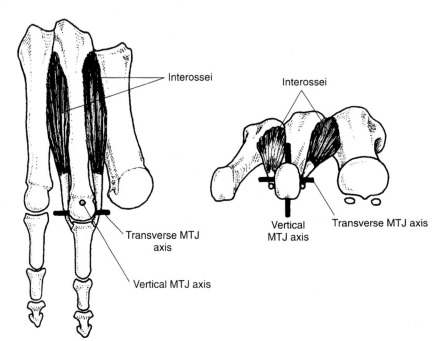

Figure 1.56.   Interossei. The tendons of the seven interossei muscles (there are four dorsal and three plantar interossei) pass very closely to the transverse metatarsophalangeal joint *(MTJ)* axes and are therefore able to exert a mild plantarflectory force at these axes. However, their tendons possess significant lever arms to the vertical metatarsophalangeal joint axes that thereby allow for the development of equally strong adductory/abductory moments. These moments are resolved into a compressive force necessary for transverse plane stabilization of the lesser metatarsophalangeal joints.

MC, Orion WP, Weed JH. Normal and Abnormal Function of the Foot. Los Angeles: Clinical Biomechanics, 1977. The interested reader is encouraged to refer to this text for a more detailed discussion of these and other muscles.)

References

1. Subotnick S, Jones R. Normal anatomy. In: Subotnick S (ed). Sports Medicine of the Lower Extremity. New York: Churchill Livingstone, 1989: 75.
2. Root MC, Orion WP, Weed JH. Normal and Abnormal Function of the Foot. Los Angeles: Clinical Biomechanics, 1977.
3. Harris GF. Analysis of ankle and subtalar motion during human locomotion. In: Stiehl JB (ed). Inman's Joints of the Ankle. Ed 2. Baltimore: Williams & Wilkins, 1991: 75.
4. Hicks JH. The mechanics of the foot. I. The joints. J Anat 1954; 88: 345–357.
5. Barnett CH, Napier JH. The axis of rotation on the ankle joint in man. Its influence upon the form of the talus and the mobility of the fibula. Anatomy 1952; 86: 1–8.
6. Wyller T. The axis of the ankle joint and its importance in subtalar arthrodesis. Acta Orthop Scand 1963; 33: 320–328.
7. Lundberg A, Svensson OK, Nemeth G, et al. The axis of rotation of the ankle joint. J Bone Joint Surg 1989; 71B: 94–99.
8. Inman VT, Ralston JH, Todd F. Human Walking. Baltimore: Williams & Wilkins, 1981.
9. Lambrinudi C. New operation on drop foot. Br J Surg 1927; 15: 193–200.
10. Bruckner J. Variations in the human subtalar joint. J Orthop Sports Phys Ther 1987; 8: 489–494.
11. Elftman H, Manter J. The evolution of the human foot, with especial reference to the joints. J Anat 1936; 70: 56–67.
12. Inman VT, Mann RA. Biomechanics of the foot and ankle. In: Mann RA (ed). DuVries' Surgery of the Foot. Ed 4. St. Louis: CV Mosby, 1978.
13. Engsberg JR, Andrews JG. Kinematic analysis of the talocal-

caneal/talocrural joint during running support. Med Sci Sports Exerc 1987; 3: 275–284.

14. Manter JT. Movements of the subtalar and transverse tarsal joints. Anat Rec 1941; 80: 397–409.

15. Green DR, Whitney AK, Walters P. Subtalar joint motions. J Am Podiatr Med Assoc 1979; 69: 83.

16. Root ML, et al. Axis of motion of the subtalar joint. J Am Podiatr Med Assoc 1966; 56: 149.

17. Bojsen-Moller F. Calcaneocuboid joint and stability of the longitudinal arch of the foot at high and low gear push-off. J Anat 1979; 129: 165–176.

18. Isman RE, Inman VT. Anthropometric studies of the human foot and ankle. Biomechanics Laboratory, University of California, San Francisco and Berkeley, Technical Report 58. San Francisco: The Laboratory, 1968.

Chapter Two

Ideal Motions during the Gait Cycle

The gait cycle is the basic reference in the description of human locomotion. One full gait cycle consists of the period of time between successive ipsilateral heel strikes; it begins when the heel initially makes ground contact and ends the moment the same heel strikes the ground with the next step (1). Note that although a small percentage of the population makes initial ground contact at the mid or forefoot, this chapter will refer only to the biomechanical events associated with the more commonly seen gait pattern in which the heel is the initial point of ground contact. Notice in Figure 2.1 the gait cycle is divided into stance and swing phases, which typically occupy 62% and 38% of the gait cycle, respectively (2).

When a person is walking, the gait cycle lasts approximately 1 second (1). As a result, stance phase occurs in 0.6 seconds and swing phase in 0.4 seconds. Because the distal end of the kinetic chain is fixed by ground reactive forces during stance phase, motions during this portion of the gait cycle are referred to as closed chain motions. In contrast, swing phase motions are referred to as open chain motions as the distal end of the kinetic chain is freely mobile. Also, because of the complexity of stance phase motions, this portion of the gait cycle has been subdivided into contact, midstance, and propulsive periods (Fig. 2.2). The timing and primary events associated with each portion of the gait cycle are discussed in the following paragraph.

STANCE PHASE MOTIONS

Contact Period

The contact period begins at heel strike (HS) and ends at full forefoot load (FFL). As illustrated in Figure 2.2, the contact period takes place during the first 27% of stance phase (or 18% of one full gait cycle) and typically lasts between 0.1 and 0.15 seconds (3). (Keep in mind that there is much variation in the percentages and timing of all phases.) In regards to the initial impact forces during the contact period, Katoh et al. (4) note that during a typical heel strike while walking, a person's ground-reactive forces average 110%, 15%, and 10% body weight in the vertical, forward, and medial directions, respectively.

At the moment that heel strike occurs, the hip is ideally flexed 30°; the knee is almost fully extended; the ankle is slightly dorsiflexed; the subtalar joint is slightly supinated; and the midtarsal joint is fully pronated about its oblique axis and supinated (inverted) about its longitudinal axis (Fig. 2.3).

As the foot proceeds through its contact period, a combination of ground-reactive forces (which are initially applied to the posterolateral heel) and inertial forces (the pelvis and lower extremity continue their internal rotation, which began during early swing phase) causes the ankle to plantarflex and the subtalar joint to pronate. Plantarflexion of the ankle is resisted by eccentric contraction of the anterior compartment musculature (5). These muscles play an important role in absorbing shock as they smoothly lower the forefoot to the ground, thereby minimizing trauma to the plantar soft tissues. Interestingly, Radin and Paul (6) state that joint motion controlled by muscles lengthening under tension is the primary kinematic process responsible for shock absorption. The ankle continues to plantarflex throughout the first 70% of the contact period, reaching a maximally plantarflexed position of 10° (Fig. 2.4). At that time, ground-reactive forces beneath the forefoot cause the ankle to dorsiflex slightly (i.e., the ankle is still plantarflexed 5° by the end of the contact period). The contact period ends with full forefoot load (FFL), which occurs when the opposite leg enters its swing phase, thereby transferring full body weight to the stance phase leg.

Throughout the entire contact period, the subtalar joint is pronating from the slightly supinated position present at heel-strike. Normally, the subtalar joint will pronate only during the contact period, with various authors (2, 7, 8) describing normal pronatory ranges that vary between 4 and 12° from neutral (the discrepancy between these figures being related to variation in orientation of the subtalar joint axis of motion).

An extremely important clinical consideration is that subtalar joint pronation is both directly and indirectly responsible for shock absorption. The importance of this action is emphasized when one considers the repetitiveness of the gait cycle and the magnitude of impact forces, i.e., each foot strikes the ground between 10 and 15 thousand times daily (9), absorbing the equivalent of 639 metric tons of pressure (10). Root et al. (2) stress the significance of this information by noting that any condition preventing the normal range of subtalar joint pronation will result in pathological amounts of stress being transmitted up the leg, into the pelvis and lumbar spine. It is of note that Fredrich (11) stated that these forces travel through the body at a speed of 200 mph.

The subtalar joint is able to effectively dampen these forces, primarily because the talus moves into an adducted and plantarflexed position as the subtalar joint pronates (12)

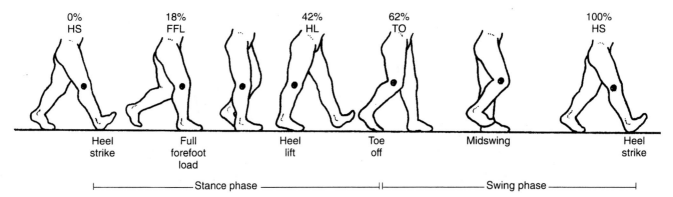

Figure 2.1. **Gait cycle of the right leg.** Stance phase begins at heel-strike *(HS)* and ends when the great toe leaves the ground. Swing phase continues until the heel again strikes the ground. The length of stride, which refers to the distance between successive ipsilateral heel strikes, is approximately 0.8 times a person's body height, and the average cadence is approximately 115 steps/min (slightly lower for men and higher for women [1]). It should be emphasized that there is marked individual variation in stride length and cadence, as each person seems to choose a gait pattern that is metabolically most efficient.

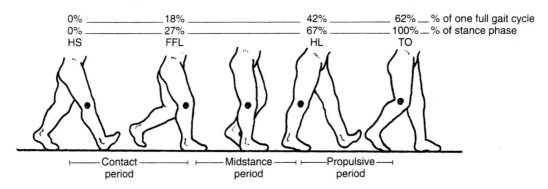

Figure 2.2. **The various periods of stance phase.** *HS,* heel strike; *FFL,* full forefoot load; *TO,* toe off.

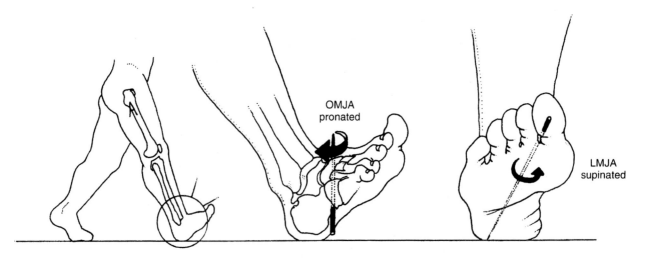

Figure 2.3. **Ideal joint positions present at heel strike.** *OMJA,* oblique midtarsal joint axis; *LMJA,* longitudinal midtarsal joint axis.

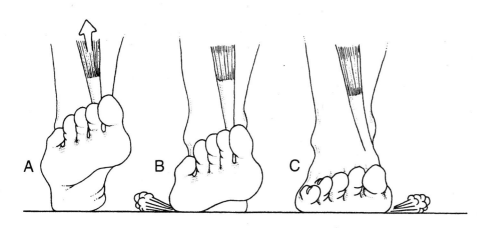

Figure 2.4. Ankle plantarflexion during early and midcontact period is resisted by eccentric contraction of the anterior compartment muscles (*arrow* in A). Approximately 40% of the way through contact period (**B**), the fifth metatarsal head strikes the ground. The forefoot is then smoothly loaded from lateral to medial with the entire forefoot making ground contact approximately 70% of the way through the contact period (**C**).

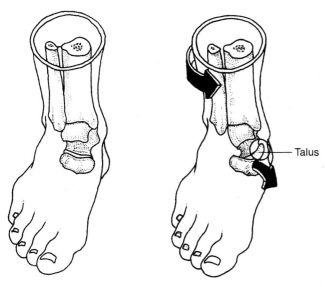

Figure 2.5. Subtalar joint pronation causes the talus to adduct and plantarflex.

(Fig. 2.5). These combined talar motions allow for shock absorption via two distinct mechanisms.

First, talar plantarflexion directly allows for shock absorption as it results in a lowering of the ankle mortise (Fig. 2.6). This motion markedly reduces impact forces by allowing the supporting musculature more time to dampen the body's momentum. This demonstrates an important concept regarding the dissipation of forces: less force will be absorbed by the tissues when the force is absorbed over a longer period of time. An analogous action is seen when a baseball player catches a fastball. If the player pulls his glove towards his body at the moment of impact, less force will be absorbed by the player's hand. If the same fastball were caught with the catcher's elbows locked and his shoulders stiff, the force absorbed by the hand would markedly increase (potentially producing injury) as forces would now be absorbed in a shorter period of time.

Subtalar joint pronation also indirectly allows for shock absorption as the adducting talus internally rotates the tibia, thereby allowing the knee to flex; i.e., the knee is not a pure

ginglymus joint: internal rotation of the tibia is a necessary prerequisite for knee flexion (Fig. 2.7). Flexion of the knee allows the quadriceps musculature more time to dampen impact forces, thereby lessening the potential for injury.

In addition to its role in shock absorption, subtalar joint pronation is also essential for surface adaptation, as it allows for an added range of midtarsal joint motion by improving the alignment of the talonavicular and calcaneocuboid axes (Fig. 2.8). Phillips and Phillips (13) demonstrated that this parallelism of axes produces an additional 11.6 degrees of midtarsal motion (which occurs primarily about the oblique midtarsal joint axis). This added range of motion allows for an improved deflection of the medial longitudinal arch that is essential for shock absorption and surface adaptation. Ker et al. (14) also note that deflection of the medial arch provides a natural energy return mechanism in which approximately 17 joules of energy are stored in the stretched muscles and ligaments of the arch (primarily the plantar fascia, the long and short plantar ligaments, and the spring ligament), only to be returned during the latter half of stance phase in the form of elastic recoil. The authors compare this to a bouncing rubber ball and claim that enough strain energy is stored in the arch to make running more efficient.

Throughout the contact period, the midtarsal joint remains pronated about its oblique axis and supinated (inverted) about its longitudinal axis. These positions are maintained initially by tension in the anterior compartment muscles as they eccentrically contract in an attempt to decelerate plantarflexion of the ankle after heel-strike: eccentric contraction of tibialis anterior inverts the forefoot about the longitudinal midtarsal joint axis while eccentric contraction of extensor digitorum longus and peroneus tertius pronates the forefoot about the oblique midtarsal joint axis. Once the plantar forefoot contacts the surface, ground-reactive forces act to maintain the midtarsal joint in its fully pronated position about the oblique axis (which now has an increased range thanks to subtalar pronation) and its fully inverted position about its longitudinal axis.

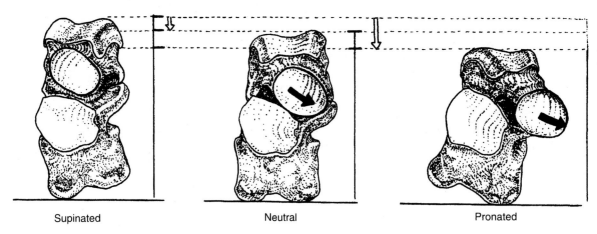

Supinated   Neutral   Pronated

Figure 2.6.   Anterior view of the right talus and calcaneus.

Figure 2.7. Inferior view of the right knee. The medial femoral condyle is situated further forward than the lateral condyle *(x)*. Internal rotation of the tibia (as supplied by the adducting talus) allows the medial tibial plateau to glide posteriorly **(A)**, thereby allowing for flexion of the knee **(B).** This rotational activity occurs simultaneously with a rolling/gliding motion as forward momentum of the pelvis pushes the femur anteriorly on the tibia, which is maintained in a relatively fixed position by ground-reactive forces. (Partially modified from Hoppenfeld S: Physical Examination of the Spine and Extremities. New York: Appleton-Century-Crofts, 1976.)

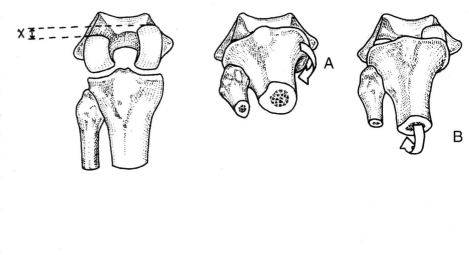

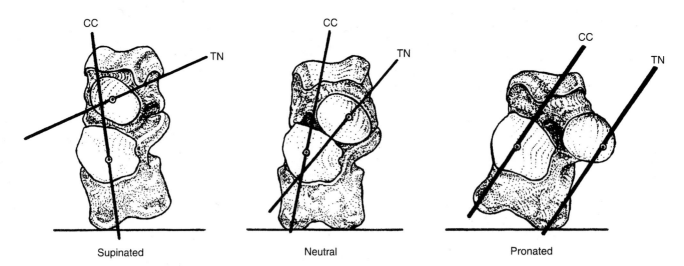

Supinated   Neutral   Pronated

Figure 2.8.   Anterior view of the right talus and calcaneus. Note the parallelism of the talonavicular *(TN)* and calcaneocuboid *(CC)* joint axes as the subtalar joint pronates.

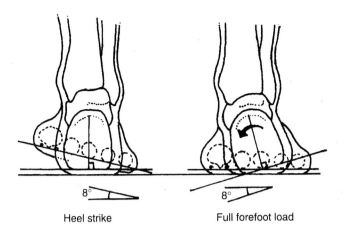

Figure 2.9. Subtalar joint pronation brings the inverted forefoot to the ground during the contact period.

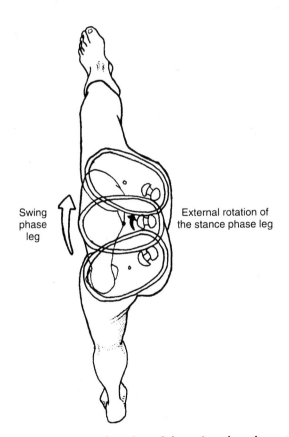

Figure 2.10. Forward motion of the swing phase leg externally rotates the stance leg, which in turn supinates the subtalar joint. Mann (15) emphasizes the role the adductors play in producing external rotation of the stance leg by noting that their firm attachment to the anterior pelvis and posterior femur allows these muscles to act as effective lever arms capable of translating the forward momentum of the swinging thigh into external rotation of the stance leg femur.

Notice in Figure 2.9 the forefoot remains inverted approximately 8° to the rearfoot throughout the contact period and the medial forefoot is brought to the ground via continued subtalar joint pronation. Mann et al. (15) claim that the final range of subtalar joint pronation available during the contact period is limited by, in order of importance, the congenital placement of the axes of the subtalar and midtarsal joints, the geometry of their articulating surfaces, and by their connecting ligaments. Apparently, the muscles play a relatively insignificant role in limiting subtalar pronation.

Midstance Period

Midstance period begins at full forefoot load and ends at heel lift. It is the longest period, occupying 40% of stance phase and lasting approximately 0.24 seconds (3). Throughout the majority of this period, the subtalar joint is maintained in a fully pronated position. However, as ground reactive forces beneath the heel begin to lessen toward the end of midstance, the subtalar joint begins to supinate as the foot attempts to convert itself from the mobile adaptor necessary during the contact period to the rigid lever necessary for the propulsive period. It partially accomplishes this task by taking advantage of the forward momentum of the contralateral lower extremity: the forward momentum of the swing phase leg externally rotates the pelvis (white arrow in Fig. 2-10), which then externally rotates the weight-bearing leg (black arrow in Fig. 2-10). Since the leg and talus behave as a closed kinetic chain during midstance, external rotation of the weight-bearing leg causes the talus to abduct, which in turn supinates the subtalar joint. This motion helps stabilize the tarsals by decreasing the parallelism of the midtarsal joint axes. All of these actions are assisted by various muscular interactions that will be discussed in more detail at the end of this section.

Shortly after the end of midstance, the subtalar joint should have supinated back to its neutral position, i.e., the head of the talus should be directly behind the navicular. In order for this to occur, the midtarsal joint must possess an adequate range of eversion about its longitudinal axis. To understand why this midtarsal motion is necessary, try to picture the following events: As the subtalar joint is supinating, the entire foot is inverting. Since body weight maintains the medial foot on the ground, inversion of the rearfoot can only occur if the medial aspect of the forefoot plantarflexes while the lateral aspect of the forefoot dorsiflexes (see Fig. 2-11). This motion occurs about the longitudinal midtarsal joint axis and constitutes eversion about that axis.

Ideally, the midtarsal joint will allow only enough motion for the rearfoot to reach vertical. At that time, the forefoot will hopefully "lock" against the rearfoot as the superior border of the pronating cuboid comes into contact with the dorsal border of the overhanging calcaneus (16). This sudden approximation of the calcaneocuboid joint represents an osseous locking mechanism that is maintained by tension in the various restraining ligaments. Continued motion, either subtalar joint supination or midtarsal joint pronation, is not

Figure 2.11. Posterior view of the right foot. The forefoot compensates for subtalar joint supination by everting about the longitudinal midtarsal joint axis.

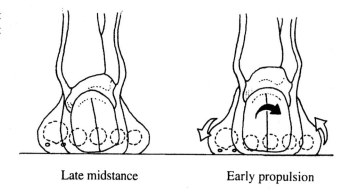

Late midstance   Early propulsion

Figure 2.12. Identifying the midtarsal joint locking position. One hand maintains the head of the talus directly behind the navicular while the opposite thumb dorsiflexes the fourth and fifth metatarsal heads to the point of firm resistance.

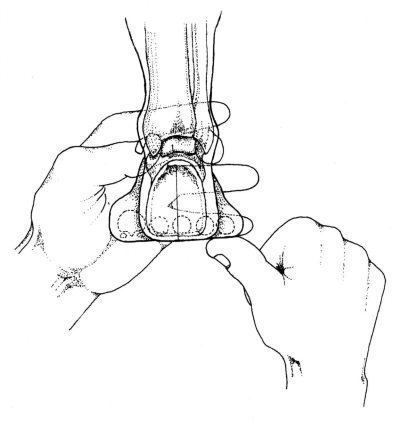

possible without overwhelming the restraining ligaments and subluxating the calcaneocuboid joint (2).

The osseous locking of the forefoot against the rearfoot at the calcaneocuboid joint is a necessary prerequisite for normal gait, as it minimizes muscular strain by allowing for a smooth transfer of accelerational forces through a locked lateral column (17). Basmajian and Deluca (5) stated that muscles should be considered only as a dynamic reserve for stabilization, as they cannot provide the support afforded by a well-designed skeletal system. Failure of the calcaneocuboid joint to lock into its close-packed position would result in a shifting of the tarsals as vertical forces are transferred from rearfoot to forefoot after heel lift occurs: the foot would behave as a flexible lever arm that is, of course, ineffective in the transfer of forces.

It is interesting that the feet of lower primates lack a midtarsal locking mechanism (16). While this makes for a less effective propulsion, the unrestrained range of midtarsal eversion is invaluable in the grasping of objects such as tree branches. Evolution of the foot required remodeling of the calcaneocuboid joint as functional needs shifted towards a faster, more efficient propulsive period. Of note, Basmajian and Tuttle (18) refer to a possible osseous locking mechanism present in the wrist and hands of African apes. If present, this locking mechanism would explain the minimal activity present in the forearm musculature during periods of knuckle walking.

Clinically, the locking position of the calcaneocuboid joint is easily determined by placing the subtalar joint of the prone patient in a neutral position and applying a firm dorsiflectory force to the fourth and fifth metatarsal heads (Fig. 2.12). This dorsiflectory force duplicates the application of ground-reactive force during early propulsion and gives the examiner an accurate picture of the forefoot/rear-

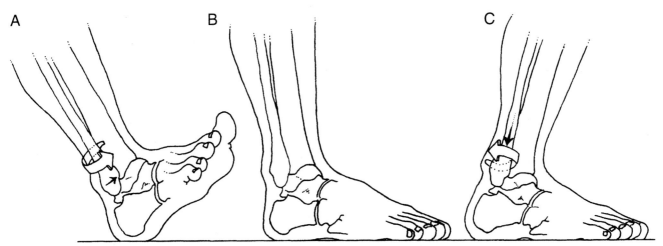

Figure 2.13. As the ankle plantarflexes during the contact period, the fibula shifts anteriorly and internally rotates an insignificant amount. However, during late midstance/early propulsion, the fibula drops inferiorly approximately 2.4 mm as it externally rotates as much as 3.7 degrees (3l). This movement is secondary to forces placed upon the fibula and interosseous membrane by active contraction of the peronei, tibialis posterior and flexor hallucis longus muscles. The downward movement acts to stabilize the ankle by increasing the depth of the mortise.

foot relationship present when the midtarsal locking mechanism engages.

As noted earlier, the calcaneocuboid joint will ideally lock when the sagittal bisection of the rearfoot is perpendicular to the ground or, as in this case, when the plantar forefoot is parallel to the plantar rearfoot. This locking position, in addition to stabilizing the forefoot against the rearfoot, also serves to improve the functional alignment between the achilles tendon and the calcaneus and protects against lateral instability of the ankle mortise by decreasing dependency on the lateral compartment musculature.

By the end of the midstance period, the ankle is dorsiflexed 10° (forward momentum of the body coupled with simultaneous knee extension throughout midstance allows the ground-reactive forces applied beneath the forefoot to dorsiflex the ankle), the subtalar joint is moving toward its neutral position, and the midtarsal joint is fully pronated about both axes, i.e., the midtarsal joint has remained fully pronated about its oblique axis throughout midstance although its available range of motion has significantly decreased due to subtalar joint supination. Because ankle dorsiflexion displaces the naturally wider anterior talus upwardly, the syndesmotic distal tibiofibular articulation may gap as much as 1.5 mm anteriorly (19) as the distal fibula externally rotates and moves inferiorly (Fig. 2.13).

Propulsive Period

The propulsive period begins the moment heel lift occurs and ends with toe off. This period occupies the final 33% of stance phase and lasts approximately 0.2 seconds. Although it appears to be a simple process, the actions responsible for producing heel lift are many. Firstly, the forward momentum of the torso displaces the center of mass directly over the forefoot, thereby minimizing the vertical forces responsible for maintaining ground contact at the heel (Fig. 2.14A). Secondly, continued contraction of the soleus and deep posterior compartment muscles acts to limit the range of ankle dorsiflexion by decelerating the forward momentum of the proximal tibia. This action allows the forward momentum of the center of mass to be applied directly towards lifting the heel (Fig. 2.14B). Lastly, the gastrocnemius muscle plays a particularly important role by simultaneously flexing the knee while plantarflexing the ankle. These combined actions serve to lift the knee upward and forward (which allows for an improved range of heel lift) while also assisting with hip flexion (Fig. 2.14C). Because of this, gastrocnemius indirectly allows for improved ground clearance during swing phase.

Once the heel has left the ground, the foot must safely channel large amounts of vertical forces (which peak during early propulsion) through locked and stable articulations. As stated by Root et al. (2), if the proximal articulations are not stabilized against the distal articulations, they will be placed into motion (and potentially injured) by forces acting on the foot. The foot is able to protect itself by again taking advantage of the external shank rotation supplied by the forward momentum of the opposite swing phase leg. Because the closed kinetic chain ends at the metatarsal heads after heel lift occurs, the continued external leg rotation will supinate the subtalar joint beyond its neutral position (ground reactive forces no longer maintain the calcaneus in a fixed position so that it is free to move with the rotating talus) while markedly supinating the forefoot about the oblique midtarsal axis: the entire rearfoot pivots medially as it abducts and dorsiflexes about the OMJA (Fig 2.15). Notice in this illustration how the external leg rotation creates a screw-like motion at the midfoot that greatly increases arch height, thereby converting the foot into a rigid lever.

Supination about the oblique axis of the midtarsal joint is aided by contraction of the intrinsic muscles originating from the medial calcaneus (particularly abductor hallu-

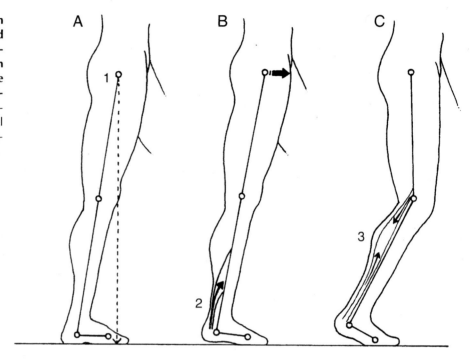

Figure 2.14. Heel lift results from the combined actions of the forward momentum of body mass *(1)*, muscular deceleration of ankle dorsiflexion *(2)*, and active flexion of the knee produced by gastrocnemius contraction *(3)*. Note that ***Panel B*** is for purposes of demonstration only as heel lift should normally occur with gastrocnemius actively flexing the knee.

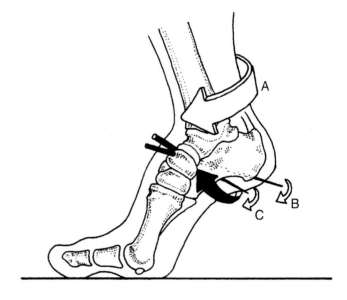

Figure 2.15. External leg rotation (A) acts to supinate the subtalar joint (B) while simultaneously supinating the forefoot about the oblique midtarsal joint axis (C). These motions increase arch height (black arrow), thereby stabilizing the various articulations of the midfoot.

cis) and by what is known as the windlass effect of the plantar fascia: dorsiflexion of the toes after heel lift draws the plantar fascia around the metatarsal heads, which acts to pull the anterior and posterior pillars of the longitudinal arch together (Fig. 2.16). This approximation of the rearfoot and forefoot allows for continued supination about the oblique

midtarsal joint axis with its concomitant increase in arch height.

While considerable stability is afforded by the increased arch height, the foot could not be considered a rigid lever were it not for the continued forefoot pronation about the longitudinal midtarsal joint axis. During early propul-

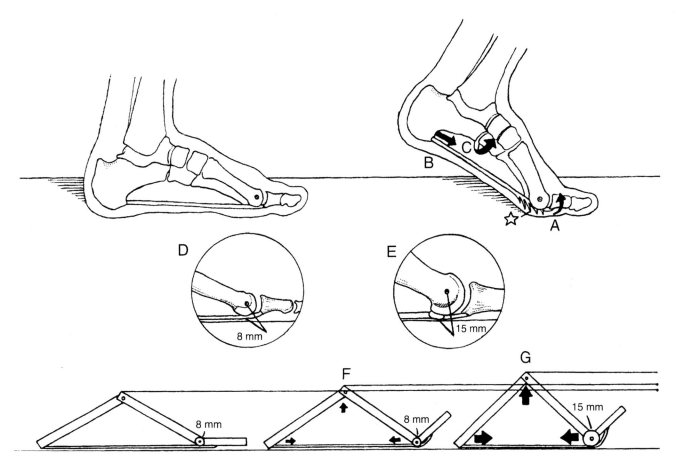

Figure 2.16. The windlass effect of the plantar fascia. During the propulsive period, ground-reactive forces are dorsiflexing the toes, which acts to draw the plantar fascia around the metatarsal heads **(A)**. This action results in the approximation of rearfoot and forefoot **(B)** and allows for the increased arch height necessary for stability **(C)**. The amount of pull generated by the plantar fascia is directly related to the distance between the transverse axis of the metatarsophalangeal joint and the passage of the plantar fascia: the greater the distance, the greater the pull placed upon the plantar fascia as the digit dorsiflexes. For example, the average lesser metatarsal has an average of 8 mm between its transverse axis and the passage of the plantar fascia **(D)** while the first metatarsal, with its larger head and the presence of sesamoid bones (which the plantar fascia invest) has a distance of nearly 15 mm between the transverse axis and the plantar fascia **(E)** (16). As a result, dorsiflexion of the first digit produces a much greater tractioning effect on the plantar fascia than any of the lesser digits (compare **F** and **G**). In order to resist the greater tensile load, the plantar fascia has its strongest attachment distal to the first metatarsal head. The plantar fascia also has strong attachments to the skin beneath the metatarsal heads **(star),** which prevents sliding on the skin as posterior shear forces are applied during the propulsive period (16).

sion, the calcaneocuboid locking mechanism is maintained by forceful contraction of the soleus muscle, which is simultaneously plantarflexing the ankle and inverting the subtalar joint. While ankle plantarflexion allows for a forward acceleration of body mass, subtalar joint inversion allows ground-reactive forces to dorsiflex the fourth and fifth metatarsals, thereby locking the lateral column.

The effectiveness of the soleus muscle in maintaining the midtarsal locking mechanism is only temporary, as early in propulsion the range of ankle plantarflexion places the soleus in such a shortened position that is unable to generate sufficient force to invert the calcaneus and can therefore no longer maintain the midtarsal locking mechanism (2). At this time, the continued forceful contraction of per-

oneus longus (which passes beneath the cuboid in the peroneal groove) acts to dorsiflex and evert the cuboid, thereby maintaining the close-packed position of the calcaneocuboid joint (Fig. 2.17).

An important consideration regarding the propulsive period function of the lateral column is that because the fourth and fifth metatarsals are shorter than the remaining metatarsals, the lateral column is unable to maintain ground contact during mid and late propulsion and is therefore unable to assist with the forward acceleration of body mass during these portions of the propulsive period. Locking of the calcaneocuboid joint at this time continues to serve a purpose, as it affords peroneus longus and brevis an effective lever arm as they now function to direct body weight

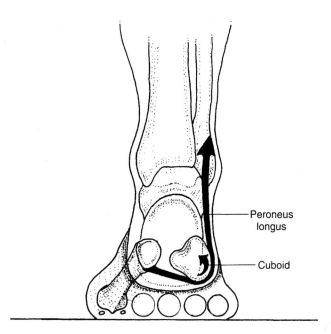

Figure 2.17. Concentric contraction of peroneus longus during early and mid propulsion serves to lift (dorsiflex and evert) the cuboid, thereby locking the midtarsal joint.

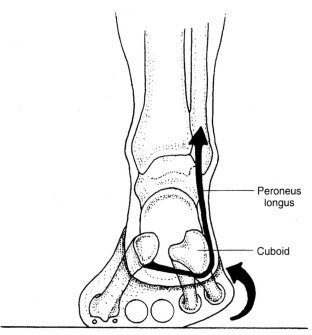

Figure 2.18. Because of their shorter stature, the fifth metatarsal leaves the ground approximately 33% of the way through the propulsive period with the fourth metatarsal leaving shortly thereafter (20). At that time, continued contraction of the lateral compartment musculature serves to shift body weight medially towards the opposite foot *(arrow)*, which is just beginning its contact period.

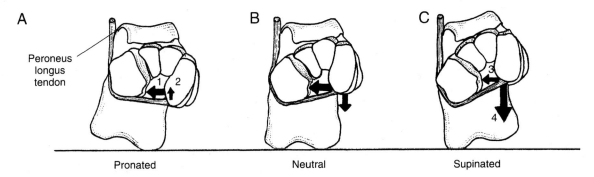

Pronated   Neutral   Supinated

Figure 2.19.   The effect of subtalar positioning on peroneus longus function. When the subtalar joint is pronated **(A)**, the nearly horizontal angle of approach afforded peroneus longus allows for the production of a strong posterolateral compressive force *(1)* and a mild dorsiflectory force about the first ray axis *(2)*. As the subtalar joint moves into a progressively more supinated position **(B** and **C)**, the posterolateral compressive force is lessened *(3)*, as the more vertical approach of the peroneus longus tendon allows for the development of a strong plantarflectory force about the first ray axis *(4)*.

medially towards the opposite foot by everting the entire lateral column (Fig. 2.18). This medial shift of body weight is necessary to maintain a straight gait pattern and to allow the final transfer of vertical forces to occur off the medial forefoot, which is better equipped to handle these forces, as the first metatarsal is twice as wide and four times as strong as any of the other metatarsals (21).

Because of its passage under the cuboid and eventual insertion into the base of the first metatarsal and medial cuneiform, peroneus longus has the interesting ability to transfer body weight medially while simultaneously stabi-

lizing the medial forefoot so it may better tolerate these forces. This stabilizing action is related to the improved angle of approach afforded the peroneal tendon as the subtalar joint is supinating (Fig. 2.19).

The improved ability of peroneus longus to function as a first ray plantarflexor is extremely important during the propulsive period, as the increased height of the medial longitudinal arch coupled with the normal parabolic curve of the metatarsal heads (i.e., the first metatarsal is normally shorter than the second metatarsal [9]) necessitates that the first ray actively plantarflex in order to maintain ground contact. In addition to the obvious importance of maintaining ground contact so as to resist ground-reactive forces, active plantarflexion of the first metatarsal allows for the dorsal-posterior shifting of the first metatarsophalangeal joint's transverse axis that is necessary for the hallux to reach its required range of 65° dorsiflexion (Fig. 2.20).

The combined actions of peroneus longus as an evertor of the lateral column and a plantarflexor of the first ray allow for what Bojsen-Moller (16) refers to as a high gear

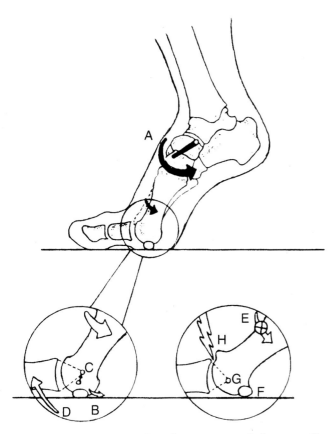

Figure 2.20. Because the first metatarsal is normally shorter than the second metatarsal, it must actively plantarflex in order to maintain ground contact during the propulsive period (A). As the first metatarsal plantarflexes, the metatarsal head glides posteriorly along the sesamoids (B), which allows for a dorsal-posterior shift of the transverse axis of the first metatarsophalangeal joint (C). This new axis allows for an unrestrained range of hallux dorsiflexion (D). Failure of the first metatarsal to plantarflex during propulsion (E) inhibits the posterior glide of the metatarsal head on its sesamoid (F), which in turn prevents the dorsal-posterior shift of the transverse axis. The hallux is now forced to dorsiflex about the original axis (G). This results in a "jamming" of the dorsal cartilage (H) with its characteristic resorption of subchondral bone and dorsal lipping of the first metatarsal head. The increased range of hallux dorsiflexion associated with first metatarsal plantarflexion can be demonstrated on yourself simply by everting your forefoot (off-weight-bearing) and noting the range of hallux dorsiflexion. Repeat the measurement with the forefoot fully inverted (which dorsiflexes the first metatarsal) and note the marked decrease in motion.

push-off. By everting the lateral column, peroneus longus allows the final transfer of body weight to occur through the transverse axis of the metatarsal heads (Fig. 2.21). Use of the transverse axis supplies the ankle plantarflexors with a longer and more effective lever arm for accelerating body mass forward. Failure of peroneus longus to evert the lateral column would allow for continued supination of the subtalar joint with the final push-off occurring as a rolling action through the oblique axis of the metatarsal heads. Because the oblique axis has a shorter lever arm to the ankle axis (the oblique axis is 15–20% closer to the ankle axis than the transverse axis), it allows for a less efficient propulsion that is referred to as a low gear push-off. Bojsen-Moller (16) states that use of the transverse axis via peroneus longus contraction represents the final evolutionary change in the process of producing a fast, efficient propulsion.

During the final portion of the propulsive period, the foot will ideally be supinated about the oblique midtarsal and subtalar joint axes. Also, the forefoot will remain fully pronated about the longitudinal midtarsal joint axis. This axis is maintained in a pronated position during late propulsion as extensor digitorum longus and peroneus tertius are vigorously contracting in preparation for the swing phase of gait. The final transfer of forces should occur through the hallux, which has been stabilized throughout the propulsive period by vigorous contraction of flexor hallucis longus. The

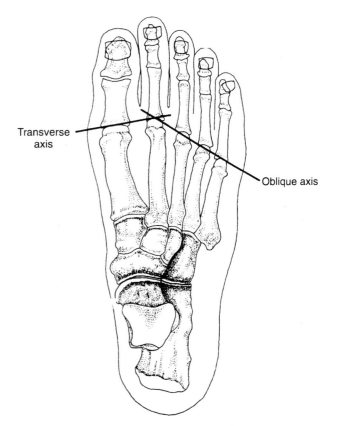

Transverse axis

Oblique axis

Figure 2.21. The transverse and oblique axes of the metatarsal heads.

entire lower extremity has continued to externally rotate throughout propulsion and into the swing phase of gait (1).

SWING PHASE MOTIONS

The swing phase, which begins at toe off and ends at heel-strike, occupies 38% of the gait cycle and lasts approximately 0.4 seconds (1, 2). The primary function of the foot and ankle during this phase is to allow enough dorsiflexion for the forefoot to clear the ground by midswing and to position the articulations so the supporting musculature may more effectively dampen impact forces as the next heel-strike occurs. Apparently, as demonstrated with infants, neuromotor control of swing phase motion is instinctive while control of the lower extremity during stance phase is a learned response (22).

During early swing phase, ground clearance of the forefoot is produced by forceful contraction of the muscles that flex the knee and hip and by concentric contraction of the anterior compartment musculature (which, as mentioned, begin contracting during late propulsion in preparation for swing phase). Since the ankle reaches its maximally plantarflexed position shortly after toe off, the anterior compartment muscles have less than 0.2 seconds to overcome inertial forces and dorsiflex the forefoot into a safe position by midswing. Because extensor digitorum longus and peroneus tertius are the first anterior compartment muscles to contract (2), the foot, in addition to dorsiflexing at the ankle, will immediately pronate about the oblique midtarsal and subtalar joint axes. (These muscles possess significant lever arms for pronating these axes.) The dorsiflectory components of these pronatory motions assist the dorsiflexing ankle in allowing for improved ground clearance.

Almost immediately after extensor digitorum longus and peroneus tertius contract, tibialis anterior and extensor hallucis longus begin contracting, thereby markedly increasing the dorsiflectory movement created at the ankle. Root et al. (2) claim that extensor hallucis longus is the strongest ankle dorsiflexor during early swing phase. Tibialis anterior, by virtue of its insertion on the first metatarsal and medial cuneiform, also acts to improve ground clearance by dorsiflexing the first ray during early swing phase (Fig. 2.22). Notice in this illustration how the forefoot is maintained in an everted position about the longitudinal midtarsal joint axis during early and midswing phase by continued contraction of extensor digitorum longus and peroneus tertius. The dorsiflectory motion of the first ray, in addition to improving ground clearance, also serves to enhance the efficiency of extensor hallucis longus as an ankle dorsiflexor, as it results in an anterior/inferior shift of the first metatarsophalangeal joint's transverse axis (Fig. 2.23).

By the time midswing has occurred, the ankle is dorsiflexed to a near neutral position; the subtalar and midtarsal joints are pronated (the midtarsal joint is pronated about both axes); and the first ray is dorsiflexed and inverted. These combined actions, when coupled with knee and hip flexion, allow for maximum amounts of ground clearance.

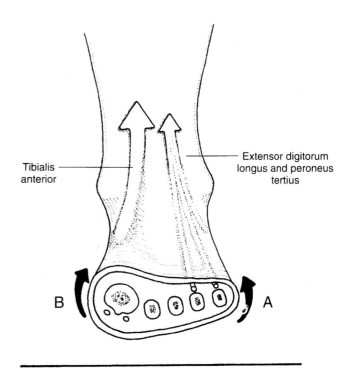

Figure 2.22.   During early swing phase, the lateral branches of extensor digitorum longus and peroneus tertius actively pronate the forefoot (A) while tibialis anterior, in addition to dorsiflexing the ankle, actively dorsiflexes and inverts the first ray (B), thereby allowing for improved ground clearance.

Shortly after the forefoot has cleared the ground, muscles of the swing leg have a relatively quiet period during which motion is maintained by inertial forces generated during propulsion and early swing (5). Just prior to heel-strike, the anterior compartment muscles simultaneously contract in anticipation of dampening the impact forces associated with the contact period.

Because of their relationships with the various axes, tibialis anterior and extensor digitorum longus produce mild dorsiflexion at the ankle, with tibialis anterior markedly inverting the forefoot while extensor digitorum longus and peroneus tertius assist with ankle dorsiflexion and pronation of the forefoot about the oblique midtarsal joint axis. Of note, Basmajian and Deluca (5) stated that tibialis anterior acts as an ankle dorsiflexor during early swing phase and an inverter of the forefoot during late swing phase. By positioning the foot with the ankle dorsiflexed, the forefoot inverted, and the subtalar joint slightly supinated, the pre-tensed muscles of the foot and leg are now prepared to effectively dampen ground-reactive forces associated with stance phase. It is interesting that with sprint running and anticipated falls, other shock-absorbing muscles (gastrocnemius, vastus lateralis, gluteus maximus, etc.) become hyperactive prior to heel-strike as they pre-tense in an effort to dampen more effectively the perceived increase in ground-reactive forces (23).

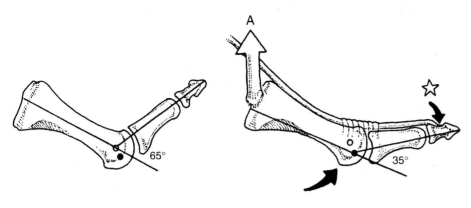

Figure 2.23. Dorsiflexion of the first ray by tibialis anterior *(A)* shifts the first metatarsophalangeal joint's transverse axis back to its original position *(black dot)*, thereby limiting the range of hallux dorsiflexion possible, i.e., only 35° of dorsiflexion are available about the new axis. The plantarflectory motion of the hallux improves the efficiency of extensor hallucis longus as an ankle dorsiflexor by stabilizing its insertion on the distal phalanx *(star)*.

DETERMINANTS OF THE GAIT CYCLE

In addition to the previously described actions present during the gait cycle (e.g., shock absorption, surface adaptation, forward acceleration of the center of mass, etc.), it is also important that the body move through each cycle with a series of smoothly coordinated structural interactions that act to minimize muscular strain. It is for this reason that Saunders et al. (24) refer to locomotion as "the translation of the center of mass through space along a path requiring the least expenditure of energy."

For example, if an individual were to walk with the knees locked and the pelvis stiff, the body's center of mass would move through a series of abruptly intersecting arcs that would greatly increase the metabolic cost of locomo-

tion, as the muscles would be forced to accommodate these angular displacements. Further strain would be placed on the supporting muscles as they attempt to absorb, then accelerate, these forces as the exaggerated curves reverse direction.

In order to minimize the metabolic cost of locomotion, each person incorporates specific actions that effectively decrease angular displacement of the body's center of mass. These actions, or determinants, are listed as follows: pelvic rotation; pelvic tilt; knee flexion/extension during stance phase; hip-knee-ankle interactions; and lateral pelvic displacement. The following illustrations, which were adapted from Saunders et al. (24), demonstrate how each determinant effects translation of the center of mass through space.

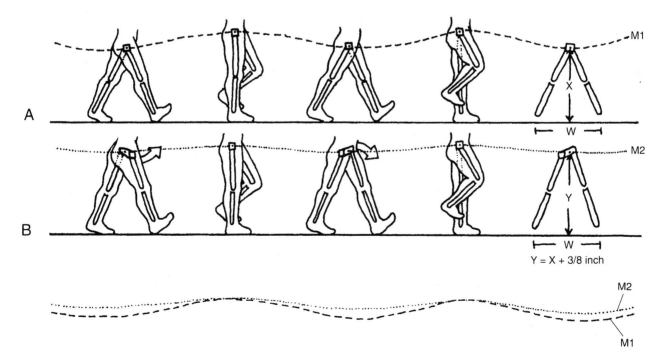

Figure 2.24. Pelvic rotation. Panel A represents a lateral view of the gait cycle without pelvic rotation while **Panel B** incorporates pelvic rotation *(arrows)*. Notice that *height X* in **A** is lower than *height Y* in **B** as rotation of the pelvis in **B** decreases the amount of hip flexion/extension necessary to achieve the same stride length *(W)*. This in turn decreases the vertical drop during double-limb support by approximately 3/8 inch, which effectively flattens the pathway for the center of mass *(M2 vs. M1)*.

Figure 2.25. Pelvic tilt. Eccentric contraction of the hip abductors during midstance lowers the pelvis on the side of the swing leg *(arrows in* **B***).* This decreases vertical displacement of the center of mass by approximately 1/8 inch.

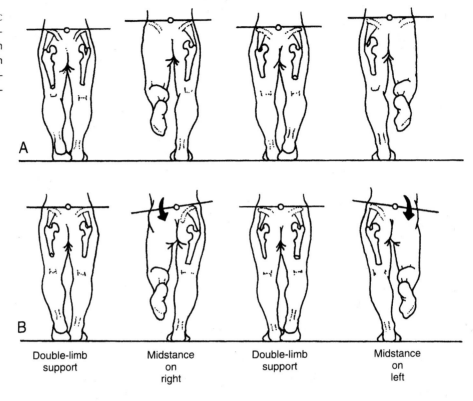

Double-limb support   Midstance on right   Double-limb support   Midstance on left

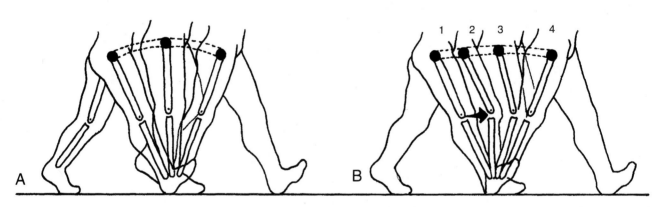

Figure 2.26. Knee flexion/extension during stance phase. **Part A** represents stance phase lower extremity motion without knee flexion while **Part B** represents the same leg with knee flexion/extension. Notice that when the lower extremity is straightened throughout stance phase, the center of mass describes a path along the arc of a circle, with the length of the lower extremity being the radius of the circle. This arc is effectively flattened by knee flexion during early stance *(1–3),* which prevents excessive elevation of the center of mass, and by knee extension during late stance *(3–4),* which prevents excessive lowering of the center of mass. Stance phase knee motions decrease vertical oscillation by approximately 1/8 inch.

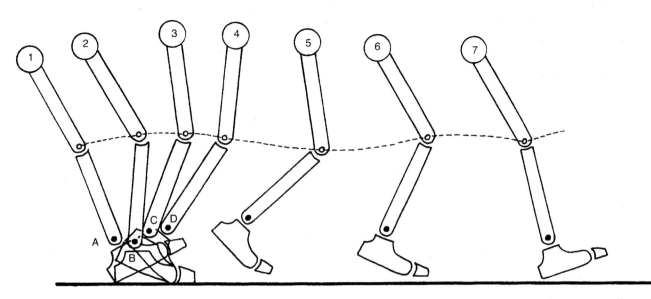

Figure 2.27. Hip, knee, and ankle interactions. As heel-strike occurs, the anterior compartment muscles eccentrically contract to slowly lower the stance leg to the ground *(A and B)*. This action, coupled with simultaneous knee flexion, maintains a smoother course for the center of mass during the contact period *(1–2)*. Forceful ankle plantarflexion during the propulsive period markedly elevates the leg *(B–D)* and is responsible for the maintenance of an almost straight pathway for the center of mass during late stance phase *(3–4)*. Flexion of the knee and hip during swing phase *(5–7)* allows for sufficient ground clearance despite lowering of the pelvis that is normally occurring on the swing leg side. If the knee and hip were unable to move through adequate ranges of motion, the individual would most likely compensate by circumducting the swing leg. This action greatly distorts movement of the center of mass and is metabolically very expensive to perpetuate.

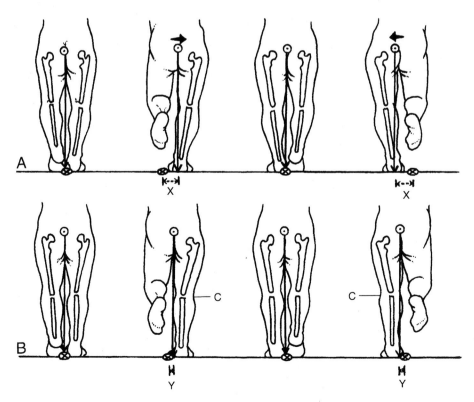

Figure 2.28. Lateral pelvic displacement. In order to maintain balance during the gait cycle, the weight-bearing leg adducts, and the swing leg abducts. This allows the center of mass to be displaced laterally over the supporting leg **(Panel A, X)**. If the lower extremity were perfectly straight (as in **Panel A**), the degree of lateral deviation necessary to maintain balance is significant. This markedly increases workload placed on the hip abductors and peroneals as these muscles attempt to accelerate the center of mass medially during late midstance and early propulsion. Fortunately, most people possess a slight degree of genu valgum *(C)* that minimizes the degree of lateral displacement by allowing for a more approximated base of gait *(Y)*. A mild genu valgum also allows the tibia to move through the gait cycle in a near vertical position **(Panel B)**.

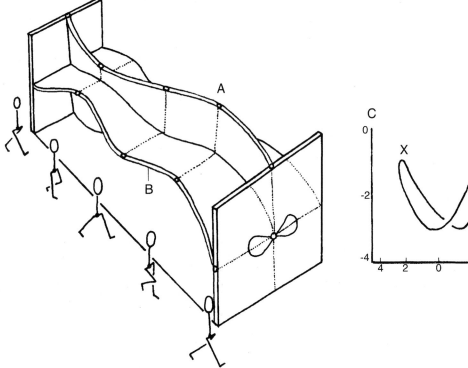

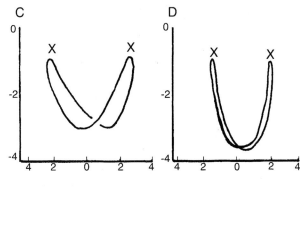

Figure 2.29. Final translation of the center of mass during a single stride. Lateral and vertical displacements are represented by **A** and **B,** respectively. Notice that these displacements are pure sine waves, with the frequency of vertical displacement being exactly twice that of the lateral displacement. **C** represents the projection of these displacements (which have been greatly exaggerated) onto a plane perpendicular to the body's line of progression. Because peak vertical displacements are reached slightly before peak lateral displacements, this curve represents a slightly distorted "lazy eight." At higher speeds of walking **(D),** the amplitude of lateral displacement is decreased, and the lateral and vertical displacements peak at the same time. As a result, the perpendicular displacement of the center of mass more closely resembles a "U." Note that even at maximal vertical displacement *(X),* the center of mass never reaches the level it would assume during static stance (which is represented by *O).* Forward acceleration of the center of mass, at both high and low speeds, is greatest at the low points of vertical displacement (i.e., during double-limb support) and least at the high points (i.e., during midstance period). Another way of saying this is that kinetic energy is greatest at the low points whereas potential energy is greatest at the high points. The brief periods of acceleration/deceleration present during the gait cycle are difficult to observe but become readily apparent as an individual walks across a room with a full bowl of hot soup: In order to avoid spilling the soup, the person will place the advancing leg directly under the center of mass, thereby avoiding the deceleration period that normally occurs between early contact and late midstance.

GRAPHIC SUMMARY OF THE GAIT CYCLE

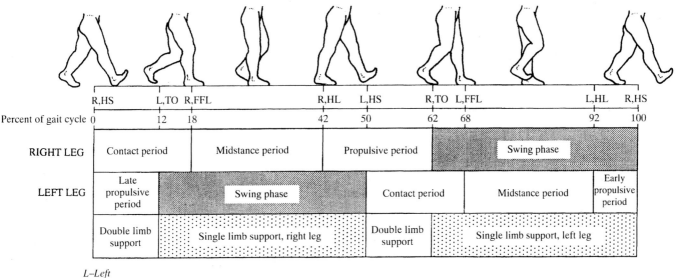

L–Left
R–Right
HS–Heel strike
FFL–Full forefoot load
HL–Heel lift
TO–Toe off

Figure 2.30.   Double-limb support. The feet simultaneously contact the ground twice during one full gait cycle: from 0–12% and from 50–62% (i.e., the first and last 12% of stance phase). During the first 12%, the opposite leg is completing its propulsive period, and during the final 12%, the opposite leg is beginning its contact period. It should be emphasized that the time spent in double-limb support decreases drastically as the individual's speed increases so that when running, there is no double-limb support, and each single-limb support stance phase is followed by a brief airborne period in which neither foot contacts the ground.

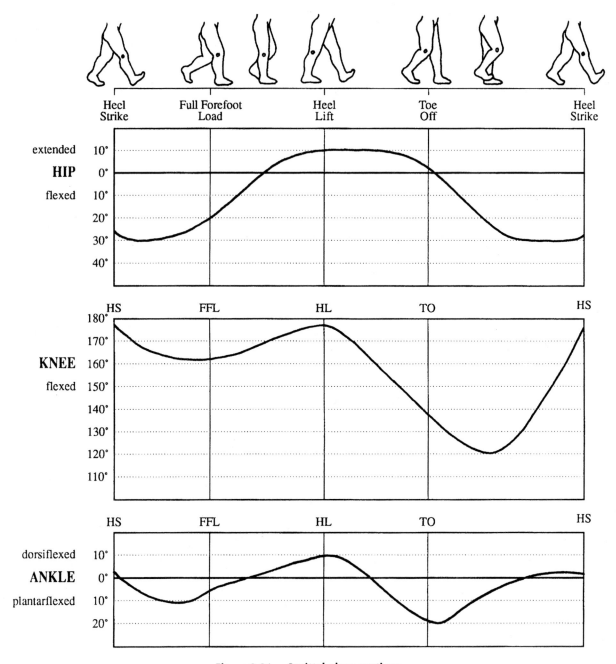

Figure 2.31.   Sagittal plane motions.

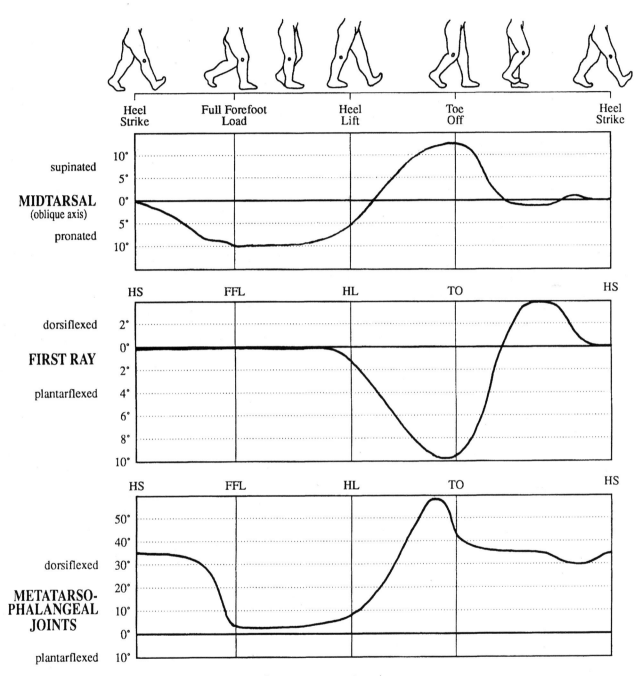

Figure 2.31—*continued*

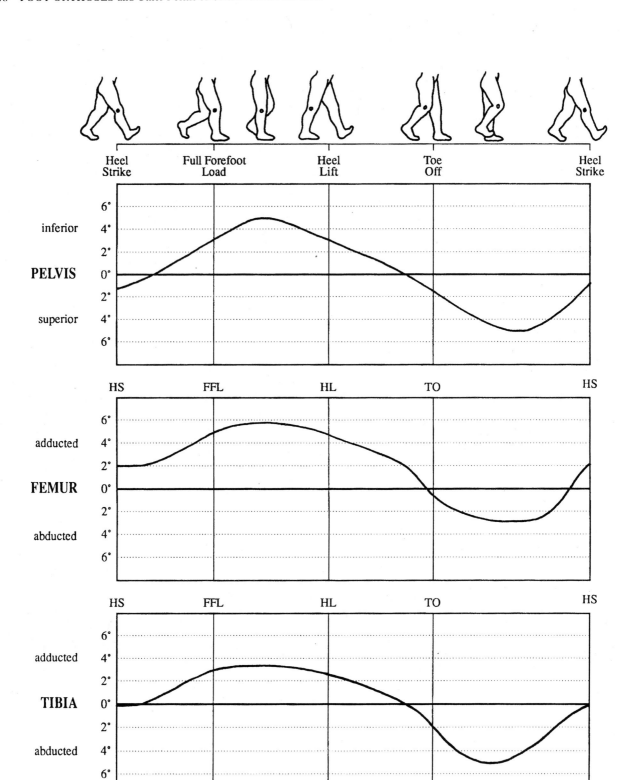

Figure 2.32.   Frontal plane motions.

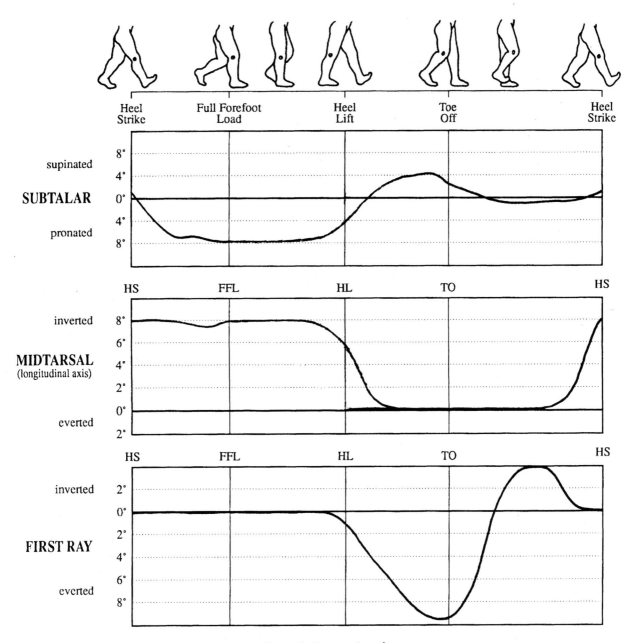

Figure 2.32—*continued*

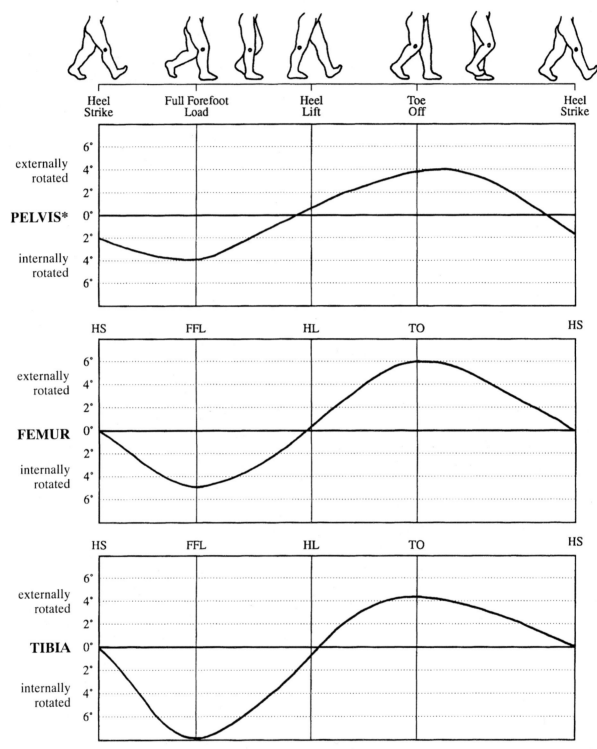

Figure 2.33. Transverse plane motions. *Although the pelvis in this graph is internally rotated only 2° at heel-strike, as higher speeds of locomotion are reached the pelvis may be maximally internally rotated at heel-strike, thereby allowing for an increased length of stride. Note that ipsilateral rotation of the pelvis is countered by contralateral rotation of the torso with the shift in motion occurring at about the eighth thoracic vertebra.

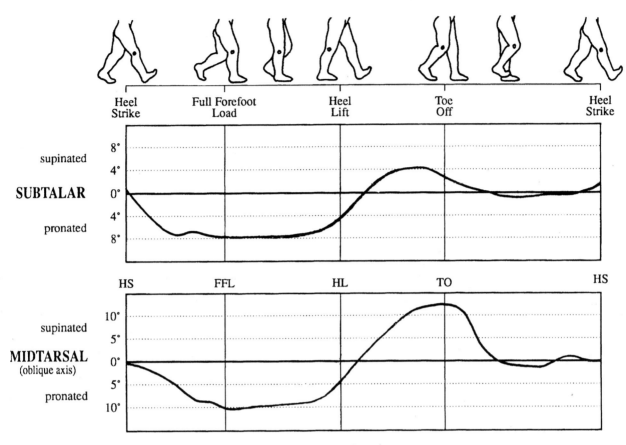

Figure 2.33—*continued*

SUMMARY OF MUSCLE FUNCTION DURING THE GAIT CYCLE

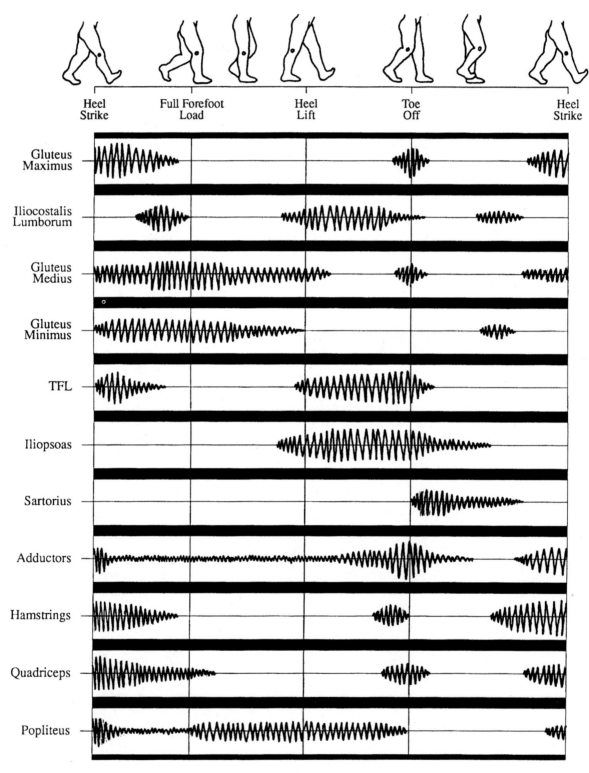

Figure 2.34.   Muscle function. *TFL* = tensor fasciae latae. (*Based on information from Basmajian (5), Inman et al. (1), Root et al. (2), Mann (15), Lyons (25), and others (26–30).)

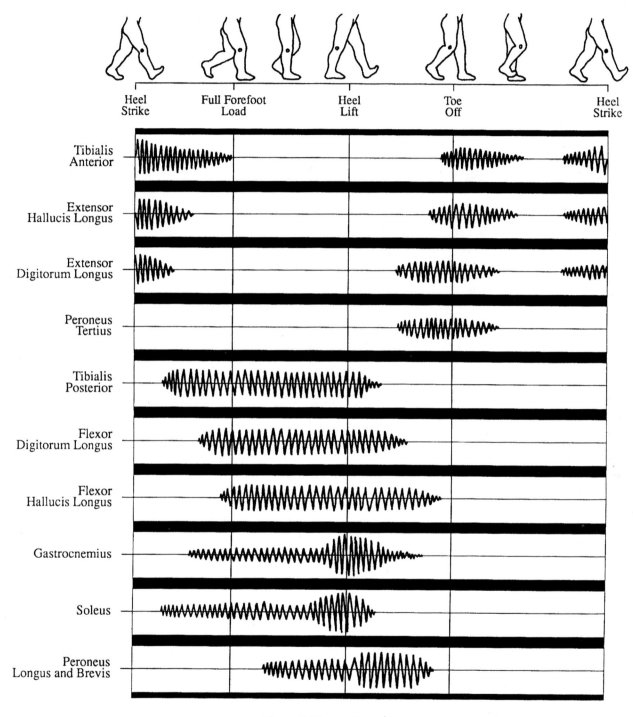

Figure 2.34—*continued*

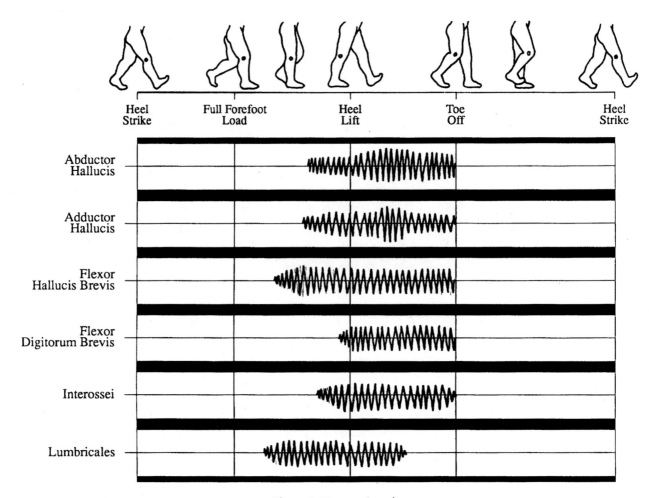

Figure 2.34—*continued*

Gluteus Maximus

This muscle contracts during late swing and early stance phase to decelerate flexion and initiate extension at the hip (although it may also mildly assist with abduction of the hip). Basmajian and Deluca (5) demonstrated that during terminal stance (toe off), the middle fibers of gluteus maximus display a brief burst of activity. Contraction at this time possibly allows these fibers to assist gluteus medius with abducting the swing phase leg. Lyons et al. (25) noted that the angles of approach afforded the various sections of this muscle allow its lower portions to act as hip extensors while the upper portions act as hip abductors. Interestingly, Duchenne (26) downplays the significance of gluteus maximus during relaxed walking by noting that complete paralysis of this muscle has minimal effect on gait.

Iliocostalis Lumborum

Because iliocostalis is the most lateral of the erector spinae musculature, it is able to assist in maintaining frontal plane stability of the pelvis during transitions from double-

limb support to single-limb support. Peak activity is seen during the early and midpropulsive periods (5). Contraction at this time prevents an exaggerated lowering of the ipsilateral pelvis as the contralateral gluteus medius (which prevents lowering of the swing phase leg) does not demonstrate peak activity until the end of the ipsilateral propulsive period. Waters and Morris (27) noted a brief burst of activity during the latter half of swing phase, as this muscle possibly contracts to assist the weakening contralateral gluteus medius in raising the ipsilateral pelvis in preparation for heel-strike.

Gluteus Medius

Gluteus medius is the primary frontal plane stabilizer of the pelvis. It begins contracting during late swing and continues throughout midstance and into propulsion. Peak activity occurs during early midstance as this muscle vigorously contracts to prevent excessive lowering of the contralateral pelvis (which is entering its swing phase). Basmajian and Deluca (5) noted a brief burst of activity in the anterior fibers of gluteus medius during toe off; contraction of these fibers possibly assists with abducting and internally rotating the femur during early swing phase.

Gluteus Minimus

This muscle functions agonistically with gluteus medius during early stance phase. The brief burst of activity during midswing most likely allows for continued internal rotation of the femur.

Tensor Fasciae Latae

Because of its insertion into the anteroproximal iliotibial band, contraction of tensor fasciae latae during the contact period acts to balance the force placed on the iliotibial band by simultaneous contraction of gluteus maximus (which has the greatest percentage of its fibers inserting into the posteroproximal iliotibial band). Contraction of tensor fasciae latae during contact period therefore prevents posterior displacement of the band and supplies gluteus maximus with a stable insertion. Tensor fasciae latae also contacts during late propulsion and early swing, during which it demonstrates its greatest activity as it assists iliopsoas with flexing the hip.

Iliopsoas

The iliopsoas muscle demonstrates peak activity during terminal stance and early swing phase, during which it assists the adductors, tensor fasciae latae, rectus femoris and sartorius with flexing the hip.

It appears that the momentum gained by rapid thigh flexion during early swing phase may play an important role in forward acceleration of the center of mass during late swing phase (15).

Sartorius

Sartorius is active only during swing phase with peak activity shortly after toe off. Because of its origin on the anterior superior iliac spine (ASIS) and insertion on the proximal anteromedial tibia, this muscle is able to assist with flexion of the knee and hip while simultaneously internally rotating the tibia during the first half of swing phase.

Adductors

The adductors as a group demonstrate peak activity during toe off, at which time they flex the hip and possibly assist with internally rotating the swing phase femur. These muscles again contract during late swing as they pre-tense in anticipation of ground-reactive forces. Although there is much individual variation in the behavior of the adductors (1), Basmajian and Deluca (5) noted that with the exception of a brief quiet period at midswing, adductor magnus fires

constantly throughout the gait cycle. Also, it is possible that the more horizontal sections of the adductors assist the contralateral swing phase pelvis with externally rotating the femur during the ipsilateral midstance period (15) (refer back to Fig. 2.10).

Hamstrings

The hamstrings demonstrate peak activity during the terminal portion of swing phase, during which they decelerate forward motion of the rapidly extending leg. These muscles continue to contract through the majority of the contact period, at which time they assist the gluteus maximus with decelerating flexion and initiating extension of the hip joint. Interestingly, Hollinshead and Jenkins (28) noted that because the distal semimembranosus releases fibrous attachments to the posterior horn of the medial meniscus, it is able to prevent impingement by drawing the medial meniscus posteriorly as the knee flexes.

With regard to propulsive period activity, Basmajian and Deluca (5) claim that in some individuals semitendinosus demonstrates a mild burst of activity during late propulsion, when it may act to assist gastrocnemius with flexing the knee. Elliot and Blanksby (29) noted that with running, all of the hamstring muscles maintain high levels of activity during the propulsive period, when they function as powerful knee flexors and moderate hip extensors.

Quadriceps

The quadriceps pre-tense during late swing phase and demonstrate peak activity during the early contact period, during which time they forcefully contract to decelerate knee flexion. These muscles continue to contract until the center of mass passes in front of the knee (1). A brief and less forceful burst of activity is seen during late stance and early swing phase as rectus femoris acts to assist with hip flexion (particularly at faster speeds) and the quadriceps act as a group to decelerate the range of knee flexion associated with early swing.

Popliteus

The popliteus muscle is a stance phase muscle that demonstrates a slight peak of activity at heel-strike with another more sustained peak through midstance and propulsion. During the contact period, popliteus concentrically contracts to assist the posterior cruciate ligament in preventing an excessive forward glide of the femur on the tibia and possibly assist the subtalar joint with producing internal rotation of the tibia. During the midstance period, this muscle eccentrically contracts to assist gastrocnemius with decelerating extension at the knee. During the propulsive period, popliteus again concentrically contracts, perhaps to assist with producing the rapid range of external femoral rotation necessary for knee flexion, i.e., throughout the propulsive period, the knee is flexing while the tibia is externally rotating. Because these motions conflict with the normal coupled motions associated with knee flexion (the tibia should be internally rotating as the knee flexes), the femur must rotate faster and further than the tibia for knee flexion to occur. The greater range of external femoral rotation allows the normal coupled motions to occur, as even though the tibia continues to externally rotate, it constantly remains internally rotated relative to the more externally rotated femur.

Tibialis Anterior, Extensor Hallucis Longus, Extensor Digitorum Longus, and Peroneus Tertius

The anterior compartment musculature demonstrates peak activity immediately after heel-strike. During the contact period, these muscles decelerate ankle plantarflexion (which allows for a smooth lowering of the forefoot to the ground), with tibialis anterior maintaining the forefoot in an inverted position about the longitudinal midtarsal joint axis during the early and midcontact periods. (Ground-reactive forces maintain this inverted position during the late contact period). These muscles are normally inactive during midstance and again contract during terminal stance. (Although Mann [15] noted that with running, the anterior compartment muscles remain active during midstance, during which they function to accelerate the body by pulling the proximal tibia over the fixed foot.)

Because extensor digitorum longus and peroneus tertius are the first anterior compartment muscles to contract during the propulsive period (2), they are able to dorsiflex the ankle while simultaneously maintaining the forefoot in a pronated position about the oblique midtarsal joint axis. (Extensor digitorum longus also acts to maintain a compressive force on the lesser metatarsophalangeal and interphalangeal joints, which prevents clawing of the digits.)

The terminal stance, early swing phase contraction of tibialis anterior also assists with ankle dorsiflexion, but its insertion on the medial cuneiform and first metatarsal allows it to produce simultaneous dorsiflexion and inversion of the first ray. The extensor hallucis longus muscle acts to maintain tension on the hallux during late stance and early swing, when it behaves as the strongest ankle dorsiflexor.

The anterior compartment muscles usually demonstrate a brief period of inactivity shortly after midswing, which is followed by simultaneous contraction of all of these muscles during terminal swing (5). This simultaneous late swing phase activity allows for mild dorsiflexion of the ankle and metatarsophalangeal joints with extensor digitorum longus and peroneus tertius reestablishing the forefoot in a pronated position about the oblique midtarsal joint axis. The late swing phase activity of tibialis anterior produces

marked inversion of the forefoot about the longitudinal midtarsal joint axis.

Tibialis Posterior, Flexor Digitorum Longus, and Flexor Hallucis Longus

Tibialis posterior functions primarily during the contact and midstance periods at which time it eccentrically contracts to decelerate subtalar pronation. Basmajian and DeLuca (5) state that tibialis posterior provides little assistance with plantarflexing the ankle at heel lift and its role at midstance appears to be a "restraining one" to prevent the foot from everting excessively. The long digital flexors play important roles during terminal midstance, as they assist with heel lift by decelerating the forward momentum of the proximal tibia (see Fig. 2.14).

The digital flexors continue contracting throughout most of the propulsive period, during which they forcefully maintain the digits against the ground and assist abductor hallucis with supinating the foot about the oblique midtarsal joint axis. Unlike flexor digitorum longus and flexor hallucis longus, tibialis posterior demonstrates its most clinically significant activity during the contact period, when it functions as the strongest decelerator of subtalar joint pronation and internal leg rotation (2).

Gastrocnemius and Soleus

Both soleus and gastrocnemius demonstrate peak activity during terminal midstance, at which time they function to produce heel lift. Soleus prevents forward motion of the proximal tibia (which decelerates and eventually stops ankle dorsiflexion) while gastrocnemius flexes the knee and plantarflexes the ankle (which actually initiates heel lift). The femoral origin of gastrocnemius also allows this muscle to maintain a constant flexion tension on the knee throughout midstance, thereby preventing hyperextension injury.

Another important action of these muscles occurs during contact period, during which soleus decelerates internal rotation of the tibia while gastrocnemius decelerates internal rotation of the femur (2). These dual activities help minimize the buildup of torsional strains at the knee during the contact period. Soleus continues to contract through midstance and into early propulsion, when, in addition to assisting with heel lift, it serves to supinate the subtalar joint, externally rotate the tibia, and stabilize the lateral forefoot against the ground (which maintains the locked lateral column).

Gastrocnemius also continues to contract throughout midstance and into propulsion, during which it assists with subtalar joint supination and external femoral rotation. An important consideration is that the rapid ankle plantarflexion and knee flexion produced by gastrocnemius during the initiation of heel lift impart a forward and upward momentum to the knee that greatly assists the hip musculature with producing hip flexion and thereby allows gastrocnemius to assist directly with ground clearance by midswing.

Peroneus Longus and Brevis

During the midstance period, peroneus longus and brevis create a pronatory force at the subtalar joint (brevis more so than longus) that partially resists the supinatory forces generated by the superficial and deep posterior compartment musculature. This antagonistic action decelerates the speed of subtalar joint supination and allows the subtalar joint to return smoothly to its neutral position by late midstance.

Contraction of peroneus longus also acts to stabilize articulations of the midfoot as this muscle works synergistically with tibialis posterior to create a compressive force on the tarsals: peroneus longus applies an abductory and posterior force at its insertion while tibialis posterior applies an adductory and posterior force at its insertion. These forces are resolved into a straight compressive force that prevents splaying of the tarsals during late midstance and early propulsion.

The peroneus brevis muscle is also able to create a stabilizing compressive force as it pulls the fifth metatarsal into the cuboid and the cuboid into the calcaneus, thereby stabilizing the lateral column.

The peroneals continue to contract throughout the majority of the propulsive period, during which peroneus longus plantarflexes the first ray (which improves ground contact and allows for the dorsal-posterior shift of the first metatarsophalangeal joint's transverse axis) while peroneus longus and brevis act together to evert the locked lateral column (thereby transferring body weight medially and allowing for a high gear push-off). Because the peroneals have such short lever arms to the ankle axis, they only slightly assist with ankle plantarflexion during propulsion. Peroneus brevis does, however, have a significant lever arm to the oblique midtarsal joint axis and is therefore able to decelerate supination smoothly about this axis during the propulsive period.

Abductor and Adductor Hallucis

The abductor and adductor hallucis muscles function during the propulsive period to stabilize the proximal phalanx of the hallux against the ground. (They maintain a plantarflectory tension on the first metatarsophalangeal joint.) These muscles are also responsible for transverse plane stabilization of the hallux, as they act to create equal and opposite rotational components of force on the proximal phalanx (which resolve into pure compressive force).

Because of its origin on the proximal phalanx and insertion into the distal metatarsals, the transverse head of adductor hallucis (transverse pedis) has the primary function of preventing the metatarsals from splaying as it pulls medially on the metatarsal heads from its stable anchor on the proximal phalanx. Failure of abductor and adductor hallucis (oblique head) to compress/stabilize the first metatarsophalangeal joint during the propulsive period makes it impossible for the transverse pedis muscle to prevent splaying of the metatarsals as its unstable origin is set into motion.

Because abductor hallucis has a significant lever arm and angle of approach to both the first ray and oblique midtarsal joint axes, it functions as an important plantarflexor of the first ray (it assists peroneus longus in this action) and supinator about the oblique midtarsal joint axis (it is assisted in this action by flexor hallucis longus, flexor digitorum longus, flexor digitorum brevis, and quadratus plantae).

Flexor Hallucis Brevis and Flexor Digitorum Brevis

By virtue of its tendinous investment of the sesamoids, flexor hallucis brevis is a powerful stabilizer of the proximal phalanx. This muscle functions with flexor hallucis longus to create a compressive force at the first metatarsophalangeal joint and to maintain the hallux against the ground during propulsion. Flexor digitorum brevis has a similar role in that it functions with flexor digitorum longus to compress the metatarsophalangeal joints of the second through fifth rays and allows the lesser digits to maintain an effective ground contact during the propulsive period. Unlike flexor hallucis brevis, flexor digitorum brevis assists in producing a strong supinatory force about the oblique midtarsal joint axis during propulsion.

Interossei and the Lumbricales

The interossei function during late midstance and propulsion to maintain transverse plane stability at the second through fifth metatarsophalangeal joints and to compress the proximal phalanx against the metatarsal heads. The lumbricales have the interesting ability to compress the intermediate and distal interphalangeal joints while also maintaining the lesser digits against the ground by creating a plantarflectory force about the metatarsophalangeal joints (2). Because the lumbricale tendons pass medially to the metatarsophalangeal joints, they are also able to generate a mild adductory force to resist the abductory shear force associated with ground contact. Since the tendons of the interossei pass below the transverse axis of the metatarsophalangeal joints, they act as plantarflexors of the proximal phalanx and, in conjunction with the lumbricales, play an important role in maintaining extensor rigidity of the digits during midstance and propulsion.

References

1. Inman VT, Ralston HJ, Todd F. Human Walking. Baltimore: Williams & Wilkins, 1981.
2. Root MC, Orion WP, Weed JH. Normal and Abnormal Function of the Foot. Los Angeles: Clinical Biomechanics, 1977.
3. Scranton PE, et al. Support phase kinematics of the foot. In Bateman JE, Trott AW (eds). The Foot and Ankle. New York: Thieme-Stratton, 1980.
4. Katoh Y, Chao EYS, Laughman RK. Biomechanical analysis of foot function during gait and clinical applications. Clin Orthop 1983; 177: 23–33.
5. Basmajian JV, Deluca CJ. Muscles Alive: Their Functions Revealed by Electromyography. Ed 5. Baltimore: Williams & Wilkins, 1985: 377.
6. Radin EL, Paul IL. Does cartilage compliance reduce skeletal impact loads? The relative force attenuating properties of articular cartilage, synovial fluid, periarticular soft tissues and bone. Arthritis Rheum 1970; 13: 139–144.
7. Subotnick SI. Biomechanics of the subtalar and midtarsal joints. J Am Podiatr Assoc 1975; 65: 756.
8. Wright DG, Desai SM, Henderson WH. Action of the subtalar and ankle joint complex during the stance phase of walking. J Bone Joint Surg 1964; 46A: 361.
9. Bojsen-Moller F. Anatomy of the forefoot, normal and pathologic. Clin Orthop Related Res 1979; 142: 10.
10. Magee D. Orthopedic Physical Assessment. Philadelphia: WB Saunders, 1987: 317.
11. Fredrich EC (ed). Sport Shoes and Playing Surfaces. Champaign, IL: Human Kinetic Publishers, 1984.
12. Hoppenfeld S. Physical Examination of the Spine and Extremities. New York: Appleton-Century-Crofts, 1976.
13. Phillips RD, Phillips RL. Quantitative analysis of the locking position of the midtarsal joint. J Am Podiatr Assoc 1983; 73: 518–522.
14. Ker RF, Bennett MB, Bibby SR, Kester RC, Alexander R. The spring in the arch of the human foot. Nature 1987; 325: 147–149.
15. Mann RA. Biomechanics of running. In Pack RP (ed). Symposium on the Foot and Leg in Running Sports. St. Louis: CV Mosby, 1982: 26.
16. Bojsen-Moller F. Calcaneocuboid joint and stability of the longitudinal arch of the foot at high and low gear push off. J Anat 1979; 129: 165–176.
17. Hicks JH. The mechanics of the foot. I. The joints. J Anat 1954; 88: 345–357.
18. Tuttle R, Basmajian JV. Electromyography of knuckle-walking: results of four experiments on the forearm of Pan gorilla. Am J Phys Anthropol 1972; 37: 255–266.
19. Close JR. Some applications of the functional anatomy of the ankle joint. J Bone Joint Surg 1956; 38A: 761–781.
20. Schwartz RF, Heath AL. A quantitative analysis of recorded variables in the walking pattern of normal adults. J Bone Joint Surg 1964; 46A: 324–334.
21. Hutton WC, Dhanedran M. The mechanics of normal and hallux valgus feet: a quantitative study. Clin Orthop 1981; 157: 7–13.
22. Elftman H, Manter J. The evolution of the human foot, with especial reference to the joint. J Anat 1936; 70: 56–67.
23. Mero A, Komi P. Electromyographic activity in sprinting at speeds ranging from sub-maximal to supra-maximal. Med Sci Sports Exerc 1987; 19: 266–274.
24. Saunders JB, Inman VT, Eberhart HT. The major determinants in normal and pathological gait. J Bone Joint Surg 1953; 58B: 153.
25. Lyons K, Perry J, Gronley JK. Timing and relative intensity of the hip extensor and abductor muscle action during level and stair ambulation. Phys Ther 1983; 63: 1597–1605.
26. Duchenne GBA. Physiologie des Movements. Philadelphia and London: WB Saunders, 1949 (originally published 1867).
27. Waters RL, Morris IM. Electrical activity of muscles of the trunk during walking. J Anat 1972; 111: 191–199.
28. Hollinshead WH, Jenkins DB. Functional Anatomy of the Limbs and Back. Ed. 5. Philadelphia: WB Saunders, 1971: 270.
29. Elliott BC, Blanksby BA. The synchronization of muscle activity and body segment movements during a running cycle. Med Sci Sports Exerc 1979; 11: 2–27.
30. Glancy J. Orthotic control of ground reactive forces during running (a preliminary report). Orthot Prosthet 1984; 3: 12–40.
31. Johnson JE. Shape of the trochlea and mobility of the lateral malleolus. In: Stiehl JB (ed). Inman's Joints of the Ankle. Ed 2. Baltimore: Williams and Wilkins, 1991: 16-17.

Abnormal Motion during the Gait Cycle

In order for the previously described ideal movement patterns to occur, several parameters for norm must exist:

1. When the individual stands in his or her normal base of gait, the lower leg should be perpendicular to the ground ($\pm 2°$).
2. When the subtalar joint is maintained in its neutral position and the calcaneocuboid joint is locked in its close-packed position (Fig. 3.1), the vertical bisection of the calcaneus should parallel the vertical bisection of the distal tibia and fibula ($\pm 2°$), the plantar forefoot should be perpendicular to the vertical bisection of the calcaneus, and the plantar metatarsal heads should all rest on the same transverse plane.
3. The distal extensions of the metatarsal heads should form a smooth parabolic curve.
4. The lower extremities must be of equal length.
5. The various articulations of the lower extremity and pelvis should move through specific minimum ranges of motion.
6. Neuromotor coordination must be intact, and the periarticular tissues must provide ample proprioceptive information.
7. The supporting muscles must possess adequate strength, power, and endurance.
8. The articular architecture should protect against excessive and/or abnormal motions.
9. Ontogeny must allow for the formation of a relatively straight lower extremity (in both the frontal and transverse planes) and for the development of a functional medial longitudinal arch.

As one must expect, whenever there are specific guidelines identifying the norm, there are bound to be situations in which individuals deviate from these outlined parameters. In fact, individual variation in the shape of the articular surfaces and/or defects in the triplanar development of the osseous structures are so common that deviation from one or more of these outlined parameters is the rule rather than the exception. As will be demonstrated, de-

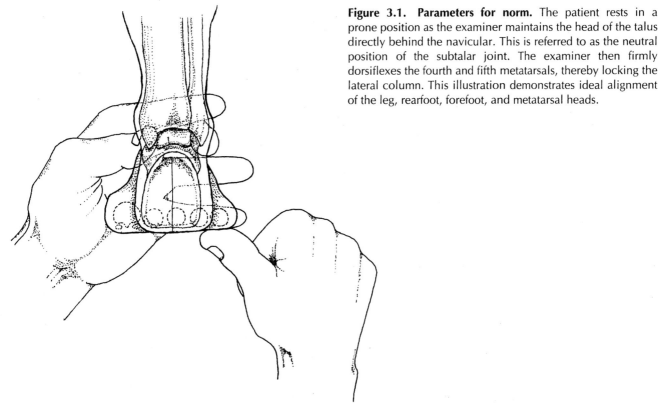

Figure 3.1. Parameters for norm. The patient rests in a prone position as the examiner maintains the head of the talus directly behind the navicular. This is referred to as the neutral position of the subtalar joint. The examiner then firmly dorsiflexes the fourth and fifth metatarsals, thereby locking the lateral column. This illustration demonstrates ideal alignment of the leg, rearfoot, forefoot, and metatarsal heads.

parture from even one of these parameters will result in some type of biomechanical malfunction. The following sections will review the pathomechanics associated with deviation from each of the described parameters.

REARFOOT VARUS DEFORMITY

By far, the most common deviation from the outlined parameters defining norm is the rearfoot varus deformity. This deformity represents an osseous malformation in which the tibia has formed in a bowed position (Fig. 3.2), and/or the subtalar joint has formed in such a way that the calcaneus is excessively inverted when the foot is maintained in its neutral position (Fig. 3.3). As a result of this deformity, the lower leg is typically unable to assume a perpendicular position during heel strike.

Because the rearfoot varus deformity represents the combined degrees of tibiofibular varum and subtalar varum, deformity greater than the ideal of 4° (a 2° variance for subtalar varum plus a 2° variance for tibiofibular varum) is extremely common. In one epidemiological study of the various foot types, McPoil et al. (1) found a rearfoot varus deformity exceeding 4° in 98.3% of the individuals measured. Because of this, it is more appropriate to refer to a straight lower leg as the ideal rather than the norm.

The etiology of the rearfoot varus deformity is related to a failure of the tibia and/or calcaneus to straighten from their infantile positions (2) (Fig. 3.4). In regards to subtalar varum, the calcaneus normally derotates 3 to 4° during early childhood. If for any reason the calcaneus does not derotate, or if derotation is incomplete, a subtalar varum will result (2, 3). In addition to subtalar derotation, the tibia must also straighten from its infantile position. The graph in Figure 3.5 demonstrates typical frontal plane development during the growth years.

While pathological genu varum may result from various metabolic/hereditary disorders, a much more common cause is Blount's disease. This disease is divided according to age into infantile (1–3 years) and adolescent (8–15 years) forms, with the infantile form up to five times more common (5). Although described as an osteochondrosis, Blount's disease appears to result from abnormal compressive forces along the medial tibial growth plate and not from avascular necrosis (6, 7). Numerous investigators feel that the juvenile form of Blount's disease may actually result from early walking when physiologic varum is at its

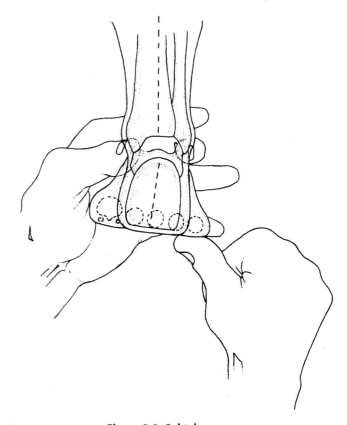

Figure 3.3. Subtalar varum.

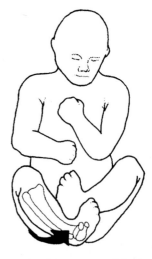

Figure 3.4. As a result of in utero positioning during the third trimester, the tibias are bowed (arrow), and the calcanei are inverted.

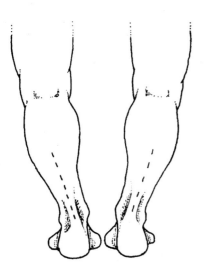

Figure 3.2. Tibiofibular varum.

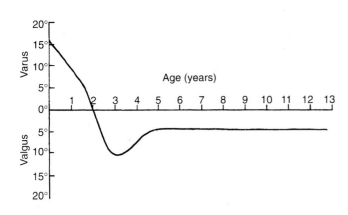

Figure 3.5. Development of the tibiofemoral angle. Note the physiologic transition from genu varum to valgum during the early years of growth. This graph is based on clinical and radiographic measurements of more than 1400 children. (Adapted from Salenius P, Vankka E. The development of the tibiofemoral angle in children. J Bone Joint Surg 1975; 57A: 259–261.)

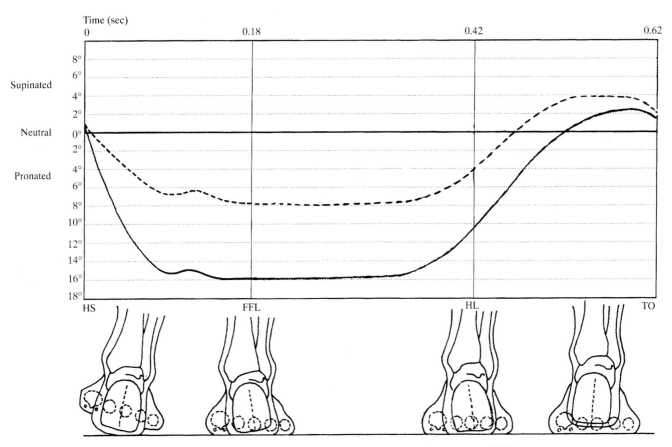

Figure 3.6. Stance phase motions with a rearfoot varus deformity *(solid line).*

peak (8–10). It has been suggested that the application of vertical forces in the presence of a large genu varum may sufficiently compress the medial tibiofemoral compartment so that growth at the medial tibial physis is inhibited (which is consistent with the Heuter-Volkmann principle). The resulting angular deformity only serves to amplify the compressive forces, thereby increasing the malformation. Cook et al. (11) developed a biomechanical model to demonstrate that a 20° tibial varum in a 2-year-old child would create sufficient force to retard physiological growth. This theory is consistent with the clinical observation that children from the West Indies and Africa, where early walking during infancy is common, typically present with a marked physio-

logical varum (12). Kling (13) stated that while the true etiology of Blount's disease remains uncertain, there is consensus that stress and growth combine to produce progressive varus deformity.

Pathomechanics

Because of the excessively inverted position of the rearfoot, initial ground contact occurs along the posterolateral edge of the calcaneus. To compensate for this deformity, the subtalar joint must pronate excessively just to bring the medial condyle of the calcaneus to the ground (Fig. 3.6). Note that the degree of subtalar pronation is directly related to the degree of the deformity, e.g., a person with an 8° tibiofibular varum coupled with a 4° subtalar varum must pronate 12° in order for the medial heel to make ground contact. Unfortunately, this fairly large range of subtalar pronation does not represent the final range of contact period subtalar joint pronation. Because the forefoot remains inverted about the longitudinal midtarsal joint axis during contact period (this position is maintained by eccentric contraction of tibialis anterior), the subtalar joint must continue to pronate an additional 6–8° in order to bring the medial forefoot to the ground.

The graph in Figure 3.6 shows that the rearfoot varus deformity produces dysfunction of the subtalar joint primarily during the contact period, as this joint most often returns to a stable position by mid propulsion. The contact period pronation associated with the rearfoot varus deformity may produce injury partly because the overall range is so large and partly because the subtalar joint moves through this exaggerated range in less than 0.15 seconds (14). Numerous studies have demonstrated that excessive subtalar joint pronation may sufficiently alter the stresses in bone, muscle, and ligament to cause a wide variety of injuries (15–17). (Excessive subtalar joint pronation is defined as calcaneal eversion equal to or greater than 13° [18].)

It is of clinical interest that recent research has demonstrated that the angular velocity of subtalar joint pronation may play a more important role in the development of various injuries than previously believed (19). This is a particularly important consideration since the subtalar joint frequently reaches its peak angular displacement during the first 50% of the contact period (20). By applying this information to the rearfoot varus deformity illustrated in Figure 3.6, you will notice that the subtalar joint pronates through an initial range of approximately 16° during the first 0.08 seconds of contact period. Because the subtalar joint acts as a directional torque transmitter converting frontal plane motion at the calcaneus into axial rotation of the shank and lower extremity (21), the tibia, in this situation, will internally rotate 16° in 0.08 second. (The tibia will rotate even more if a high subtalar joint axis is present.)

The rapid, sometimes extreme range of motion associated with subtalar joint compensation for a rearfoot varus deformity is capable of generating tremendous amounts of torque. These forces must be effectively dampened within fractions of a second, thousands of times per day, if the individual is to remain injury-free. A series of potential injuries associated with the rearfoot varus deformity are illustrated in Figure 3.7.

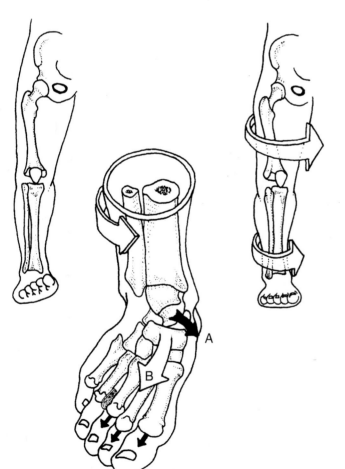

Figure 3.7. Potential injuries associated with excessive subtalar pronation. As the subtalar joint pronates to compensate for a rearfoot varus deformity, the talus is forced to adduct and plantarflex an excessive amount **(A)** while the calcaneus simultaneously everts. These actions markedly strain the calcaneonavicular ligament (the spring ligament) and the plantar talonavicular joint capsule. Over time, these exaggerated movements can lead to a pathologic laxity of these tissues. In addition, excessive subtalar pronation may damage the plantar fascia and/or soft tissues of the forefoot, as the talus is displaced anteriorly approximately 1.5 mm with every 10° of calcaneal eversion (30). Manter (30) likens this to the forward motion of a right-handed screw placed directly along the subtalar joint axis: As the calcaneus everts, the screw tightens, thereby pushing the talus anteriorly. While this forward motion is insignificant in an average foot, it may play a critical role in the pathomechanics associated with excessive subtalar joint pronation, as the anterior displacement of the talus causes the navicular and first three rays to move forward and abduct relative to the fourth and fifth rays **(B)**. The forward motion of the medial column irritates the medial plantar fascia, as it places a tensile load on this tissue that may exceed its functional ability to elongate, i.e., the plantar fascia is relatively inelastic. This would result in an increased tractioning of the plantar fascia's periosteal attachment, which could potentially lead to the development of a heel spur. The abductory movement of the medial column may also be responsible for injury, as it creates a compressive force at the junction of the medial and lateral column. This may lead to chronic intermetatarsophalangeal bursitis with an interdigital neuritis (31).

In addition to producing various injuries in the foot, excessive subtalar joint pronation may be responsible for a wide range of injuries along the entire kinetic chain. For example, it has been documented that excessive subtalar pronation is causally related to shin splints (15, 19) (shin splints being defined as pain along the medial distal two-thirds of the tibia). Also, Matheson et al. (22) demonstrated that excessive subtalar pronation predisposes to lower tibial stress fractures, possibly because the distal tibia, with its relatively low polar moment of inertia (23), is unable to tolerate the increased torsional strains associated with excessive talar adduction.

The excessive internal tibial rotation may also be responsible for medial knee injury, as the medial tibial plateau is forced into rapid posterior glide beneath the medial femoral condyle. This movement strains the medial meniscus and the medial joint capsule and may produce chronic pes anserine bursitis. (It should be noted that Lutter [24] was able to relate 77% of 213 knee injuries to faulty mechanics of the foot.)

While most authorities feel excessive subtalar pronation most frequently produces medial knee injury (25), Noble (26), in a study of 100 individuals diagnosed with iliotibial band friction syndrome, concluded that excessive subtalar joint pronation was a significant etiological factor in the development of that injury. Apparently, the excessive internal tibial rotation "drags" the distal iliotibial band over the lateral femoral epicondyle, thereby predisposing to this friction syndrome.

Another point of interest relates to retropatella pain with excessive subtalar joint pronation. Although it has been frequently noted that excessive pronation increases the Q angle, thereby predisposing patients to retropatella arthralgia (27), this is only true during static stance, when the cruciate ligaments maintain the extended knee in a locked position. When the knee is flexed (as it is during contact period), the tibia internally rotates further than the femur, thereby decreasing the Q angle (28). This may be responsible for medial retropatella injury, as Huberti and Hayes (29) demonstrated that a reduction in the Q angle will, approximately 50% of the time, result in a reduction of pressure beneath the lateral patella facet with a redistribution of this pressure elsewhere (thereby increasing the potential for chondromalacia at these points). Perhaps this is why Kegerreis et al. (28) stated that excessive subtalar joint pronation is as causally related to the plical band syndrome as an increased Q angle is related to extensor mechanism dysfunction.

The final postural considerations associated with excessive subtalar joint pronation can be directly related to the increased range of internal femoral rotation (Fig. 3.8).

In Figure 3.8, excessive internal rotation of the femur (A) may produce injury as it increases tensile strain on the insertion of gluteus maximus (B) and may therefore be responsible for chronic strain of that tendon. Also, the greater

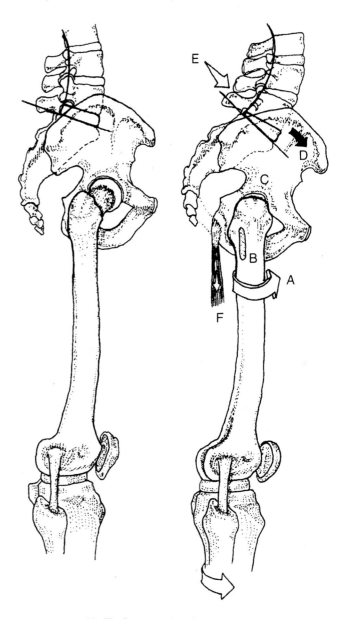

Figure 3.8 (A-F) Postural effects associated with excessive subtalar pronation. (See text.)

trochanteric bursa is more prone to injury as the proximal femur rotates through a greater arc of motion. This acts to increase shear forces on this bursa, which is located between the greater trochanter and proximal iliotibial band. Of much greater clinical significance is the effect that internal femoral rotation has on the pelvis. Internal rotation of the femur displaces the femoral head posteriorly (C), which in turn causes the entire pelvis to tilt anteriorly (D). This may produce a wide range of injuries as the sacral base angle is increased, the intervertebral discs become wedged posteriorly, and the spinous processes are approximated as the lumbar lordosis increases (E). Also, the anterior tilting of the pelvis tractions the hamstring origin (F) which, because tendinous slips from biceps femoris are continuous with the sacrotuberous ligament, may predispose to sacro-coccygeal dysfunction.

Classic Signs and Symptoms Associated with the Rearfoot Varus Deformity

Because the various structural/kinetic deviations from the outlined norm produce very specific patterns of compensation, Langer and Wernick (32) have described a list of classic signs and symptoms associated with each of the various deformities. Remember that this list reflects only the most frequently seen signs and symptoms and does not apply to all cases (especially when one considers that various combinations of deformities may exist together):

1. A medium height to the medial longitudinal arch off-weight-bearing with only a slight lowering of the arch upon weight-bearing (Fig. 3.9).

2. Mild-to-moderate callus formation under the second and third metatarsal heads. Because the subtalar joint is pronated at the beginning of propulsion, the articulations of the foot remain unlocked, and the first metatarsal is unable to bear weight effectively. As a result, a disproportionate amount of weight is shifted to the second and third metatarsal heads, which predisposes to pain and a diffuse hyperkeratotic lesion.

3. Exaggerated shoe wear along the lateral heel.

4. Retrocalcaneal bursitis or pump bump (Fig. 3.10). This bursa may be chronically irritated as it is sheared between the skin (which is maintained in a somewhat fixed position by the lateral heel counter) and the overly mobile calcaneus.

5. Morning heel pain. It has been documented (34, 35) that a rearfoot varus deformity can produce microdamage to the various tissues inserting on the plantar calcaneus (particularly the plantar fascia and abductor hallucis muscle).

During periods of prolonged rest, an inflammatory edema may accumulate within the limited confines of the connective tissue septa. This inflammatory reaction may produce enough swelling to compress neighboring nerve fibers, thereby producing pain (36). This pain will be lessened after brief periods of walking as movement improves venous and lymphatic drainage, thereby decreasing intracompartmental pressures.

6. Hammering of the fifth digit. If the subtalar joint is maintained in a pronated position during propulsion (as it is with a large rearfoot varus deformity), the pull of flexor digitorum longus is displaced medially, thereby predisposing to hammering of the fifth digit.

7. Chronic myositis/tendinitis of the musculature responsible for decelerating subtalar pronation. Tibialis anterior and posterior, flexor digitorum longus, flexor hallucis longus, and the triceps surae musculature all may be chronically strained, as they are forced to decelerate subtalar pronation through larger ranges at faster speeds (19, 37).

8. Symptoms associated with exaggerated torsion of the lower extremity, i.e., stress fracture of the distal tibia, medial retropatella arthralgia, pes anserine bursitis, greater trochanteric bursitis, etc. (see Figs. 3.6 and 3.7).

Orthotic Management for the Rearfoot Varus Deformity

Keeping in mind that the rearfoot varus is an osseous deformity that cannot be changed short of surgically straightening the bowed structure, the goal of treatment must be to decrease the need for compensatory subtalar pronation by designing an orthotic that will accurately accommodate the deformity. This is partially accomplished

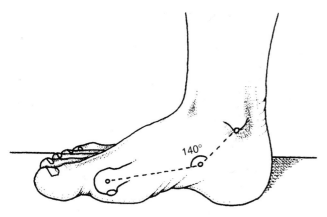

Figure 3.9. Appearance of the medial longitudinal arch with a rearfoot varus deformity. Because categorizing the medial arch as high, medium, or low is so subjective, Dahle et al. (33) recommended measuring the angle formed between the distal medial malleolus, the navicular tuberosity, and the metatarsal head. If the resultant angle approaches 180°, the arch is considered high; an angle between 130 and 150° is considered medium; and an angle nearing 90° is considered low. It should be noted that this method is far from ideal and that, with practice, subjective interpretation may be more reliable.

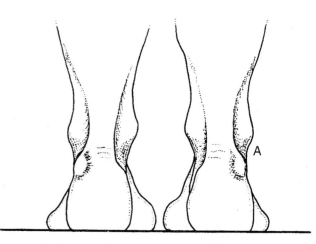

Figure 3.10. The achilles "pump-bump" (A).

by placing a varus wedge or post under the medial foot. The post basically acts to bring the surface to the patient's medial foot, rather than forcing the patient to pronate in order to bring the medial foot to the surface (Fig. 3.11).

Use of a rearfoot varus post to bring the surface to the deformity represents a basic tenet of orthotic design: A well-made orthotic does not necessarily shift the bony structures from a visually malaligned to an aligned position; rather, it acts to custom contour a surface that, when possible, allows for noncompensated movement patterns, with all joints functioning about their neutral positions (neutrality being defined as maximal congruency at the talonavicular articulation with the calcaneocuboid joint maintained in a close-packed position).

The ability of the varus post to control subtalar motions has been demonstrated by Cavanagh et al. (20). By using high-speed cinematography and force-plate analysis, they were able to demonstrate that the addition of a varus post not only decreased the overall range of subtalar pronation but also produced a marked reduction in the angular velocity in which pronation occurred. In addition, force-plate analysis revealed a marked decrease in medial shear forces at the time of initial ground contact. Mann (38) demonstrated that use of a medial support would bring about a decrease in eversion of the calcaneus and internal rotation of the tibia. The author emphasized that altering the

transverse rotation of the tibia may correct clinical symptoms at the knee and hip.

The observation that varus posts decrease the range and speed of subtalar pronation has been supported by other investigators (39, 40). In fact, Smart et al. (41) were so impressed with the ability of the varus wedge to control the range and speed of subtalar motion that they recommended use of a 12- to 15-mm wedge in all casual and athletic shoe gear (although this angle seems somewhat excessive, as the average orthotic is not posted at more than 4° varus, i.e., 7 mm). Schoenhaus and Jay (42) stated that the rearfoot varus post should never exceed 7° (13 mm), as an angle greater than this would produce lateral instability, thereby predisposing the patient to inversion sprain of the ankle.

In addition to the control afforded by the varus post, subtalar motions can also be modified by making certain changes in the shape of the orthotic shell (which ends just prior to the metatarsal heads). In order to accurately mold this shell (which may be made from a variety of materials), a foot impression must be taken with the subtalar joint maintained in its neutral position. The positive model of this impression is then altered by adding plaster to the medial longitudinal arch, the calcaneal incline angle and, if nonweight-bearing impression techniques have been used, the plantar circumference of the heel (Fig. 3.12).

The addition of plaster allows for normal displacement of the plantar soft tissues during ground contact and, more importantly, it allows for only that range of subtalar and midtarsal (oblique axis) pronation necessary to absorb shock: the medial aspect of the orthotic shell (particularly the calcaneal incline angle) creates a physical block that disallows exaggerated pronation. By varying the amount of plaster applied to the positive model, the practitioner may allow (or disallow) any range of subtalar motion desired.

In situations in which the degree of deformity greatly exceeds the degree of the posting angle, a more generous amount of plaster must be added to the positive model, as the subtalar joint will be moderately pronated prior to con-

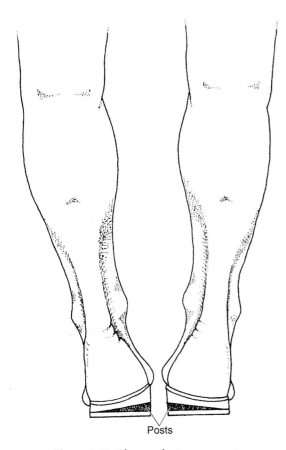

Figure 3.11. The rearfoot varus post.

Posts

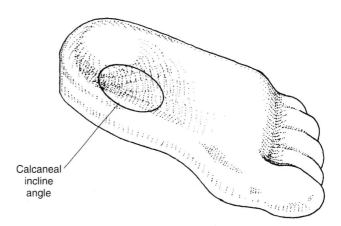

Calcaneal
incline
angle

Figure 3.12. A plantar medial view of a positive model. The *shaded areas* represent location of the additional plaster.

tacting the shell. For example, if a 15° rearfoot varus is treated with an orthotic shell posted in 4° varus, the subtalar joint will have pronated 11° prior to striking the shell. As a result, the contour of the medial arch will have significantly lowered from the neutral position prior to contacting the shell. If this were not taken into consideration by adding greater amounts of plaster to the positive model, the soft tissues beneath the medial arch (particularly near the calcaneal incline angle) would be chronically contused as they collided with the inadequately lowered orthotic shell.

Additional information regarding fabrication of the orthotic shell and the various posting techniques will be discussed in the laboratory preparation section.

The clinical efficacy of orthotics that allow for neutral subtalar positioning has been well documented (17, 39, 43–45). In fact, in a study of 53 patients receiving neutral position orthotics, Donatelli et al. (46) stated that 96% of these individuals reported relief from pain with 70% being able to return to their previous level of activity. By combining an accurately contoured shell with a post angle that lessens the need for compensatory subtalar pronation, an orthotic has the ability to improve functional alignment of the subtalar joint, thereby lessening potential strain along all aspects of the kinetic chain.

ALIGNMENT OF THE REARFOOT AND FOREFOOT

As mentioned, the calcaneocuboid joint should lock in its close-packed position with the vertical bisection of the rearfoot perpendicular to the plantar surface of the forefoot. Unfortunately, this is not always the case as individual variation in triplanar ontogeny of the tarsals may allow the plantar forefoot to be maintained in either an inverted or everted position when the calcaneocuboid locking mechanism is engaged. If the plantar forefoot locks in an inverted position relative to the plantar rearfoot, it is referred to as a forefoot varus deformity (Fig. 3.13). Conversely, if the plantar forefoot locks in an everted position, it is referred to as forefoot valgus deformity (Fig. 3.14).

As expected, the forefoot varus and valgus deformities produce very different patterns of compensation. The forefoot varus deformity will be discussed first, as it is usually the more destructive.

FOREFOOT VARUS DEFORMITY

Although the forefoot varus deformity is present in less than 9% of the population (1), the individual possessing this foot type is frequently seen in a clinical setting as the forefoot varus is responsible for many knee, hip and pelvic disorders. Strauss (47) originally described this deformity in 1927, attributing it to a failure of the talar neck to derotate from its infantile inverted position (Fig. 3.15). Although most authorities continue to blame talar neck deformity, McPoil et al. (48) recently disproved this theory, suggesting that the forefoot varus deformity results from osseous abnormality in the talonavicular and/or calcaneocuboid joints, not from variation in the talar head or

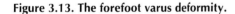

Figure 3.13. The forefoot varus deformity.

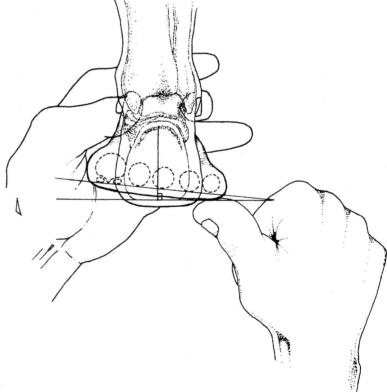

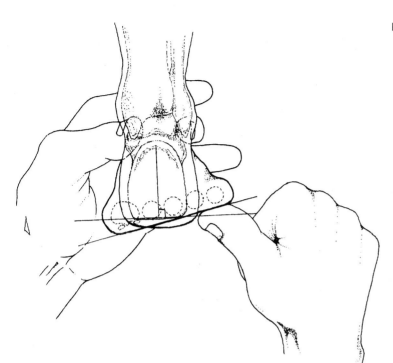

Figure 3.14. The forefoot valgus deformity.

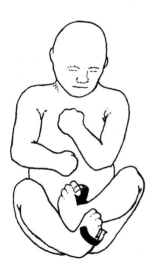

Figure 3.15. The forefeet are maintained in an inverted position during the third trimester.

neck. Regardless of its origin, the inverted forefoot should have ideally derotated back to a neutral position by age 5 (49).

Pathomechanics

To compensate for the constantly inverted position of the forefoot, the subtalar joint is forced to pronate through extreme ranges of motion just to bring the medial forefoot to the ground (Fig. 3.16). This exaggerated range of subtalar pronation causes the talus to shift medially relative to the calcaneus, which in turn supplies body weight with a much more effective lever arm for maintaining the subtalar joint in a pronated position. This creates a vicious cycle in that the range of subtalar pronation necessary to compensate for the forefoot deformity during contact period allows body weight to maintain the pronated position throughout midstance and early propulsion.

The increased range of subtalar pronation present during the contact period predisposes to the same types of injuries seen with a rearfoot varus deformity. However, exaggerated subtalar pronation throughout midstance and propulsion makes this deformity particularly destructive, as it disallows locking of the calcaneocuboid joint and creates a series of conflicting motions between the knee and talus. Because the talus is held in an adducted position by the pronated subtalar joint (this position is maintained by the superimposed body weight), the external rotational moment created by the swing phase leg is unable to generate a force strong enough to abduct the talus. As a result, the torsional forces associated with this external rotational moment must be temporarily stored in the stance phase lower extremity (Fig. 3.17). The release of these stored torsional forces is frequently evidenced by a sudden "abductory twist" of the rearfoot the moment the heel lift occurs; i.e., because ground-reactive forces no longer maintain the plantar heel, the entire rearfoot is free to snap medially, as though released from a loaded spring. Clearly, the development of such torsional forces has the potential to do much damage.

Because a chain is most likely to give at its weakest link, the prolonged application of these forces will most often produce a pathological laxity of the involved joint capsules, particularly the knee. Coplan (50) corroborated

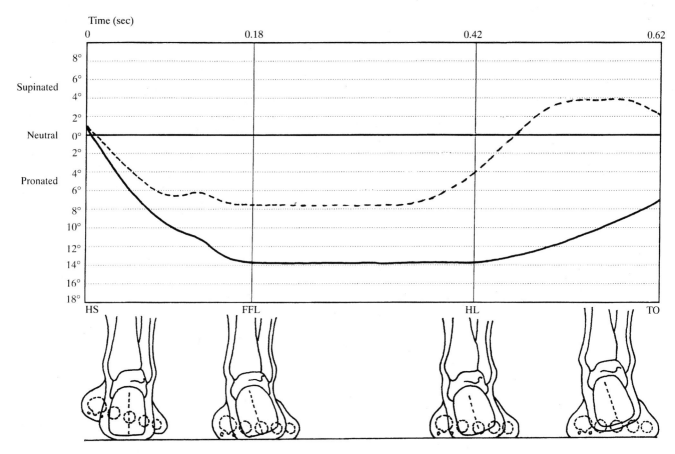

Figure 3.16. Stance phase motions with a forefoot varus deformity (solid line). *HS* = heel strike; *FFL* = full forefoot load; *HL* = heel lift; *TO* = toe off.

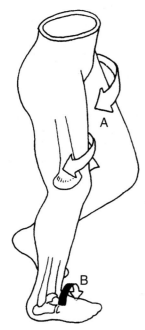

Figure 3.17. When a forefoot varus deformity is present, the external rotatory moment created by the swing phase leg (A) is unable to generate a force sufficient to shift the subtalar joint from its fully pronated position (B).

this theory by noting that individuals possessing excessive ranges of subtalar pronation were more likely to display significantly greater ranges of tibiofemoral rotation, particularly as the knee approaches full extension (its normal position of function as torsional strains peak during late midstance). In her study, which was done off weight-bearing, the mean range of tibial rotation when the knee was flexed 5° was 11.4° for the normal group and 18.5° for the pronating group. She speculated that the opposing rotary torques present during the late midstance period produced laxity of the tissues that normally limit knee rotation.

Another potential injury that may result from these conflicting motions occurs when the anteromedial talar dome collides into the articular surface beneath the medial malleolus (Fig. 3.18). Repeated compression of these two surfaces may eventually lead to chronic synovitis and/or chondromalacia of the talar dome (star).

Possibly the most detrimental aspect of excessive subtalar pronation throughout late midstance is that it disallows the normal coupled motions necessary for knee extension, i.e., because the knee is not a pure ginglymus joint, the tibia must externally rotate for the knee to smoothly extend. (The knee can extend without external tibial rotation, but this is a subluxatory rather than a smooth

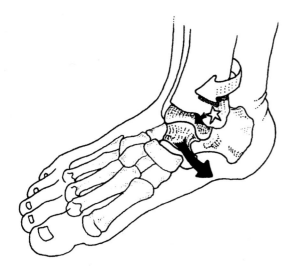

Figure 3.18. Conflicting talar and tibial motions during late midstance period. *star* = the point of compression between the anteromedial talar dome and the articular surface beneath the medial malleolus.

motion.) Excessive subtalar pronation during late midstance presents a biomechanical dilemma in that the tibia is maintained in an internally rotated position as the knee extends.

Tiberio (51) mentioned that the body might solve this dilemma by means of a process he referred to as compensatory internal femoral rotation (CIFR). If the femur were able to reverse its usual direction so as to internally rotate during midstance, normal coupled knee motions would be restored, provided the femur could internally rotate farther than the fixed tibia. The greater range of internal femoral rotation would result in the tibia being in an externally rotated position relative to the femur, thereby restoring coupled motions. Unfortunately, while CIFR solves one biomechanical problem, it creates another as the internally rotating femur drives its lateral femoral condyle into the respective patella facet. Tiberio (51) suggested that CIFR, if present, could be an important etiological factor in the development of lateral retropatella arthralgia.

While excessive subtalar pronation during midstance predisposes to injury because of conflicting movement patterns between the leg and talus, continued subtalar pronation through the propulsive period may be even more destructive, as it maintains a parallelism of the midtarsal axes. The continued parallelism of these axes essentially produces an unlocking of the articulations at a time when maximum stability is needed. This results in a pathological shifting of the tarsals, as ground-reactive forces peak during early propulsion: the foot is forced to behave as a flexible lever arm rather than as the rigid beam necessary to withstand vertical forces.

In addition to the instability produced by the parallelism of axes, the talonavicular joint is mechanically less stable when the subtalar joint is pronated. As Mann (38) pointed out, the concavoconvex configuration of this joint

allows for increased stability only when forces are channeled through it with the subtalar joint near neutral (Fig. 3.19). Because the chronically adducted position of the talus associated with the forefoot varus deformity disallows this saddle joint relationship, the talus is allowed to shift plantarly, medially, and anteriorly as ground-reactive forces peak.

Manter (30) claimed that the anterior displacement of the talus widens the gap between the navicular and sustentaculum tali and is responsible for creating laxity of the ligaments that bridge this gap (primarily the calcaneonavicular ligament and the deep portion of the bifurcate ligament). Because these ligaments are important stabilizers of the midtarsal joint, their laxity will allow for increased ranges of midtarsal motion, particularly about the oblique axis. This acts to perpetuate and even amplify the instability as the forefoot is allowed to abduct and dorsiflex through greater ranges, eventually allowing for the collapse of the medial longitudinal arch. This in turn enables the subtalar joint to pronate through progressively larger ranges of motion, constantly supplying body weight with a more effective lever arm to maintain the calcaneus in a fully everted position.

Glancy (52) theorized that prolonged calcaneal eversion will create permanent elongation of the subtalar supinators, which eventually limits the ability of these muscles to store elastic energy during early stance phase. As Cavagna et al. repeatedly demonstrated (53, 54), the power of concentric contraction (which is necessary to return the pronated subtalar joint to neutral) is seriously compromised when the muscle is not prestretched. If the resting lengths of the subtalar supinators have been sufficiently overex-

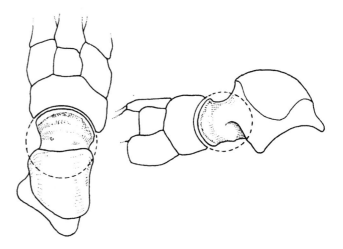

Figure 3.19. Superior and lateral views of the right talonavicular joint. Loading of the neutral subtalar joint increases talonavicular stability as the convex head of the talus settles neatly into the concave navicular. (Adapted from Mann RA. Biomechanics of running. In: Pack RP (ed). Symposium of the Foot and Leg in Running Sports. St. Louis: Mosby, 1982: 28.)

tended by prolonged calcaneal eversion, they will be unable to return the pronated subtalar joint to its neutral position as their ability to store and return plastic energy is lost. As a result, a cycle of excessive subtalar pronation, soft tissue elongation, muscular dysfunction, and continued subtalar pronation is perpetuated. This cycle may eventually end with subluxation of the unstable articulations.

The chronically everted heel associated with forefoot varus deformity may produce other injuries as it tractions the tibial nerve and can compress various branches of the calcaneal nerves at several sites. The medial and lateral plantar nerves may be compressed against the sharp fascial edge of the abductor hallucis muscle (55) (Fig. 3.20), while branches of the lateral plantar nerve and the nerve to abductor digiti quinti may be compressed between the plantar aponeurosis, intrinsic foot muscles, and the calcaneus (56) (Fig. 3.21).

A valgus heel may also produce injury to the plantar fascia, as the adducted talus inhibits the normal propulsive period supination that occurs about the oblique midtarsal joint axis. This negates the approximation of the anterior and posterior pillars associated with the windlass mechanism (refer back to Fig. 2.16), and the tensile strain developed in the plantar fascia is transferred directly into that tissue's periosteal attachment on the medial calcaneal tubercle. Over time, the prolonged traction may produce inflammatory erosive changes with proliferation of new bone, i.e., calcaneal spur formation (57).

Smith (58) stated that the tremendous shear loads created by the pull of the plantar fascia against the medial calcaneal condyle creates a cyclic loading at the junction of the medial condyle and the corpus calcaneum that is capable of producing microcortical fracture at this site. The author claims that this stress-induced microfracture has the potential for unstable crack propagation that might ultimately

lead to comminuted fracture. This is consistent with information provided by Williams et al. (59), as they demonstrated that 60% of 52 painful heels showed increased uptake of technetium-99 isotope at the calcaneum.

Possibly the most important factor limiting propulsive period stability in the forefoot varus deformity is the inability of peroneus longus to stabilize the first ray when the subtalar joint is pronated. As previously mentioned, subtalar pronation alters the angle of approach afforded peroneus longus to the first ray axis, making it ineffective as a first ray plantarflexor. Because ground-reactive forces are normally transferred to the medial forefoot during propulsion (Fig. 3.22), the first ray must be effectively stabilized by a mechanically efficient peroneus longus if it is to resist application of these forces.

Failure of peroneus longus to stabilize the first ray will result in a dorsal shifting of the first metatarsal as ground-reactive forces are applied. (The first ray will actually dorsiflex and invert.) This eventually leads to the formation of a hypermobile first ray that is unable to assist with the transfer of forces during propulsion (Fig. 3.23). As a result, greater amounts of pressure are borne by the second and third metatarsal heads, which predisposes to metatarsal stress fractures and hyperkeratotic lesions beneath the central metatarsal heads. In fact, Hughes (60) demonstrated that individuals with forefoot varus deformity are 8.3 times more likely to develop a stress fracture/reaction than those with normal measurements.

Root et al. (3) mention that propulsive period pronation of the subtalar joint (with the associated dorsal shifting of the hypermobile first ray) will predispose the first

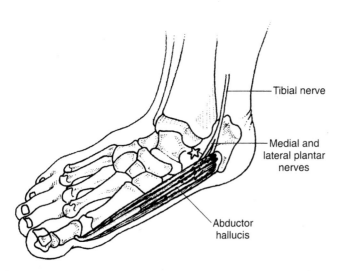

Figure 3.20. Calcaneal eversion may produce compression of the medial and lateral plantar nerves.

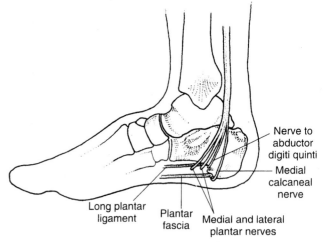

Figure 3.21. Branches of the lateral plantar nerve and the nerve to abductor digiti quinti may be compressed between the abductor hallucis and quadratus plantae muscles (not illustrated). Compression may also occur as these nerves pass near the medial tubercle of the calcaneus, where they may be subject to pressure from a calcaneal spur or local inflammation associated with plantar fasciitis.

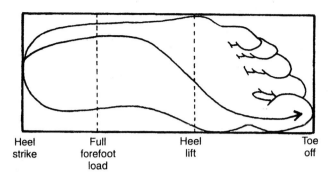

Figure 3.22. Normal progression of forces during stance phase. Because the center of mass is shifting laterally over the foot during the first half of stance, the force curve is maintained along the lateral column. Medial displacement of the center of mass by gluteus medius and the peroneals during the latter half of stance shifts the force curve through the first metatarsal, which is firmly stabilized by peroneus longus. (Adapted partially from Root MC, Orion WP, Weed JH, et al. Normal and Abnormal Function of the Foot. Los Angeles: Clinical Biomechanics, 1977.)

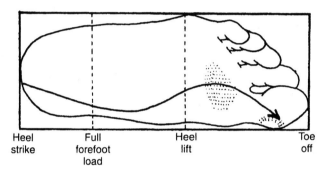

Figure 3.23. Progression of forces with the forefoot varus deformity. Exaggerated subtalar pronation immediately displaces the force curve toward the medial heel and arch. Because peroneus longus is unable to stabilize the first ray, the force curve shifts toward the central metatarsal heads. During propulsion, the curve returns to the hallux, as the individual with this foot type frequently terminates propulsion by rolling off the medial aspect of the hallux. (Adapted partially from Root MC, Orion WP, Weed JH, et al. Normal and Abnormal Function of the Foot. Los Angeles: Clinical Biomechanics, 1977.)

metatarsophalangeal joint to different deformities, depending on the alignment of the metatarsals (Fig. 3.24): If metatarsus rectus is present, the metatarsophalangeal joint is prone to developing hallux limitus/rigidus; if metatarsus adductus is present, the metatarsophalangeal joint is prone to developing hallux abductovalgus.

The pathomechanics associated with each of these deformities will be reviewed, beginning with hallux limitus/rigidus.

When the subtalar joint remains pronated during

propulsion, ground-reactive forces maintain the first metatarsal in an elevated position (Fig. 3.25). This is detrimental to the first metatarsophalangeal joint, as it disallows the normal plantarflectory range at the first ray necessary for the dorsal-posterior shifting of the first metatarsophalangeal joint's transverse axis (Fig. 3.26). As a result, the hallux is only able to reach the range of dorsiflexion available about the original axis. Because this range is typically less than 35°, the dorsal cartilage of the phalanx quickly collides with the dorsal cartilage of the first metatarsal head (Fig. 3.27). Root et al. (3) mentioned that the repeated compression of cartilage in younger individuals results in characteristic proliferative changes along the dorsal first metatarsal head's articular surface. In older individuals (i.e., older than 30), the repeated trauma may produce degenerative changes throughout the metatarsophalangeal joint. Over time, the range of motion available to the first metatarsophalangeal joint will gradually lessen (referred to as hallux limitus) and may eventually become ankylosed (hallux rigidus).

The biomechanical factors producing hallux limitus/rigidus will only occur if the metatarsals are in a rectus pattern or if the angle of the metatarsus adductus is less than 10° (3). If the metatarsus adductus is 11° or

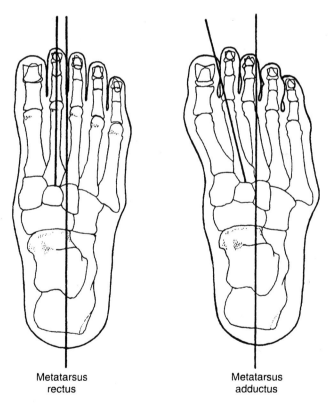

Figure 3.24. With the foot in a neutral position, the long axis of the second metatarsal shaft may be either straight (metatarsus rectus) or adducted (metatarsus adductus) relative to the long axis of the rearfoot. Note that regardless of the metatarsal's position, the toes always parallel the longitudinal bisection of the rearfoot.

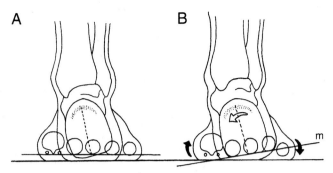

Figure 3.25. The everted position of the rearfoot in part A maintains the forefoot in its fully inverted position about the longitudinal midtarsal joint axis. Because the range of rearfoot eversion associated with the forefoot varus frequently exceeds the range of longitudinal midtarsal joint inversion (which is approximately 8°), the plantar forefoot can only maintain ground contact if the first metatarsal dorsiflexes and inverts while the fifth metatarsal plantarflexes and everts **(B).** Note that because the second through fourth metatarsals lack their own axis for frontal plane motion, they remain fully inverted about the longitudinal midtarsal joint axis *(m).*

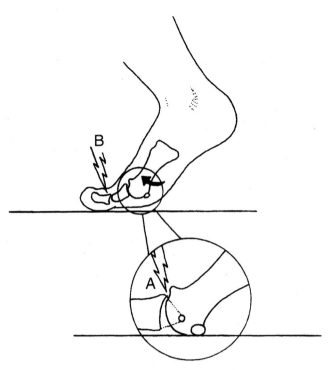

Figure 3.27. As the hallux reaches its full range of motion available about the original axis, the dorsal phalanx collides with the metatarsal head (A). If the propulsive period were to continue, the first interphalangeal joint may be forced into compensatory hyperextension **(B).**

greater, the transverse plane position of the metatarsals allows for the development of hallux abductovalgus. Root et al. (3) described four stages in the development of hallux abductovalgus that are outlined as follows.

As mentioned, an unstabilized first metatarsal will dorsiflex and invert as ground-reactive forces peak during early propulsion. Because the hallux plantarflexors are vigorously contracting during early propulsion in order to stabilize the great toe against the ground, the hallux is held in a fixed position and is therefore unable to move with the first metatarsal. Since the first metatarsophalangeal joint lacks an axis to allow frontal plane motion (refer back to Fig. 1.30), inversion of the first metatarsal against the immobilized hallux creates a torsional strain capable of subluxing the metatarsophalangeal joint. In the first stage of hallux abductovalgus, the metatarsophalangeal joint instability created by the dorsiflexing and inverting first metatarsal allows the transverse pedis muscle to shift the proximal phalanx laterally (Fig. 3.28).

This shifting of the hallux is destructive, as it laterally displaces the sesamoids from their plantar first metatarsal grooves and eventually leads to mechanical erosion of the articular crest (Fig. 3.29). Because this crest serves as a guiding flange for the sesamoids (which allow the abductor and adductor hallucis musculature to develop equal rotatory moments), its destruction provides the adductor hallucis

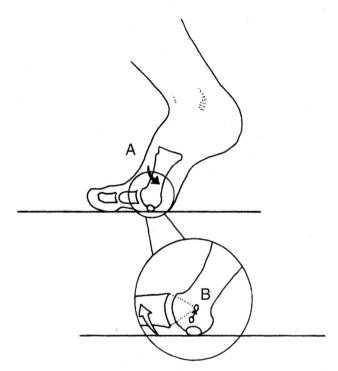

Figure 3.26. Plantarflexion of the first ray (A) allows for a dorsal-posterior shifting of the first metatarsophalangeal joint's transverse axis (B). This shift is necessary for the hallux to achieve the full range of dorsiflexion necessary for a normal propulsion (i.e., 65°).

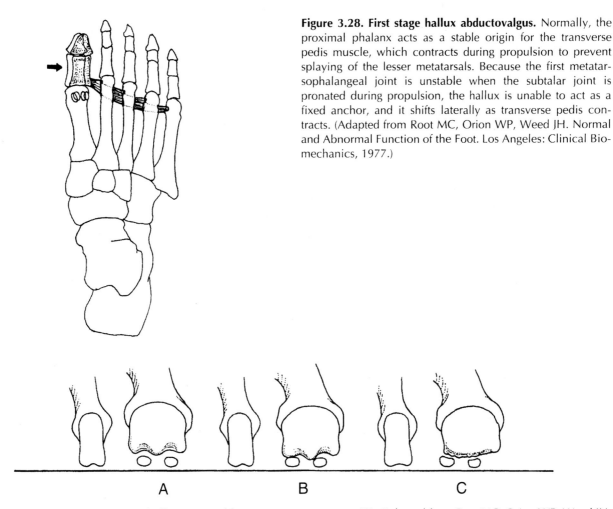

Figure 3.28. First stage hallux abductovalgus. Normally, the proximal phalanx acts as a stable origin for the transverse pedis muscle, which contracts during propulsion to prevent splaying of the lesser metatarsals. Because the first metatarsophalangeal joint is unstable when the subtalar joint is pronated during propulsion, the hallux is unable to act as a fixed anchor, and it shifts laterally as transverse pedis contracts. (Adapted from Root MC, Orion WP, Weed JH. Normal and Abnormal Function of the Foot. Los Angeles: Clinical Biomechanics, 1977.)

Figure 3.29. The sesamoids are typically separated by an osseous crest along the plantar first metatarsal head (A). Subtalar pronation during propulsion dorsiflexes and inverts the first metatarsal **(B),** which allows for gradual erosion of the osseous crest **(C).** (Adapted from Root MC, Orion WP, Weed JH. Normal and Abnormal Function of the Foot. Los Angeles: Clinical Biomechanics, 1977.)

muscle with a much longer lever arm to the vertical first metatarsophalangeal joint axis, allowing that muscle to overwhelm the antagonistic abductor hallucis.

These actions allow for the second stage of hallux abductovalgus (which quickly follows the first stage and may even occur simultaneously if a large metatarsus adductus is present) as the shifting hallux also displaces the long flexor and extensor tendons laterally relative to the vertical axis of the first metatarsophalangeal joint. This allows these tendons (along with adductor hallucis muscle) to produce transverse plane subluxation of the hallux (Fig. 3.30). If a rectus foot type had been present, this pattern of compensation would not have occurred, as lateral displacement of the sesamoids (and long tendons) is minimized by the well-aligned longitudinal axes of the first metatarsal shaft and the hallux.

Throughout the second stage, abduction of the hallux causes the first metatarsophalangeal joint to widen medially and compress laterally. This eventually results in osseous

adaptation of the first metatarsal head as bone is added to its distal medial aspect and absorbed along the lateral articular margin of the distal and dorsal first metatarsal head. These osseous changes most often occur in the juvenile foot and are consistent with Heuter-Volkmann and Delpeches principles, i.e., increased or decreased pressure on a physis will, respectively, decrease or increase bone growth.

In the third stage of deformity, compressive forces produced by muscular contraction on the abducted hallux produce a retrograde adductory force on the first ray (Fig. 3.31). This produces even greater deformity of the first metatarsophalangeal joint and results in the formation of a primus metatarsus adductus with its characteristic cuneiform split (c.s. in Fig. 3.31). Root et al. (3) noted that the marked displacement of the hallux in stage 3 requires the formation of a new articular surface on the first metatarsal head in order to accommodate the abducted hallux. They stated that a "functional adaptation of bone creates a new triplane axis for the first metatarsophalangeal

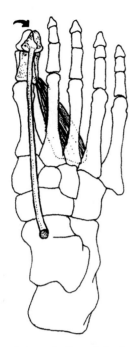

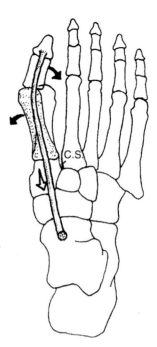

Figure 3.30. Second stage hallux abductovalgus. The lateral shifting of the hallux in Stage 1 supplies adductor hallucis and the long flexor and extensor tendons with a significant lever arm to abduct the hallux. If this occurs during growth years, functional adaptation of bone quickly follows. (Adapted from Root MC, Orion WP, Weed JH. Normal and Abnormal Function of the Foot. Los Angeles: Clinical Biomechanics, 1977.)

Figure 3.31. Third stage of hallux abductovalgus. The laterally displaced muscles and tendons in Stage 2 will continue to abduct the hallux only until the distal phalanx presses into the neighboring digit. At that time, a retrograde rotary moment is reflected back into the first metatarsal, forcing it into a position of adduction (referred to as metatarsus primus adductus). (Adapted from Root MC, Orion WP, Weed JH. Normal and Abnormal Function of the Foot. Los Angeles: Clinical Biomechanics, 1977.)

joint which is used throughout the range of hallux dorsiflexion. The original transverse plane axis is still present, but only for hallux motion in the plantarflexion range."

The progression of deformity typically ends during the third stage of hallux abductovalgus as the individual, because of pain or instability, learns to avoid bearing weight on the hallux by developing an apropulsive gait pattern (i.e., lifting the heel and forefoot simultaneously). If the hallux continues to bear weight, the fourth and final stage of deformity will follow. This stage is characterized by complete dislocation of the hallux from the metatarsal head (Fig. 3.32). This dislocation can only occur if the second metatarsal loses its buttressing effect, such as when a dorsally subluxed second metatarsophalangeal joint allows the hallux to underride the digit. Because of the extreme articular instability necessary to allow dislocation, the fourth stage of deformity rarely occurs without underlying rheumatic inflammatory disease or neuromuscular disorder (3).

It should be emphasized that this outlined biomechanical model for the development of hallux abductovalgus represents only one possible etiology, as there is no single theory that can explain the myriad of forms this deformity may present with. However, numerous investigators (61–63) believe that abnormal subtalar joint pronation is the primary cause of most hallux abductovalgus deformity.

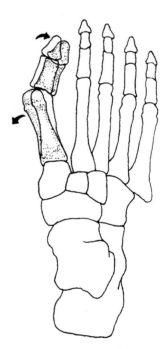

Figure 3.32. Fourth stage of hallux abductovalgus. Continued use of the hallux during propulsion eventually results in dislocation of the first metatarsophalangeal joint. (Adapted from Root MC, Orion WP, Weed JH. Normal and Abnormal Function of the Foot. Los Angeles: Clinical Biomechanics, 1977.)

Root et al. (3) even refuted the theory that hallux abducto-valgus is congenital. They strongly emphasized that it is the structural deformity that produces the destructive compensatory subtalar joint pronation that is congenital (such as the forefoot varus), not the actual metatarsophalangeal joint deformity. Root et al. (3) contend that if the propulsive period subtalar pronation were not present, hallux abductovalgus would not develop. (Although this belief seems a bit extreme since hallux abductovalgus deformity is nearly nonexistent in barefooted populations of the world [64] and may be associated with congenital anomalies such as a rounded first metatarsal head [65] and/or obliquity of the first metatarsocuneiform joint [64].)

A final consideration in the pathomechanics of the forefoot varus deformity relates to the inability of the tibialis anterior muscle to resupinate an excessively pronated subtalar joint during late swing phase. Because subtalar pronation shifts the subtalar joint axis closer to the insertion of tibialis anterior (Fig. 3.33), this muscle is frequently unable to supinate the subtalar joint in time for the next heel-strike. As a result, heel-strike occurs with the calcaneus progressively more everted. Subotnick (66) stated that failure to negotiate a phasically sound subtalar resupination during late swing phase will result in a loss of kinetic shock

absorption with eventual pronatory subluxation of the subtalar joint. The individual with a forefoot varus deformity may compensate for the lack of shock absorption by shortening the stride length (which lessens the initial impact forces) and by striking the ground with the ankle in an excessively dorsiflexed position. This position allows the anterior compartment muscles more time to assist with shock absorption as they decelerate the ankle through a larger range of plantarflexion.

Classic Signs and Symptoms Associated with the Forefoot Varus Deformity

1. A low medial longitudinal arch both on and off-weight-bearing with the heels everted during static stance.

2. Moderate-to-marked callus formation under the second, third, and sometimes fourth metatarsal heads with a "pinch" callus or tyloma under the distal medial aspect of the proximal phalanx. This pattern of callus formation follows a line along the typical progression of forces associated with propulsive period pronation (Fig. 3.23). As the tissues under the central metatarsal heads are forced to support more weight, they react with a diffuse hyperkeratosis. Because a large abductory force is placed on the hallux when the individual terminates propulsion by rolling off the medial aspect of the proximal phalanx, a shearing or pinch callus quickly develops. When seen in children, a mild hyperplasia of skin at this location may be the first sign of impending hallux abductovalgus (3).

3. Hammering of the fifth digit. In a random survey of patients requiring surgery for contracture of the fifth toe, a significant correlation was found between the presence of a forefoot varus and hammering of the fifth digit (67). The reason for this is as the forefoot varus deformity maintains the subtalar and midtarsal (oblique axis) joints in their fully pronated positions, the line of drive afforded flexor digitorum longus is altered allowing it to pull the plantar aspects of the lesser digits medially (Fig. 3.34). This medial pull (which inverts the more lateral digits) is increased as the calcaneus everts beyond perpendicular as the tendon of flexor digitorum longus is stretched by the shifting sustentaculum tali (black arrow in Fig. 3.34, B).

When the fifth digit is maintained in a varus position, a series of events occur that predispose to a hammered digit. Firstly, inversion of the proximal phalanx shifts the tendons of the lumbricales and the dorsal and plantar interossei above the transverse axis of the fifth metatarsophalangeal joint (Fig. 3.35). (Normally these tendons pass under this axis and act to plantarflex the proximal phalanx.) This new position of function allows these muscles to act as dorsiflexors of the proximal phalanx, thereby initiating a hammering of the digit. Secondly, inversion of the proximal phalanx shifts the tendon of abductor digiti quinti under the metatarsal head, making it a plantarflexor, not an abductor of the digit. As a result, the third plantar interossei is unopposed in creating medial deviation of the digit. The new re-

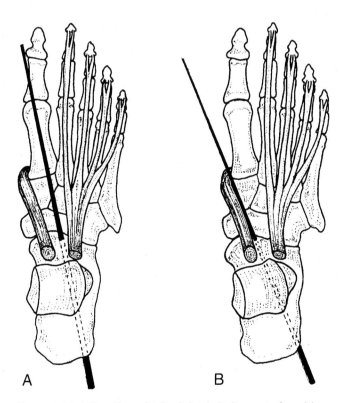

Figure 3.33. When the subtalar joint is in its neutral position (A), the tibialis anterior tendon has a significant lever arm to supinate the subtalar joint. However, when the subtalar joint is pronated **(B)**, tibialis anterior is unable to control subtalar motion, and the improved lever arm afforded extensor digitorum longus allows this muscle to maintain the subtalar joint in a pronated position throughout the entire swing phase.

Figure 3.34. The midstance and propulsive period pronation associated with the forefoot varus deformity produces abduction of the forefoot with simultaneous eversion of the calcaneus. These movements negate the normal lateral pull of quadratus plantae necessary to straighten flexor digitorum longus's angle of approach toward the digits **(A).** Instead, quadratus plantae exerts its force straight posteriorly (and may even pull posteromedially), allowing the long digital flexor to bowstring medially, drawing the more lateral digits into a varus position *(arrow 1 in upper left corner of **B***).

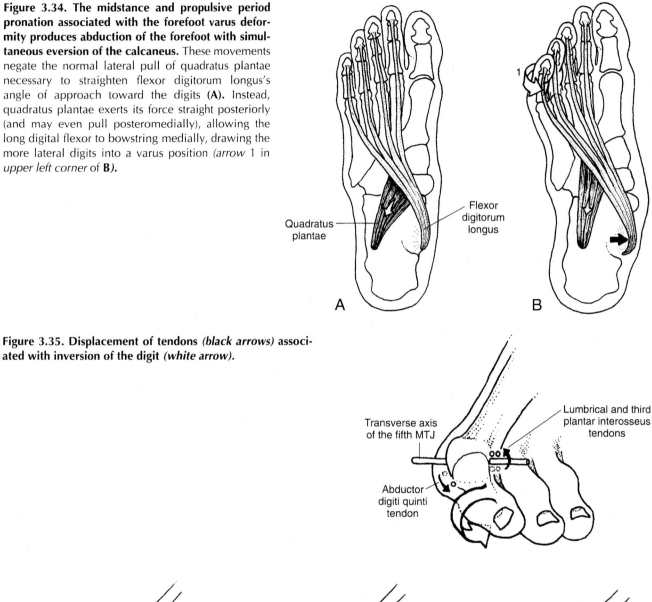

Figure 3.35. Displacement of tendons *(black arrows)* associated with inversion of the digit *(white arrow).*

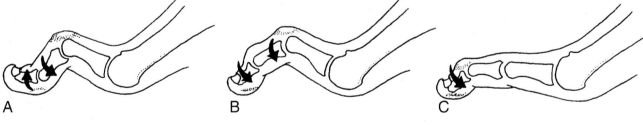

Figure 3.36. (A) Hammer toe; (B) claw toe; (C) mallet toe. Focal points of pressure and friction may produce painful calluses.

lationship these tendons have with the transverse metatarsophalangeal joint axis allows the involved musculature to maintain the proximal phalanx in a dorsiflexed and inverted position with the proximal interphalangeal joint plantarflexed. Over time, contracture develops in the respective joint capsules that perpetuates the deformity. The various types of deformity are illustrated in Figure 3.36.

4. Hallux abductovalgus or hallux limitus, depending on the angle of forefoot adductus. Ironically, the forefoot varus deformity typically does not produce bunion pain (3). Because the forefoot varus foot type moves through the propulsive period with relatively little movement between the dorsal metatarsal head and the skin (e.g., the first ray moves into a dorsiflexed and inverted position during early propulsion and then remains relatively stationary during the remainder of that period), shearing forces on the adventitious bursa (which forms over the dorsomedial aspect of the first metatarsal head during the second stage of hallux abductovalgus) are minimal. If the first metatarsal were to continue to dorsiflex and invert throughout propulsion, the bursa would be trapped between the rotating metatarsal head and the skin (which is held in a fixed position by shoe gear), and a painful bunion would result (Fig. 3.37).

5. Heel pain with possible entrapment neuropathies. A chronically everted calcaneus predisposes to entrapment neuropathies of the medial and lateral plantar nerves and the nerve to abductor digiti quinti. (These nerves are trapped with a scissors-like action between the everting calcaneus and the neighboring soft tissues.) The everted heel may also predispose to plantar fasciitis, microcortical fracture of the corpus calcaneus, and/or myositis of the abductor hallucis muscle. The increased strain placed on abductor

hallucis was demonstrated by Mann and Inman (68), as they recorded electrical activity in various intrinsic muscles in normal and flat-footed individuals (Fig. 3.38). Notice that the abductor hallucis muscle in the flat-footed individual is electrically active throughout all phases of stance, not just during the late midstance and propulsive periods. This hyperactivity is potentially injurious and most likely represents an attempt by this muscle to decrease the ligamentous strains associated with excessive subtalar and midtarsal pronation.

6. Medial achilles peritendinitis. Using high-speed cinematography, Smart et al. (41) demonstrated that prolonged pronation will produce a "whipping action or bowstring effect" on the achilles tendon. They emphasized that the forefoot varus deformity is a frequent cause of prolonged pronation and that the resultant snapping of the achilles tendon can potentiate microtears, particularly along the medial side of the tendon. Because of the extreme forces that the achilles tendon is subjected to during the

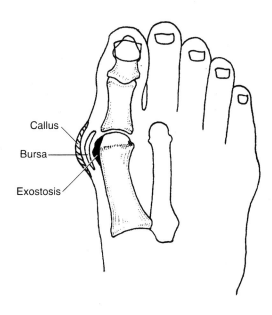

Figure 3.37. Bunion.

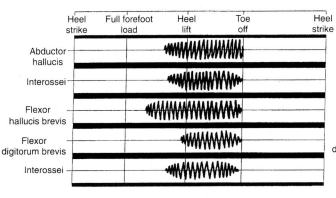

Figure 3.38. EMG activity in normal *(left chart)* and flat-footed individuals *(right chart)*. (Adapted from Mann R,

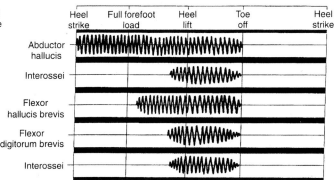

Inman VT. Phasic activity of intrinsic muscles of the foot. J Bone Joint Surg 1964; 46A (3): 469–481.)

propulsive period (ranging from 5.3 to 10 times the body weight [69]), these microtears may initiate peritendinitis and/or tendinosis and may even lead to total rupture (41).

The medial aspect of the achilles in individuals possessing the forefoot varus deformity is even prone to injury during static stance, as the everted calcaneus places a constant tensile strain on the medial aspect of the tendon. This prolonged traction produces a vascular impairment that may predispose the tendon to subsequent degenerative changes. The section of tendon approximately 2–6 cm proximal to the insertion is particularly prone to injury because of its relative avascularity.

7. *Chronic hypermobility of the ankle and/or knee joint.* The conflicting movement patterns between the talus and pelvis during propulsion create torsional strains capable of creating plastic deformity of the various restraining ligaments around the ankle and knee. The initial symptoms associated with this hypermobility may be as mild as a vague ache with occasional cavitation of the involved joint. Other injuries that may result from these conflicting motions include tibial stress fracture, retropatella arthralgia, pes anserine bursitis, and/or chondromalacia of the anterior medial talar dome (see text).

8. *Sciatica.* In a 1971 article published in the *Annals of the Swiss Chiropractors Association,* Curchod (70) claimed that 4–5% of all sciatica cases result from faulty posture of the foot, particularly when the heel is maintained in an everted position (as with the forefoot varus deformity). One possible mechanism for this is that in approximately 10% of the population, the sciatic nerve emerges from the pelvic bowl between two portions of the tendinous origin of the piriformis muscle (71). Because the pronated subtalar joint maintains the lower extremity in an internally rotated position, the piriformis muscle is constantly being tractioned, thereby predisposing to entrapment neuropathy as the sciatic nerve is compressed between the tendinous origins of the tightened piriformis muscle. While this represents one possible etiology for sciatic neuralgia, Curchod

(70) felt that the pain pattern associated with the valgus heel was not a true sciatica but actually represented a "stress syndrome" with pain in the foot, malleoli, lateral aspect of the thigh, gluteals, and the lumbar region, with concomitant anterior tilting of the ilium and contracture of the psoas muscle. He referred to this syndrome as a "false L5 sciatica" and claimed that the pain pattern may extend along the entire spine.

Orthotic Management for the Forefoot Varus Deformity

In order to treat the forefoot varus deformity properly, a negative impression must be taken that accurately captures the forefoot/rearfoot relationship when the foot is maintained in its neutral position. A positive model is made from this impression and, after the appropriate changes are made to allow for soft tissue displacement, a shell is molded along the plantar contour. An angled wedge or post is then placed under the distal medial aspect of the orthotic shell (just prior to the metatarsal heads). This post is of a height sufficient to bring the sagittal bisection of the rearfoot to vertical (Fig. 3.39).

By supporting the inverted forefoot, the post prevents pronatory compensation by the subtalar joint and allows the foot to enter the propulsive period with all of its articulations locked and stable. As with the rearfoot varus deformity, the orthotic does not change the osseous malposition; it merely accommodates the deformity by bringing a custom-molded surface to the neutral position foot.

In regard to controlling motion during terminal stance phase, a major shortcoming of the orthotic shell is that because it ends along the distal metatarsal shafts, it is only able to control motion during contact and midstance periods (i.e., when body weight is centered over the orthotic shell). For this reason Glancy (69) stated that "the foot and ankle complex is most vulnerable to injury and most difficult to control between heel lift and toe off."

Figure 3.39. (A–C) The forefoot varus post.

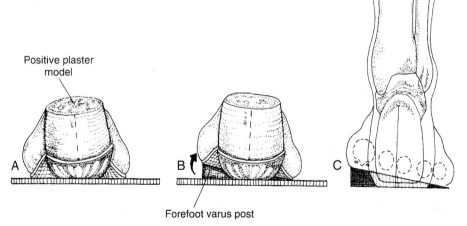

Positive plaster model

Forefoot varus post

Because the normal progression of forces passes beyond the distal metatarsal shafts during the propulsive period (they are centered over the metatarsal heads and the hallux), the orthotic shell and post become nonfunctional at a time when control is needed most. (Although the orthotic remains indirectly functional, as it places the subtalar joint in a more favorable position during midstance, thereby allowing the muscles to maintain a stable position more effectively, i.e., the contact and midstance period lever arm that maintains the subtalar joint in its fully pronated position is disallowed, thereby enabling the supporting musculature to function more effectively during late stance phase).

If a small forefoot varus deformity is present, the propulsive period pronation necessary to bring the medial forefoot to the ground typically does not produce injury, as it is well-controlled by the mechanically efficient musculature. If, however, a large forefoot varus deformity is present (i.e., greater than 4°), the added range of propulsive period pronation may produce a significant shifting of the articulations that may be responsible for injuries such as intermetatarsal bursitis, interdigital neuroma, and bunion pain (to name but a few).

The propulsive period pronation associated with a forefoot varus deformity can be prevented with what is referred to as a compressible post to the sulcus. This addition represents a continuation of the forefoot post extended beneath the metatarsal heads, ending at the sulcus (the base of the toes). This addition is made from a flexible material (usually rubber or cork) so as not to limit dorsiflexion at the metatarsophalangeal joints. The compressible post to sulcus is recommended for all forefoot deformities greater than 4°, as it prevents compensatory propulsive period pronation by allowing the orthotic to remain functional for longer periods of time.

As with casting techniques and laboratory preparation, all additions will be discussed in detail in a later section.

FOREFOOT VALGUS DEFORMITY

The forefoot valgus deformity is the most frequently seen frontal plane deformity of the forefoot. In their evaluation of 116 feet, McPoil et al. (1) noted that 44.8% of this group presented with a forefoot valgus deformity. In another study of 552 feet, Burns (72) noted that 70% of all frontal plane deformities were in valgus and that this deformity was more likely to be larger than the forefoot varus. (It should be noted that this was a symptomatic population.)

The exact etiology of the forefoot valgus deformity remains somewhat obscure, possibly because it is of multiple origins. It may simply represent a congenital anomaly in the calcaneocuboid joint that disallows the normal close-packed position. For example, in Bojsen-Moller's study of the calcaneocuboid joint (73), 8% of the cuboids evaluated

(2 of 25) lacked a calcanean process, and the corresponding articular surface on the calcaneus was flat. The calcaneocuboid joint in this situation could allow for greater ranges of forefoot eversion (i.e., forefoot valgus), as the cuboid would be allowed to glide along the flattened surface of the calcaneus. (Normally, the calcanean process serves as a pivot that the cuboid will dorsiflex and evert about until its dorsal border contacts the overhanging calcaneus.) The calcaneocuboid joint lacking the calcanean process is classified as of the plane variety, which allows for greater ranges of gliding motion, as compared to the usual concavoconvex configuration typically present.

What has become the most widely accepted theory regarding the development of the forefoot valgus deformity is described by Sglarato (74) as developmental overrotation of the talar neck. Because the forefoot valgus deformity is not seen in children, it is believed that a period of transition is needed to transform the talar neck from the varus position present at birth to the valgus position that appears by adulthood. Although the simplicity of this theory makes it tempting to accept, the work by McPoil et al. (1) has all but disproved this theory. In their study of anatomical abnormalities of the talus, they could find no correlation between the forefoot valgus deformity and the position of the talar neck. It is possible that post-mortem changes in the foot could be responsible for error in their evaluations, but this is unlikely since this was a particularly well-planned study.

The final consideration regarding the etiology of the forefoot valgus deformity relates to the formation of a pes cavus foot, i.e., *Dorland's Medical Dictionary* defines pes cavus as "an exaggerated height of the longitudinal arch of the foot, present from birth or appearing later because of contractures or disturbed balance of muscles." Because the forefoot valgus deformity is often present in the cavus foot, possible etiologies for its formation should include those etiologies associated with the development of the cavus foot, namely, congenital malformation, neuromuscular disorder, various idiopathic conditions (such as scarlet fever or diphtheria, which may produce a discrepancy in bone or muscle growth), and trauma. Since the cavus foot typically possesses limited ranges of subtalar joint motion (75) and because the heel in the cavus foot is often maintained in a varus attitude (referred to as a cavovarus foot), it is quite possible that the forefoot valgus deformity merely represents a developmental malformation necessary to compensate for the inverted and rigid rearfoot (Fig. 3.40).

In an overview of cavus deformities, Dwyer (76) stated that the majority of these deformities are associated with neuromuscular disease and the incidence of association may be as high as 95% if methods of neurological evaluation could be refined. He claimed that viral or "other factors" may produce irritating stimuli in the motor tracts of anterior horn cells capable of producing various degrees of overactivity in the invertor muscles, ranging from obvious spasm to clinically undetectable increases in muscle tone.

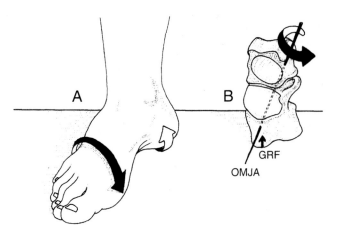

Figure 3.40. The cavus foot. An inverted heel requires valgus compensation by the forefoot (via first ray plantarflexion and eversion about the longitudinal midtarsal joint axis) if the plantar medial forefoot is to maintain ground contact *(black arrow in* **A***).* This can create a self-perpetuating cycle in that the more the forefoot everts, the more the rearfoot is allowed to invert *(white arrow in* **A***),* which exponentially increases the ability of peroneus longus to act as a first ray plantarflexor. Since closed-chain plantarflexion of the first ray creates a retrograde supinatory force at the subtalar joint, the improved mechanical advantage afforded peroneus longus may allow for progressive deformity as plantarflexion of the first ray continually tips the rearfoot into a position of increased inversion. The inverted position of the subtalar joint also acts to bring the oblique midtarsal joint axis *(OMJA)* into a more vertical position **(B).** As a result, ground-reactive forces *(GRF)* are unable to produce the pronatory forces necessary to resist the supinatory forces created by the intrinsic musculature (particularly the abductor hallucis). Because of this, the forefoot is allowed to adduct *(black arrow in* **B***),* and the deformity is amplified.

He maintained that this deformity is not congenital, that the focal central nervous system discharge initiates inversion of the heel, often in conjunction with plantar fascial contracture, and that the forefoot valgus deformity is compensatory in nature. It should be noted that Lariviere et al. (77) strongly disagreed with Dwyer. They believed that the forefoot valgus is the primary deformity, noting that surgical straightening of the inverted calcaneus, which would be successful if the rearfoot deformity were primary, has a dismal 70% failure rate.

Glancy (69) had a completely different opinion regarding the etiology of the cavus foot. He believed that because a high percentage of individuals possess cavus feet without underlying disease or disorder, this deformity must have a genetic origin and should therefore be considered a normal variant. This conclusion was supported by Bruckner (78), whose study suggested that cavus foot may be associated with a triarticulated subtalar joint.

Pathomechanics

The extent of mechanical malfunction associated with the forefoot valgus deformity depends on the size of the deformity and the rigidity of the midfoot. Thus, in order to describe the compensatory pathomechanics associated with the forefoot valgus more accurately, this deformity is divided into rigid and flexible subgroups. The rigid forefoot valgus possesses limited ranges of midtarsal and first ray motion and is only able to bring the plantar forefoot to the ground via supination of the subtalar joint (Fig. 3.41A) while the flexible forefoot valgus is able to bring the plantar forefoot to the ground via inversion about the longitudinal midtarsal joint axis and, if necessary, dorsiflexion and inversion of the first ray (Fig. 3.41B and C). In Burn's survey of various foot types (72), he found 70% of all forefoot valgus deformities to be flexible.

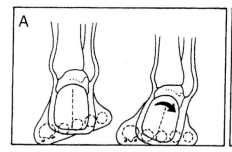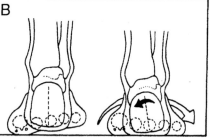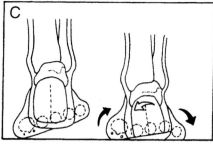

Figure 3.41. Patterns of compensation for the forefoot valgus deformity. If the forefoot deformity is rigid (A), the subtalar joint must supinate in order to bring the lateral plantar forefoot to the ground. When a flexible forefoot valgus is present **(B),** the plantar forefoot is able to make ground contact without affecting subtalar motions as long as the range of forefoot inversion is large enough to compensate for the forefoot valgus deformity. However, if the size of the deformity exceeds the range of inversion available about the longitudinal midtarsal joint axis (as in **C**), the forefoot, in its attempt to make ground contact, will invert its full range about the longitudinal midtarsal joint axis (note the central metatarsals), then continue to compensate via pronation (dorsiflexion and inversion) about the first ray axis and supination (plantarflexion and inversion) about the fifth ray axis *(arrows in* **C***).*

As Figure 3.41B and C demonstrate, the pattern of compensation in a flexible forefoot valgus deformity is dependent on the range of motion available about the midtarsal joint. In some cases, the flexible forefoot valgus deformity may possess such large ranges of longitudinal midtarsal joint inversion that the subtalar joint is allowed to pronate excessively throughout all periods of stance phase (Fig. 3.42).

While Figure 3.42 represents one possible movement pattern seen with the flexible forefoot valgus deformity, a more common movement pattern is seen in individuals pos-

sessing normal or decreased ranges of longitudinal midtarsal joint axis inversion with increased ranges of longitudinal midtarsal joint axis eversion (Fig. 3.43).

During the contact period, the individual with this range of midtarsal motion could pronate the subtalar joint only until the forefoot reaches its fully inverted position (with motion occurring at both the longitudinal midtarsal joint axis and first ray axis; see FFL in Fig. 3.44). At that time, the soft tissue-restraining mechanisms that stabilize these axes would prevent continued subtalar joint motion.

During early propulsion, this foot can usually ac-

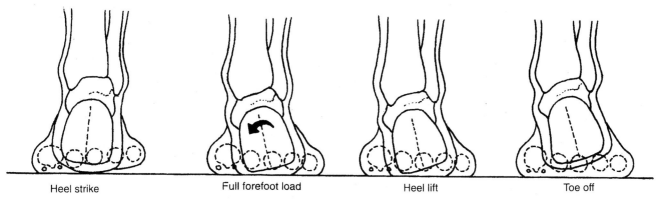

Heel strike   Full forefoot load   Heel lift   Toe off

Figure 3.42. The flexible forefoot valgus deformity possessing a large range of inversion about the longitudinal midtarsal joint axis will be allowed to pronate throughout all phases of stance.

Figure 3.43. Normally, the forefoot can evert from its fully inverted position only until the plantar forefoot reaches horizontal (A, N). However, when a flexible forefoot valgus deformity is present, the plantar forefoot is able to evert beyond horizontal while the range of inversion remains limited **(B).** (Note how the overall range of motion remains the same.)

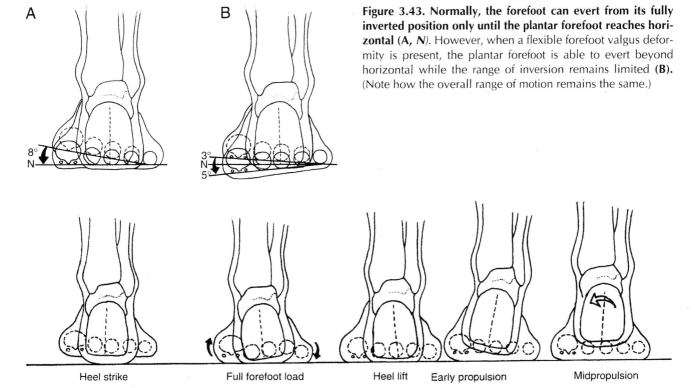

Heel strike   Full forefoot load   Heel lift   Early propulsion   Midpropulsion

Figure 3.44. Motions with a flexible forefoot valgus deformity possessing limited ranges of longitudinal midtarsal joint axis inversion. Note how the first ray at full forefoot load has dorsiflexed and inverted to allow the full range of subtalar pronation. (Normally, the first ray does not move during the contact period.)

complish a phasically sound resupination of the subtalar joint. However, because of the increased range of eversion available about the longitudinal midtarsal joint axis, the calcaneocuboid joint does not lock when the rearfoot reaches its vertical position after heel lift. If the range of available forefoot eversion is small (i.e., less than 6°), the individual may attempt to lock the lateral column during the propulsive period by inverting the rearfoot (see early propulsion in Fig. 3.44).

While this increased range of subtalar supination helps stabilize the articulations by bringing the calcaneocuboid joint into its close-packed position, it can be damaging, as it creates a lateral instability capable of producing chronic inversion sprain of the ankle mortise. To protect against this lateral instability, the individual will often invert the forefoot about the longitudinal midtarsal joint and, if necessary, the first ray axis, thereby bringing the rearfoot back to a more stable position (see midpropulsion in Fig. 3.44). Although these motions reestablish frontal plane stability of the ankle, they may be destructive, as they set the articulations of the mid- and forefoot into motion as vertical forces peak. This may lead to chronic bunion pain over the dorsomedial first and dorsolateral fifth metatarsal heads as the adventitious bursae are sheared between the skin (which is maintained in a fixed position by shoe gear) and the rotating metatarsal heads.

Also, inversion of the forefoot during propulsion prevents the normal plantarflectory motion of the first ray necessary for the dorsal-posterior shift of the first metatarsophalangeal joint's transverse axis (and may therefore be responsible for the development of hallux limitus or hallux abductovalgus) and will lessen the ability of the first metatarsal head to resist ground-reactive forces (as is evidenced by a diffuse callus formation beneath the second and third metatarsal heads.)

If the flexible forefoot valgus is greater than 6°, the excessive subtalar supination necessary to lock the calcaneocuboid joint may be evident as early as late midstance (Fig. 3.45). This premature subtalar supination increases the range of calcaneal inversion and external tibial rotation, which strains the peroneals as these muscles attempt to decelerate the exaggerated movements. As this foot enters its propulsive period, the individual initially protects against the lateral instability by inverting the forefoot about the midtarsal and first ray axes.

However, when a large forefoot valgus deformity is present, the amount of forefoot inversion needed to bring the rearfoot to perpendicular often exceeds the ranges of motion available about these axes. This being the case, the continued range of calcaneal eversion necessary to bring the rearfoot back to vertical can only occur via sudden pronation of the subtalar joint (see midpropulsion in Fig. 3.45). This of course predisposes to injury, as it unlocks all of the articulations of the foot at a time when maximum stability is essential.

While the flexible forefoot valgus deformity produces lateral instability (with its associated dysfunction) primarily during the terminal stance phase, the rigid forefoot valgus deformity, regardless of its size, will produce postural dysfunction during all portions of stance phase (Fig. 3.46).

During the contact period, the individual possessing a rigid forefoot valgus deformity will be able to pronate the subtalar joint only until the plantar forefoot makes ground contact. At that time, the subtalar joint is forced into rapid supinatory compensation (referred to as "supinatory rock") as the rearfoot tips laterally to bring the plantar forefoot to the ground (see midcontact in Fig. 3.46). If this foot had been flexible, the first ray and midtarsal joint would have compensated for the forefoot valgus deformity by allowing the entire forefoot to invert. However, because this foot possesses such limited ranges of midtarsal and first ray motion, the lateral aspect of the plantar forefoot can only make ground contact if the subtalar joint supinates.

While the pattern of compensation illustrated in Figure 3.46 is often described as classic for a rigid forefoot valgus deformity (79), clinically, it is rarely seen. More often, the individual with this forefoot deformity is able to avoid the supinatory rock by striking the ground with the rearfoot

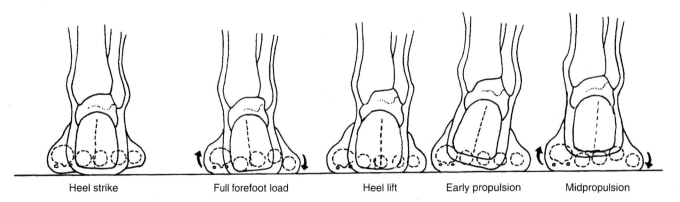

| Heel strike | Full forefoot load | Heel lift | Early propulsion | Midpropulsion |

Figure 3.45. Foot motions with flexible forefoot valgus deformity greater than 6° (posterior view of the right foot).

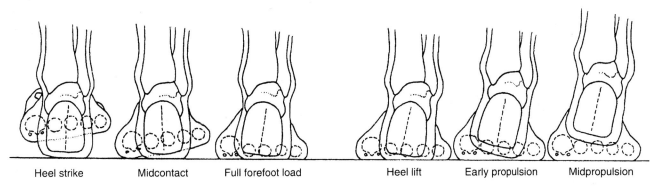

Heel strike	Midcontact	Full forefoot load	Heel lift	Early propulsion	Midpropulsion

Figure 3.46. Foot motions with a rigid forefoot valgus (posterior view of the right foot).

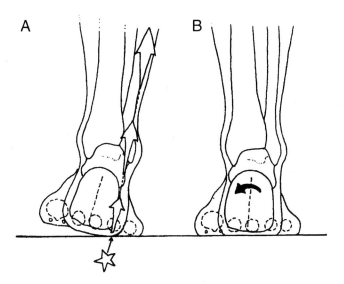

Figure 3.47. By excessively inverting the rearfoot prior to heel-strike (A), the individual with a rigid forefoot valgus deformity is allowed to pronate the subtalar joint through a larger range of motion (B), avoiding the supinatory rock that would have otherwise occurred. Unfortunately, inversion of the rearfoot during late swing phase displaces the initial point of ground contact laterally *(star)* which, because of the limited time available to absorb these forces, predisposes the lateral lower extremity to high-impact injuries. This strike pattern may explain why individuals with cavus feet are more likely to suffer from femoral stress fracture (22), greater trochanteric bursitis (25), and iliotibial band friction syndrome (24). It also explains why so many investigators believe that the rigid forefoot valgus deformity predisposes to low back pain (80) and why this foot type is often referred to as a high-impact foot.

excessively inverted (Fig. 3.47). This may be a learned response in which the subtalar joint is deliberately inverted beyond neutral in anticipation of the supinatory rock, or, more commonly, is the result of a combination rearfoot varus/forefoot valgus deformity in which the degree of rearfoot varus is equal to or exceeds the degree of forefoot valgus.

In order to minimize the destructive force impulses associated with a lateral heel-strike, many individuals with a rigid forefoot valgus deformity will strike the ground with the ankle in an excessively dorsiflexed position (16). Besides delaying the initial contact of the plantar forefoot (which allows the subtalar joint to pronate for a longer period of time) the increased amount of ankle dorsiflexion affords the anterior compartment muscles more time to assist with shock absorption as they decelerate the ankle through greater ranges of plantarflexion. Unfortunately, although this pattern of compensation may improve the foot's ability to absorb shock, it may also predispose to chronic myositis/periostitis of the anterior compartment tissues.

While the rigid forefoot valgus deformity produces high-impact symptoms during the contact period, the midstance period motions are relatively normal, with the exception that the rearfoot is maintained in an excessively inverted position. Unfortunately, this may result in chronic tenosynovitis of peroneus longus (which is tractioned behind the lateral malleolus) and may be responsible for an entrapment neuropathy of the superficial peroneal nerve where this nerve pierces the fascia between the anterior and lateral compartments (81) (Fig. 3.48).

Cangialosi and Schall (81) claim that the excessive subtalar joint supination associated with the rigid forefoot valgus deformity creates a "tautness of the nerve against its fascial window" which provides the initial stimulus for a neuropathy. They noted that the clinical signs of this mononeuropathy may range from hyperesthesia to hypoesthesia, or even anesthesia, along the distal lateral leg and dorsal foot. They also claim that palpation in the area where the nerve exits the fascial window may reveal a nodular fibrosis along the course of the nerve and that compression at this point may exacerbate the pain along the nerve's sensory distribution.

It is also possible for the rigid forefoot valgus deformity to produce entrapment neuropathy of the posterior tibial nerve. As stated by Radin (82), inversion of the heel significantly narrows the interspace between the medial calcaneus and the flexor retinaculum (i.e., the tarsal tunnel), which results in an increased compressive force placed on the posterior tibial nerve in the subretinacular space. Irrita-

Figure 3.48. The increased range of subtalar supination during the midstance period strains the lateral compartment musculature (A) and predisposes to entrapment neuropathy where the superficial peroneal nerve pierces the fascia (B). The sensory distribution of this nerve is illustrated in part **C.** *STJ axis* = subtalar joint axis.

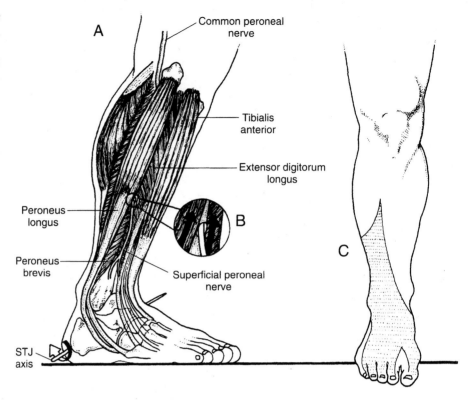

Figure 3.49. Normally, the subtalar joint pronates during late propulsion (A), which allows the final push-off to occur about the transverse metatarsal axis (which runs between the first and second metatarsal heads). Note that the plantar fascia is visibly tensed during this push-off. Conversely, when a rigid forefoot valgus deformity is present **(B),** the rigid and inverted disposition of the rearfoot disallows use of the transverse axis, and the foot is forced to roll off its oblique metatarsal axis. (These illustrations were adapted from photographs from Bojsen-Moller F. Calcaneocuboid joint and stability of the longitudinal arch of the foot at high and low gear push-off. J Anat 1979; 129: 165–176.)

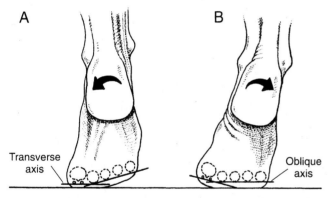

ters its propulsive period, the subtalar joint is often unable to prevent lateral instability because of the typically limited range of subtalar eversion (eversion in a cavus foot is often limited to 5° or less [75]). As a result, the subtalar joint remains supinated and the application of ground-reactive forces progresses from the lateral heel to the lateral forefoot, where the final transfer of force occurs about the oblique metatarsal axis, not the transverse metatarsal axis (Fig. 3.49).

As mentioned earlier, Bojsen-Moller (73) refers to the use of the oblique metatarsal axis as a low gear push-off because of the significantly shorter lever arm afforded this axis. He was able to study the structural interactions associated with a low gear push-off by using a large glass plate as a walking platform and then recording the various portions of the gait cycle with a high-speed camera. The photos revealed that with low gear push-off, propulsion proceeded as a rolling action over the lateral part of the ball of the foot with the leg externally rotated, the rearfoot inverted, and the forefoot adducted. As the foot moves into its final stages of propulsion, continued ground contact at the lateral forefoot forces the lesser digits into an excessively dorsiflexed position, which predisposes to Morton's neuroma (84, 85), as dorsiflexion of the lesser toes tractions the interdigital nerve against the transverse ligament (Fig. 3.50). Also, because the second through fifth metatarsal heads possess smaller radii to the plantar fascia (refer back to Fig. 2.16), dorsiflexion of the lesser digits results in only an insignificant tightening of the plantar fascia, and the stabilization afforded by the windlass mechanism is lost.

tion of the nerve at this site is further aggravated by the fact that eversion of the forefoot tractions the lateral plantar nerve, thereby creating an environment that favors the development of tarsal tunnel syndrome.

As the foot with a rigid forefoot valgus deformity en-

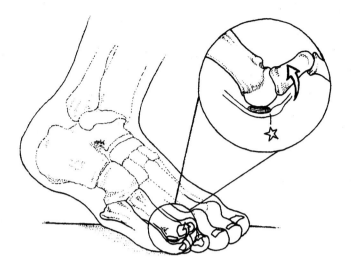

Figure 3.50. Use of the oblique metatarsal axis during the propulsive period maintains the lesser digits in a dorsiflexed position for an extended length of time *(arrow* in *inset).* This action results in a tethering of the interdigital nerve against the distal edge of the transverse metatarsal ligament *(star* in *inset).* Because the proximal portion of this nerve is fixed by attachments to flexor digitorum brevis (which fires vigorously during propulsion), the nerve is tractioned at both ends as it bends against the fibrous edge of the ligament.

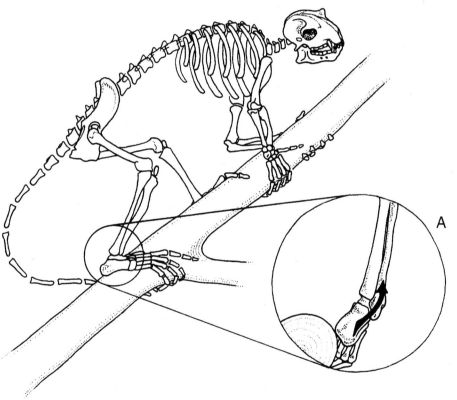

Figure 3.51. The postaxial fibular border *(black arrow* **in A) is exposed to propulsive forces in a variety of amphibians, reptiles, and tree-climbing mammals.** (Partially adapted from Carroll RL. Vertebrate Paleontology and Evolution. New York: Freeman: 469.)

This was demonstrated in Bojsen-Moller's (73) recordings in that during low gear push-off, although the medial arch became high, neither the plantar fascia nor peroneus longus could be seen to tense under the skin. Also, he emphasized that throughout low gear push-off, the rearfoot remains inverted, thereby exposing the postaxial fibular edge to larger vertical forces. He compared this lateral transfer of propulsive forces to those occurring in the hindlimbs of amphibians and reptiles and to those in the climbing foot of arboreal primates (73) (Fig. 3.51). It seems likely that this lateral displacement of propulsive forces could predispose to fibular and other lateral knee injuries.

Classic Signs and Symptoms Associated with the Forefoot Valgus Deformity

The signs and symptoms associated with the forefoot valgus deformity are dependent upon the flexibility of the midtarsal and subtalar joints and on the particular pattern in which the individual compensates for the deformity. For example, if the forefoot valgus is associated with a large range of motion about the longitudinal midtarsal joint that allows for continued subtalar pronation throughout propulsion (refer back to Fig. 3.42), the individual will display signs and symptoms similar to those of a forefoot varus deformity: hallux abductovalgus, medial achilles peritendinitis, plantar fasciitis, etc. However, if the individual possesses a flexible forefoot valgus deformity that produces a lateral instability during the propulsive period (refer back to Figs. 3.44 and 3.45), the following signs and symptoms should be expected.

1. A medium-to-high medial longitudinal arch height off-weight-bearing with a slight lowering of the arch upon weight-bearing.

2. Mild-to-moderate callus formation under the first, second, and sometimes third metatarsal heads. During the contact period, the individual with a flexible forefoot valgus deformity possessing limited ranges of longitudinal midtarsal joint axis inversion will most often be forced to dorsiflex the first ray in order to pronate the subtalar joint (refer back to Fig. 3.44). This results in an excessive loading of the plantar first metatarsal head with eventual diffuse callus formation.

The flexible forefoot valgus deformity may also produce a diffuse callus formation under the second and third metatarsal heads as during the propulsive period, the subtalar and/or midtarsal motions necessary to bring the rearfoot back to a vertical position may inhibit the normal plantarflectory motions of the first ray. This lessens the ability of the first metatarsal head to bear weight (due to the altered angle of approach afforded peroneus longus), which in turn forces the second and third metatarsal heads to support a greater percentage of ground-reactive forces (predisposing to diffuse hyperkeratosis).

3. Hallux limitus, hallux abductovalgus. If propulsive period compensation for the lateral instability includes pronation of the first ray (Fig. 3.45), a hallux limitus deformity may result as the dorsal-posterior shifting of the first metatarsophalangeal joint's transverse axis is suddenly blocked just as the hallux is reaching its peak range of dorsiflexion. If a significant metatarsus adductus is present (i.e., greater than 11°), the sudden propulsive period first ray pronation may produce subluxation of the metatarsophalangeal joint with the eventual formation of a hallux abductovalgus deformity. Because the first ray is allowed to plantarflex during early propulsion, the metatarsophalangeal joint deformity associated with the flexible forefoot valgus deformity is usually mild, i.e., the hallux abductovalgus rarely progresses beyond the second stage, and the hallux will maintain at least 45° of dorsiflexion.

4. Dorsomedial and dorsolateral bunion pain. (Note that the dorsolateral bunion is often referred to as a tailor's bunion or a bunionette). The sudden propulsive period shifting of the articulations associated with subtalar, midtarsal, and first ray compensation for the lateral instability increases the frontal plane motion of the metatarsal heads (the first metatarsal suddenly inverts while the fifth metatarsal everts; see Fig. 3.45). This increased movement produces a marked shearing of the dorsomedial and dorsolateral adventitious bursae, which are trapped between the

rotating metatarsal heads and the skin (which is held stationery by shoe gear). As a result, painful inflamed bunions are extremely common with this foot type.

5. Intermetatarsophalangeal bursitis with possible interdigital neuroma. In addition to predisposing to bunions and bunionettes, the sudden propulsive period rotation of the metatarsal heads associated with compensation for a flexible forefoot valgus deformity may produce a chronic shearing of the intermetatarsal bursae (Fig. 3.52) with eventual bursitis. While numerous authors have suggested that motion of the metatarsal heads causes a direct pinching of the interdigital nerves (this theory was originally postulated by T. G. Morton in 1876 [87]), the location of the nerve under the transverse ligament makes such direct entrapment unlikely. Rather, it has been suggested by Bossley and Cairney (88) that an interdigital neuroma results when the inflamed, swollen bursa is sufficiently displaced from its interspace to cause compression of the neurovascular bundle. They noted that during surgical exploration of a painful interspace, lateral compression of the forefoot did indeed cause the inflamed bursa to protrude from between the metatarsal heads, where it pressed against the interdigital nerve.

Apparently, no part of the nerve is protected from the compressive force, as histological findings include epi-, peri-, and endoneural fibrosis (89). The third interspace is particularly prone to injury, as it receives branches from both the medial and lateral plantar nerves and is therefore thickest at this junction (Fig. 3.53).

Clinically, it is often possible to identify a neuroma by squeezing the metatarsal heads together (which compresses the interdigital bursae), then applying pressure along the plantar surface of the affected web space. If a neuroma is present, this plantar pressure will produce an immediate increase in pain as the neuroma is compressed

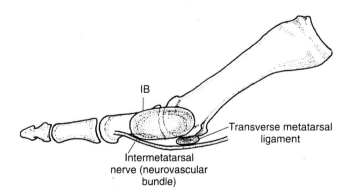

IB

Transverse metatarsal ligament

Intermetatarsal nerve (neurovascular bundle)

Figure 3.52. The intermetatarsophalangeal bursa (IB), which may be up to 3 cm long, extends between the metatarsal heads and ends distally near the center of the proximal phalanx. The exception to this occurs at the fourth and fifth interspace, where the bursa does not extend beyond the transverse metatarsal ligament, which most likely explains the rarity of symptoms at this interspace.

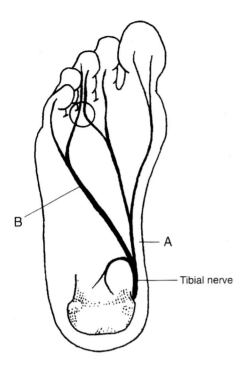

Figure 3.53. The third interspace *(circle)* receives branches from both the medial (A) and lateral (B) plantar nerves.

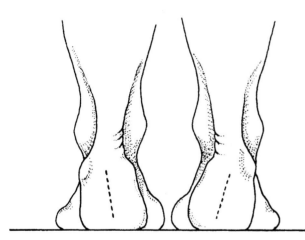

Figure 3.54. Relaxed calcaneal stance with a rigid forefoot valgus deformity.

by the distal, inferior aspect of the swollen bursa. Obviously, tight-fitting shoes would greatly amplify the symptoms associated with intermetatarsophalangeal bursitis.

6. Myositis of the lateral compartment musculature. When the flexible forefoot valgus is greater than 6°, compensatory subtalar supination and external leg rotation begin during the late midstance period (Fig. 3.45). These movements must be resisted by vigorous eccentric contraction of peroneus longus and brevis, which may predispose to chronic strain of these muscles. Peroneus brevis is also strained during the propulsive period as it attempts to stabilize against lateral instability by concentrically contracting

to pronate the subtalar joint. A chronic muscular ache in the lateral compartment may be the only symptom associated with this exaggerated muscular stabilization.

While the above-mentioned signs and symptoms have been associated with the flexible forefoot valgus deformity, a different group of injuries should be expected with the rigid forefoot valgus deformity. The classic signs and symptoms associated with the rigid forefoot valgus deformity are as follows.

1. High medial longitudinal arch, both on and off-weight-bearing, with the heels inverted during static stance (Fig. 3.54). The potential for injury is directly related to the height of the medial longitudinal arch, as high-arched people are more likely to be injured (90).

2. Moderate-to-marked callus formation under the first and fifth metatarsal heads. Because of the fixed position of forefoot eversion associated with the rigid forefoot valgus, the initial point of ground contact for the plantar forefoot often occurs directly beneath the first metatarsal head (Fig. 3.46). As there is a markedly limited range of motion available about the first ray axis, the first metatarsal is maintained in its plantar position, which subjects the skin under the first metatarsal head (particularly under the tibial sesamoid) to relatively large impact forces; a localized hyperkeratotic lesion quickly follows. As the subtalar joint compensates for the forefoot deformity by inverting the rearfoot, ground-reactive forces shift from the first metatarsal head to the fifth metatarsal head. As this foot moves into its propulsive period, its characteristic low-gear push-off causes ground-reactive forces to peak under the fifth metatarsal head, which may result in marked callus formation at that site.

3. Clawing or hammering of the digits (particularly the fourth and fifth). The larger metatarsal decline angle associated with the cavus foot forces the proximal phalanx into a dorsiflexed position (Fig. 3.55). Unfortunately, this creates a biomechanical environment that favors the formation of digital contractures, as even slight dorsiflexion of the proximal phalanx results in a superior displacement of the lumbricale and interossei tendons (Fig. 3.56). This superior displacement, if mild, will prevent these muscles from acting as metatarsophalangeal joint plantarflexors, as they will be able to create only a compressive force at this joint. If this superior displacement is sufficient, the interossei tendon will act above the transverse axis of the metatarsophalangeal joint, making this muscle a dorsiflexor of the proximal phalanx.

The extensor digitorum longus muscle, even though it has no direct attachment to the proximal phalanx, will amplify the metatarsophalangeal joint deformity by virtue of its tendinous sling that wraps around the proximal phalanx (Fig. 3.56, black arrow in B).

During a cadaveric evaluation of the digital extensor mechanism, Sarrafian et al. (91) noted that when the proximal phalanx is in a slightly dorsiflexed position, manually

Figure 3.55. The proximal phalanx in a cavus foot is maintained in a dorsiflexed position.

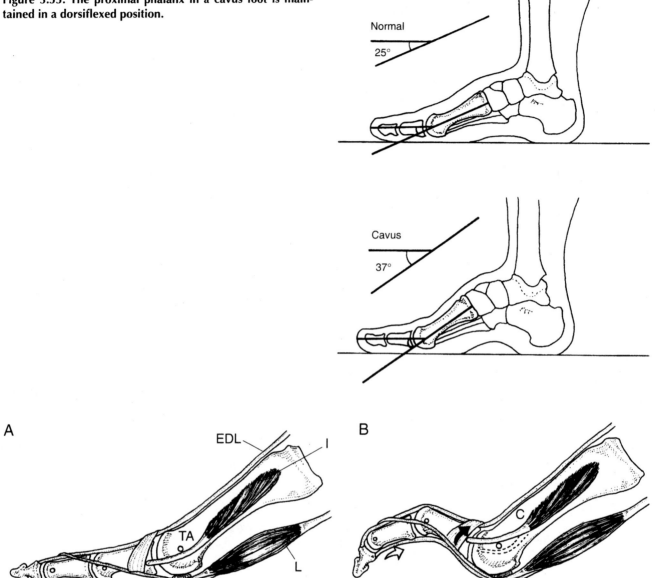

Figure 3.56. (A) Ideally, the lumbrical (L) and interossei (I) tendons will pass below the transverse axis of the metatarsophalangeal joint (TA), which allows these muscles to act as plantarflexors of the proximal phalanx. The lumbrical and extensor digitorum longus *(EDL)* tendons continue along a pathway dorsal to the interphalangeal joints, where they cre-ate the compressive force necessary to maintain the digits in full extension. **(B)** Dorsiflexion of the proximal phalanx displaces the lumbricale and interossei tendons **(C),** where in conjunction with extensor digitorum longus, they allow flexor digitorum longus to create a clawing of the interphalangeal joints *(white arrow).*

pulling the extensor digitorum longus tendon produced marked dorsiflexion of the proximal phalanx (via the sling), yet had absolutely no effect on movement at the interphalangeal joints. They stated that the extensor digitorum longus becomes an extensor of the interphalangeal joints only when the proximal phalanx is held in a plantarflexed position. In the rigid forefoot valgus deformity, the inability of the lumbricales and extensor digitorum longus to extend the interphalangeal joints allows flexor digitorum longus to act unopposed in creating flexion deformity of the interphalangeal joints. The fourth and fifth digits are particularly prone to clawing, as the low gear push-off typically seen with this deformity forces the lesser digits into a dorsiflexed position that, during propulsion, is amplified by contraction of the displaced interossei tendons. Since flexor digitorum longus fires briskly during propulsion as it attempts to maintain digital ground contact, the interphalangeal joints may suddenly claw.

Bordelon (92) noted that the proximal phalanx may be forced into extreme dorsiflexion during early swing phase as extensor digitorum longus fires to assist with ground clearance of the forefoot by midswing. Over time, contracture occurs along the dorsal metatarsophalangeal joint and plantar interphalangeal joints, which will maintain the deformity. It is of clinical significance that digital contractures displace the fat pads normally present beneath the metatarsal heads anteriorly, thereby predisposing to metatarsalgia secondary to decreased cushioning (93).

Unfortunately, Calliet (94) mentions that digital contractures are most often resistant to manual stretching techniques while Schoenhaus and Jay (79) claim that even a well-made functional orthotic is unable to reduce the degree of contracture. Consequently, the patient should be informed of a possible poor prognosis with conservative care, and recommendations should be made for modifications in shoe gear (particularly stretching sections of the toe box contacting the deformed digit).

4. Interdigital neuromas. While the flexible forefoot valgus predisposes to interdigital neuroma secondary to compression by a swollen bursa, the rigid forefoot valgus may produce injury via direct mechanical irritation of the nerve against the transverse ligament; because the interdigital nerves contain no elastin (84), they are incapable of elongating or stretching. Because of this, the excessive dorsiflexion of the lesser toes during low gear push-off will traction the nerve over the distal edge of the unyielding transverse ligament (Fig. 3.50). The repeated tethering of this nerve against the ligament may eventually lead to a proliferative reaction with reactive scarring of the nerve.

Betts (95), who originally suggested that stretching, not compression, was the cause of interdigital nerve pain, claims that the nerve in the third interspace is particularly prone to stretch injury because the proximal portions of medial and lateral plantar nerves (which later join to form this interdigital nerve) originate from opposite sides of the flexor digitorum brevis muscle and may become fixed as that muscle contracts during propulsion. This markedly increases the shearing forces under the transverse ligament, as the proximal portion of the nerve is held stationary while the distal nerve is pulled by the dorsiflexing toes.

5. Haglund's deformity with retrocalcaneal bursitis. Because the heel of the individual possessing a rigid forefoot valgus is maintained in a varus position during static stance, the superolateral portion of the calcaneus is frequently compressed into the shoe's heel counter. This is particularly troublesome when associated with enlargement of the superior portion of the os calcis (often referred to as Haglund's deformity or achilles "pump bump"; see Fig. 3.57), as repeated contact between the deformed calcaneus and the lateral heel counter may produce a localized periostitis and/or lateral achilles tendinitis.

Also, as mentioned by Bordelon (92), the enlargement of the superolateral calcaneus may be responsible for

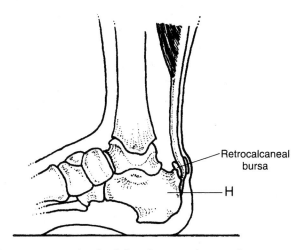

Figure 3.57. Haglund's deformity (H) refers to a bony protrusion along the posterior superior portion of the calcaneus.

chronic inflammation, with or without calcification of the retrocalcaneal bursa, which is sheared between the bony deformity and the achilles tendon.

6. Lateral achilles peritendinitis. The achilles tendon may be chronically injured even if Haglund's deformity is not present, as the excessive range of calcaneal inversion necessary to compensate for the rigid forefoot valgus deformity may greatly increase the tensile strains placed on the lateral aspects of the achilles tendon. The increased tension may seriously compromise the already inadequate blood supply present in the tendon, particularly the section 2–6 cm proximal to the calcaneal insertion.

The effect of tensile strain on tendinous blood flow was noted by Rathbun and MacNab (96) as they demonstrated that increased tension on the supraspinatus and subscapularis musculature results in a reduced filling of the vascular beds of the tendons. By applying this information to the calf, it seems quite possible that an excessively inverted calcaneus could sufficiently "strangle" the lateral achilles tendon (particularly during early propulsion, when tensile strains on the tendon may exceed 1200 lbs. [97]) to the point of producing a morbid degeneration (tendinosis) of the nearly avascular tissues.

7. Chronic tenosynovitis of peroneus longus and/or inversion sprains of the ankle mortise. The inverted position of the rearfoot, coupled with the exaggerated height of the medial longitudinal arch, acts to create a strong traction force on the peroneus longus tendon (Fig. 3.58A and B). This may produce a chronic tenosynovitis of peroneus longus and may even produce an entrapment neuropathy of the superficial peroneal nerve. In addition, because the ankle in a cavus foot possesses a higher center of mass, the compensatory inversion of the rearfoot associated with the forefoot valgus deformity is much more likely to produce chronic ankle sprain, as it creates a marked inversion instability (Fig. 3.59).

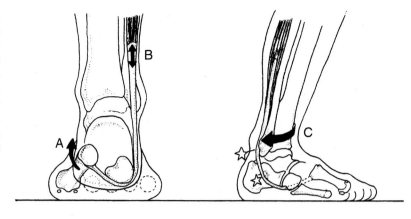

Figure 3.58. The elevated medial longitudinal arch associated with the cavus foot displaces the insertion of peroneus longus superiorly (A), thereby increasing tensile strains placed on the remainder of the muscle (B). The continued range of shank external rotation associated with a low-gear push-off **(C)** further aggravates the problem by straining the peroneus longus tendon at its passage behind the fibula and beneath the peroneal tubercle (stars).

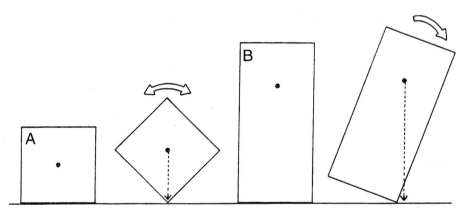

Figure 3.59. Note how block A can be tilted 45° and still not fall on its side. In **block B**, the elevated center of mass (black dot) is quickly displaced lateral to its base of support, causing it to fall. This action is analogous to how a top-heavy jeep is more likely to flip when making a fast turn.

8. Diffuse lateral ankle and knee pain. The jarring and abrupt application of vertical forces along the posterolateral heel during the contact period, coupled with the postaxial transfer of forces during the propulsive period, subjects the lateral ankle and knee to a greater potential for injury. Because the fibula normally supports only one-sixth of the total axial weight borne by the leg (98), the increase in vertical forces may produce a diffuse fibular stress reaction with the potential for cortical hypertrophy as the fibula attempts to accommodate the exaggerated workload. In addition to stressing the bone, the increased ground-reactive forces may be responsible for producing a relative laxity of the restraining ligaments at the distal tibiofibular articulation and/or joint dysfunction at the proximal tibiofibular articulation.

The propensity for lateral knee pain in individuals possessing a cavus foot was demonstrated by Lutter (24). In his study of 213 runners with a variety of knee injuries, he noted that individuals with cavus feet were much more likely to suffer from lateral joint space pain and iliobitial band friction syndrome. Lutter's (24) evaluation was particularly interesting, as he demonstrated that nearly 80% of all knee injuries could be related to faulty mechanics in the foot, with pronatory feet producing medial knee pain and cavus feet producing lateral knee pain. This finding was also corroborated by McKenzie et al. (25).

9. Chronic gluteus medius strain with possible os-
teoarthrosis of the hip. Ideally, during the late midstance and early propulsive periods, the body's center of mass reaches peak lateral displacement and is then projected medially so as to allow for the contralateral heel strike. The return of the center of mass toward midline is dependent on adequate locking of the calcaneocuboid joint, peroneus longus and brevis eversion of the lateral column and gluteus medius (and upper gluteus maximus) abduction of the hip. Because the individual with a rigid forefoot valgus typically possesses limited ranges of subtalar motion, peroneal eversion of the lateral column is often not possible, and the hip abductors must fire vigorously in an attempt to prevent continued lateral displacement of the center of mass during propulsion. The individual may learn to avoid straining the hip abductor musculature by walking with a narrowed base of gait, which decreases lateral deviation of the center of mass. Unfortunately, while the narrow base of gait reduces gluteus medius strain, it increases the risk of inversion ankle sprain and may even predispose to a greater trochanteric bursitis.

The hip joint in individuals possessing a rigid forefoot valgus is also prone to injury because the extreme range of compensatory subtalar supination necessary for the plantar forefoot to make ground contact maintains the entire lower extremity in an externally rotated position during all phases of gait. This places the head of the femur into a perpetually retrograde position while significantly reducing surface contact between the head of the femur and the acetabulum. As a result, vertical forces are now applied over a smaller surface area, which produces a proportional increase in pressure and "unmitigated shock" over the sections of the joint that have remained in contact (99). The sequela of such an increase in axial loading is an accelerated rate of articular degeneration with joint space narrowing (99). The early signs of such a lesion include a decreased range of hip abduction with x-ray evidence of subchondral sclerosis along the superior acetabular rim.

10. Low back pain. Several authors have claimed that the rigid forefoot valgus deformity is causal in the development of low back pain (3, 32, 80, 100). It has been assumed that the "shock-wave" from the sudden peak in contact period ground-reactive forces is transferred from the foot and leg, directly into the low back (3). While it has been demonstrated that the increased skeletal transients associated with the cavus foot may predispose to lateral knee pain (24) and/or stress fractures in the foot or femur (22), it has never been proven that these shock-waves predispose to low back pain. In fact, in their evaluation of 105 variables potentially responsible for low back pain, Roncarati and McMullen (101) found that individuals possessing cavus feet were actually less likely to suffer from low back pain. (The sample group in this study was 674 randomly chosen subjects.) It should be noted that Roncarati and McMullen used Feiss' line measurements to identify the cavus feet (Fig. 3.60). If they had measured the degree of forefoot valgus deformity, the range of midtarsal and subtalar motion (particularly subtalar eversion), and/or evaluated the speed of contact period subtalar pronation, they might have found a more significant correlation with low back pain.

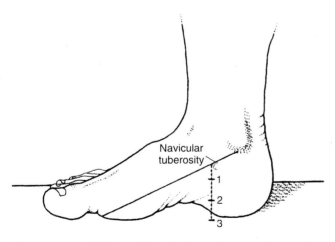

Figure 3.60. Feiss' line. A line is drawn between the inferior aspect of the medial malleolus and the distal first metatarsal. A *vertical line* is then dropped directly through the navicular tuberosity *(dotted line)* and is divided into equal thirds. A cavus foot is present if the navicular tuberosity is situated near the upper border of the first division while a pronated foot will often present with a navicular tuberosity in the second division.

It is likely that the potential for the individual with a cavus foot to develop low back pain is dependent upon how he or she compensates for the deformity: if the person walks with short strides, is relatively inactive and/or lands toe-heel, the potential for injury to the proximal structures would be greatly reduced.

Conversely, if the individual were a distance runner with a long stride and a hard heel-strike, the potential for high-impact injury would dramatically increase.

In a case history relating the cavus foot to lumbosacral facet syndrome, Builder and Marr (80) contended that the cavus foot is often responsible for low back pain, particularly when a facilitated spinal segment is present. They described a facilitated segment as "one in which the motor reflex threshold is lowered as a result of some subthreshold bombardment of the motor neurons at that level of the spinal cord." They cited the work of Denslow and Korr (102), who demonstrated electromyographically that the paraspinal musculature supplied by the facilitated or "lesioned" segment was the first to fire and the last to stop firing in response to a given stimulus anywhere in the body.

For example, mechanical stimulation of a spinous process on an unaffected spinal segment did not stimulate the musculature of that segment, but it did cause the paraspinal musculature supplied by the facilitated segment to fire. In their case history, Builder and Marr (80) describe an individual who, despite comprehensive conservative care (which included manipulation, sacro-occipital therapy along with a variety of therapeutic modalities, i.e., ultrasound, massage, and acupuncture), continued to suffer from prolonged bouts of chronic low back pain. Functional evaluation revealed a "heavy heel-strike" that produced a visible jarring of the lumbar spine. Treatment with an orthotic possessing high-density rubber padding under the heel resulted in a marginal reduction in pain during the first 2 weeks with an almost complete resolution of symptomatology by the 12th week.

The efficacy of reducing skeletal transients in persons presenting with low back pain was demonstrated in a 5-year study by Wosk and Voloshin (103) in which 382 back pain patients were treated with viscoelastic shock-absorbing inserts. An astonishing 80% of those treated reported significantly reduced pain levels with objective improvements in mobility. Because of the somewhat surprising results of this study, its authors proposed that low back pain patients are less able to attenuate the repetitive intervertebral impacts associated with walking and are therefore subjected to repeated microdamage at the troublesome S1-L5-L4 area.

By combining the results of Wosk and Voloshin's study (103) with the evaluation of low back pain correlates by Roncarati and McMullen (101), one is most likely to find that, although the cavus foot will not produce low back pain in a healthy population (and ironically may even protect against low back pain by limiting the degree of pelvic extension associated with excessive lower extremity internal rotation), it may play a significant role in perpetuating an even minor low back injury.

Orthotic Management for the Forefoot Valgus Deformity

Whether the forefoot valgus deformity is flexible or rigid, the goal of orthotic therapy is to allow neutral position function of the subtalar joint. As with the forefoot varus deformity, this is best accomplished by taking an impression of the foot that accurately captures the forefoot-rearfoot relationship when the calcaneocuboid joint is locked and the talar head is maintained behind the navicular. A positive model is then obtained from this impression, and the appropriate changes are made to allow for soft-tissue displacement upon weight-bearing and for the lowering of the medial longitudinal arch necessary for shock absorption. After these changes have been made, which are discussed more fully in the laboratory preparation section, an orthotic shell is molded along the plantar surface, ending just proximal to the metatarsal heads. An angled wedge or post is then added to the plantar anterolateral shell, bringing the bisection of the rearfoot to a vertical position (Fig. 3.61).

This post should never exceed 15°, as shoe fit becomes a problem, and the distal lateral shell might dig into the shaft of the fifth metatarsal. When a large post angle is necessary, the posting should be extended under the metatarsal heads. (As noted previously, this addition is referred to as a compressible post to sulcus). Although the extended post may produce difficulties with shoe fit, it will decrease strain on the lateral metatarsal shafts, as a greater percentage of weight will be borne by the metatarsal heads. Also, the compressible post to sulcus will allow for continued orthotic control through the propulsive period as the progression of forces remains centered over the compressible post. Without this extension, the foot with a large forefoot valgus deformity (e.g., greater than 4°) will tip laterally into supinatory compensation the moment body weight is

centered distal to the orthotic shell, i.e., early propulsion, which could result in continued symptomatology as propulsive period forces are transferred along the postaxial fibular border.

When a flexible forefoot valgus deformity is present, the shell of the orthotic (specifically, the calcaneal incline angle) will limit excessive subtalar pronation while the forefoot post will prevent lateral instability. Schoenhaus and Jay (79) claim that if initiated early enough, use of a functional orthotic will prevent severe hallux abductus and bunion formation.

When the forefoot valgus deformity is rigid, the forefoot post is invaluable during propulsion, as it assists in the development of a high gear push-off by shifting the progression of forces medially through the transverse axis of the metatarsal heads. Use of the high gear push-off will improve the windlass effect of the plantar fascia, displace the transfer of propulsive period forces away from the postaxial fibular border, and minimize stretching of the more lateral interdigital nerves as the lesser toes dorsiflex through smaller ranges of motion. The forefoot post will also be effective during the contact period as it prevents supinatory compensation by the subtalar joint, as the lateral forefoot will now be supported. (This allows for a more equal distribution of ground-reactive forces beneath the metatarsal heads that in turn lessens the potential for metatarsalgia.)

It must be stressed that even though the forefoot valgus post prevents excessive rearfoot inversion during the contact period, it is unable to provide the continued range of subtalar pronation necessary for adequate shock absorption. This is because the forefoot post should only be large enough to bring the subtalar joint to its neutral position. While overposting the lateral forefoot to induce the range of subtalar pronation necessary for shock absorption would be ideal during the contact period (assuming the subtalar joint were able to pronate this additional range), it would be detrimental to do so during early propulsion, as it would forcefully maintain the subtalar joint in a pronated position as vertical forces peak (Fig. 3.62). This situation could eventually result in a permanent elongation (plastic defor-

Figure 3.61. (A–C) The forefoot valgus post.

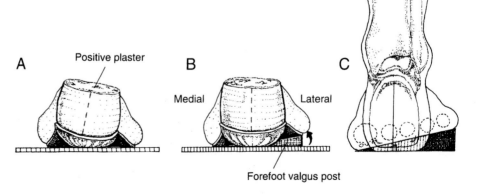

A   Positive plaster

B   Medial   Lateral

C

Forefoot valgus post

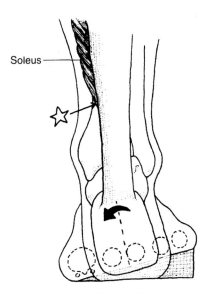

Soleus

Figure 3.62. Overposting the forefoot can produce an increased range of subtalar pronation, which would be beneficial during the contact period, as it would allow for improved shock absorption. Unfortunately, this post will maintain the calcaneus in an everted position during midstance and early propulsion, potentially producing a variety of injuries (primarily chronic soleus strain (*star*)).

mity) of the spring ligament, chronic medial achilles peritendinitis, and/or chronic strain of the soleus muscle. Soleus strain is perhaps the most common iatrogenic injury associated with overposting the lateral forefoot, as this muscle fires vigorously in an attempt to reestablish subtalar neutrality by inverting the entire foot up and over the oversized post.

The only way an individual with a rigid forefoot valgus deformity can properly absorb shock is if the subtalar joint possesses adequate ranges of subtalar pronation. Because this motion is so frequently limited in such patients, many of their high-impact symptoms will continue despite appropriate use of the forefoot post. It is for this reason that several authors claim that rigid foot types respond less favorably to orthotic therapies (79, 104). However, the rigidity of this foot type does not necessitate a poor prognosis. By aggressively manipulating inflexible articulations, the individual is often able to resume a symptom-free life-style. (Although it cannot be overstated that when the range of subtalar pronation is limited bilaterally and/or the joint's end-play is hard and abrupt, it should be suspected that the reduced range of motion is associated with a triarticulated subtalar joint in which case manipulation is contraindicated.)

Even if increasing the range of subtalar pronation is not possible, the symptomatology may still be lessened by simply inserting shock-absorbing material under the heel (or incorporating it into an orthotic), instructing the individual to walk with shorter strides and, lastly, telling the patient to wear running shoes as often as possible. McKenzie

et al. (25) advocate that individuals with cavus feet should wear slip-lasted, curve-lasted shoes with softer ethylene vinyl acetate (EVA) midsoles. Also, in order to minimize patient frustration with a treatment program, these individuals should be informed that cavus feet are typically slow to heal. In one study relating certain foot types to knee injuries in runners (105), it was noted that the cavus-related injuries required 86 days before full return to running was possible while the pronation-related knee injuries required only 46 days.

In closing, it should be emphasized that the mechanical dysfunction associated with the rigid forefoot valgus is often progressive, which makes most forms of mechanical control temporary and ever-changing. As a result, this foot type should be evaluated regularly to ensure that the most effective treatment program is being rendered. If significant changes in forefoot/rearfoot alignment do occur, the foot should be recast, and the post angles should be altered accordingly.

If conservative treatment is unable to halt the progression of this deformity, surgical intervention may be necessary. Fortunately, this is rarely the case, as the vast majority of patients respond favorably to conservative care. Schoenhaus and Jay (79) are particularly optimistic, as they claim a well-made orthotic will eliminate retro-achilles irritation, alleviate symptoms associated with the plantar callus formation (by distributing weight across all of the metatarsal heads), and reduce symptomatology associated with interdigital neuromas, lateral calf and knee pain, and sciatica. They did acknowledge that the digital contractures will not change significantly and may even progress, particularly at the fifth toe.

TRANSVERSE PLANE ALIGNMENT OF THE METATARSAL HEADS

As with the forefoot varus and valgus deformities, alignment of the metatarsal heads is checked with the foot in its neutral position. Although the literature is full of disagreement regarding the presence or absence of a transverse arch at the level of the metatarsal heads, Bojsen-Moller (106) explains this phenomenon by noting that the metatarsal shafts are curved longitudinally, with the central metatarsals extending furthest distally. He noted that these factors give a false impression of a transverse metatarsal arch while, in reality, all of the metatarsal heads are resting on the same transverse plane (Fig. 3.63). Cavanagh et al. (107) conclusively demonstrated that there is no such thing as a transverse metatarsal arch by measuring plantar pressure patterns beneath the metatarsal heads in symptom-free individuals. Because peak pressure points were greatest beneath the central metatarsal heads, they concluded that a transverse arch at the level of the metatarsal heads could not be present and that such a concept should be completely discarded.

Figure 3.63. Note how the metatarsal shafts form a transverse arch (A) while the metatarsal heads rest evenly on the ground.

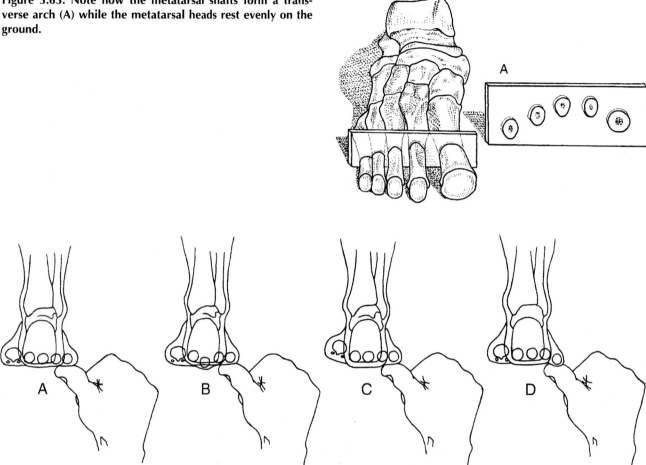

Figure 3.64. (A) Ideal alignment of the metatarsal heads; (B) a plantarflexed third metatarsal; (C) a dorsiflexed first metatarsal; (D) a plantarflexed fifth metatarsal. Note: The left hand, which would normally be maintaining talonavicular congruency, has been removed in order to improve clarity.

Figure 3.65. The proximal phalanx of a hammered or clawed digit creates a retrograde plantarflectory force (A) that maintains its respective metatarsal head in a lowered position (B). This is possible primarily because the ligaments that restrain tarsometatarsal motions are less able to resist plantarflectory than dorsiflectory motions (106).

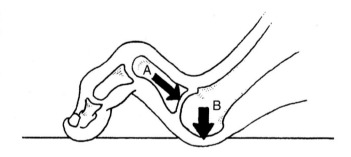

While all of the metatarsal heads should ideally be resting on the same transverse plane, there are numerous situations in which either congenital or acquired anomalies allow one or more of the metatarsal heads to deviate above or below the common transverse plane (Fig. 3.64). Bojsen-Moller (106) describes an interesting phenomenon in which a hammered second or third digit will force its respective metatarsal head into a plantarflexed position (Fig. 3.65), which may eventually result in painful plantar callosities or even ulceration due to an unequal distribution of pressures.

The ability of a malpositioned metatarsal head to affect foot function detrimentally is dependent on which of the metatarsals is involved and, more importantly, the range of motion available to that metatarsal. For example, if the third metatarsal is situated in a plantarflexed position and its metatarsal head easily shifts back to the common transverse plane of the other metatarsals, foot function will not be seriously compromised, and the risk of injury is minimal (although the plantar third metatarsal head and the neighboring intermetatarsophalangeal bursae are prone to injury as they are subjected to greater compressive and shear forces, respectively).

On the contrary, if it had been the fifth metatarsal head that had been plantarflexed and the fifth ray were rigid and unable to allow the fifth metatarsal head to return to the common transverse plane of the other metatarsals, the risk of injury would greatly increase, as the subtalar joint would be forced into compensatory pronation in an attempt to bring the medial forefoot to the ground (Fig. 3.66). This foot behaves identically to the forefoot varus deformity and is therefore subjected to the same potential injuries. Fortunately, although defects in the alignment of a lesser metatarsal may produce potentially injurious compensatory rearfoot motions, these defects are not very common.

THE PLANTARFLEXED FIRST RAY DEFORMITY

The plantarflexed first ray deformity (Fig. 3.67) is much more common and of greater clinical significance than a plantarflexed lesser metatarsal. This deformity is present in approximately 15% of the population (1) and may be either congenital or acquired. It is possible to ascertain whether a given deformity is congenital or acquired, as the congenital deformity is typically very large and the first ray in this deformity usually possesses equal amounts of dorsi and plantar motion (Fig. 3.68).

Conversely, the acquired plantarflexed first ray deformity possesses osseous or soft tissue restrictions that limit first ray movement and produce asymmetrical dorsi-plantar motions that often vary markedly between the two feet. With advancing age, it is often difficult to distinguish between congenital and acquired deformities, as age-related decreases in first ray motion may allow for asymmetrical movement patterns in the congenital deformity.

Because the congenital deformity is so large, it has a greater potential for producing injury. In fact, Root et al. (3) claimed that the congenital plantarflexed first ray is the most common cause of compensatory subtalar joint supination, and they related this deformity to the development of a cavus foot type. They stated that when a congenital plantarflexed first ray is present in a child, the first ray and longitudinal midtarsal joint axis almost always possess enough motion to compensate for this deformity (Fig. 3.69). How-

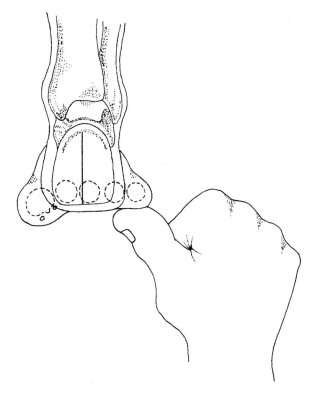

Figure 3.67. The plantarflexed first ray deformity.

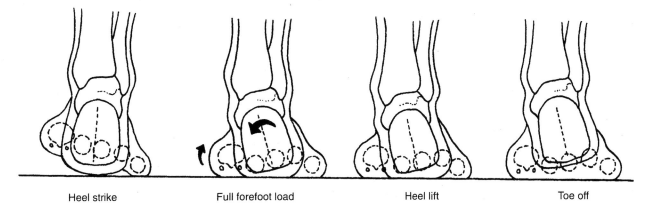

| Heel strike | Full forefoot load | Heel lift | Toe off |

Figure 3.66. A rigid plantarflexed fifth metatarsal requires compensatory subtalar joint pronation in order to bring the medial forefoot to the ground. Note that the subtalar joint is maintained in a pronated position throughout stance phase. If the fifth ray were flexible, it could have dorsiflexed and everted during the contact period, and subtalar function would not have been compromised (although the fifth ray movement would most likely result in a tailor's bunion, as the dorsolateral bursa would be repeatedly sheared between the rotating metatarsal head and the skin/shoe gear).

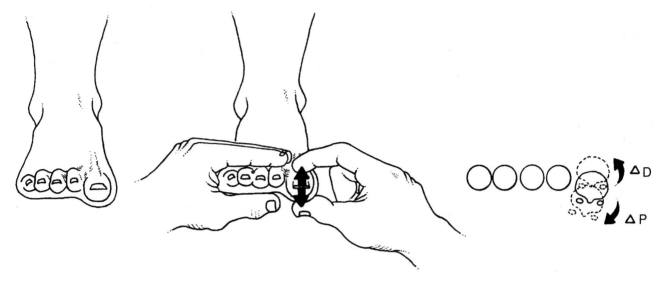

Figure 3.68. The congenital plantarflexed first ray will usually dorsiflex and plantarflex through equal ranges ($\Delta P = \Delta D$).

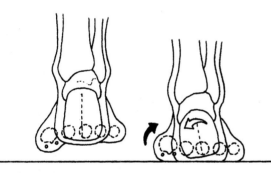

Figure 3.69. When the first ray and midtarsal joint possess adequate ranges of motion, they are able to fully compensate for the plantarflexed first ray deformity.

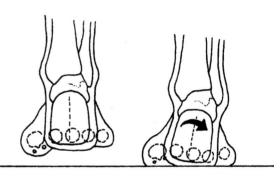

Figure 3.70. Age-related decreases in first ray and midtarsal motion force the subtalar joint into compensatory supination.

ever, as the child reaches ages 7–15, the range of motion available about these axes lessens, and subtalar joint supination is necessary to compensate for the plantarflexed first ray (Fig. 3.70).

This begins a cycle in which inversion of the rearfoot increases the mechanical advantage afforded peroneus longus, which in turn allows for an amplification of the plantarflexed first ray deformity. This increase in first ray plantarflexion creates a retrograde supinatory force that inverts the rearfoot even further and allows the oblique midtarsal joint axis to shift into a more vertical position. With the oblique midtarsal joint axis in this new position, the forefoot is allowed to adduct; the medial longitudinal arch height greatly increases; the toes claw; and a pes cavus deformity eventually forms (Fig. 3.71).

Although the acquired plantarflexed first ray deformity tends to be much smaller, it is often associated with compensatory subtalar supination and may therefore be responsible for injury to the proximal structures. A list of the

possible etiological factors associated with the acquired plantarflexed first ray deformity are as follows.

Flaccid paralysis or extreme weakness of gastrocnemius. Conditions such as polio or surgical lengthening of the achilles tendon often result in a marked weakness of the gastrocnemius muscle. (The weakness associated with surgical lengthening is only temporary.) If for any reason gastrocnemius is unable to function properly during late midstance, the long digital flexors and peroneus longus will fire vigorously in an attempt to produce heel lift. Because these muscles are such weak ankle plantarflexors, they only succeed in clawing the digits and plantarflexing the first ray. If this continues over an extended period of time, an acquired plantarflexed first ray deformity develops.

Hypertonicity of peroneus longus. Any condition that causes pain upon dorsiflexion of the first ray or inversion about the longitudinal midtarsal joint axis (such as an inflammatory reaction at the first tarsometatarsal articulation or a cuboid that has undergone subluxation) will result

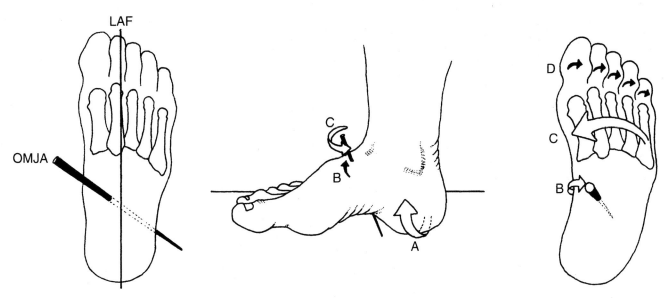

Figure 3.71. Inversion of the rearfoot (A) brings the oblique midtarsal joint axis into a more vertical position (B), which allows the forefoot to adduct (C). Since the toes always parallel the longitudinal axis of the foot *(LAF),* adduction of the forefoot will result in a proportional abduction (with resultant

clawing) of the digits **(D).** It is of note that the acquired plantarflexed first ray, which is much more common, never requires enough subtalar joint supination to adduct the forefoot about the oblique midtarsal joint axis *(OMJA)* or severely claw the toes (3).

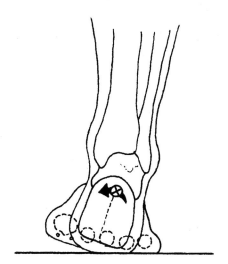

Figure 3.72. An uncompensated rearfoot varus. The subtalar joint is fully pronated, and the medial condyle of the calcaneus has not made ground contact.

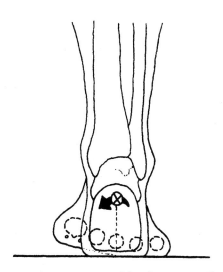

Figure 3.73. An uncompensated forefoot varus. The subtalar joint is fully pronated, and the plantar medial forefoot has not made ground contact.

in a protective tonic spasm of peroneus longus. Because of its attachment to the base of the first metatarsal and medial cuneiform, an acquired plantarflexed first ray may quickly form. The hypertonic peroneus longus is readily identified, as it rapidly pronates the foot during swing phase.

Flaccid paralysis or extreme weakness of tibialis anterior. Weakness of this muscle would allow the antagonistic peroneus longus to plantarflex the first ray.

Presence of an uncompensated rearfoot or forefoot varus deformity. When the subtalar joint in a rearfoot

varus foot type lacks the range of eversion necessary to bring the medial calcaneus to the ground, it is referred to as an uncompensated rearfoot varus (Fig. 3.72). Similarly, when the subtalar joint in an individual possessing a forefoot varus foot type is unable to bring the medial forefoot to the ground, it is referred to as an uncompensated forefoot varus (Fig. 3.73).

Although these foot types are discussed in a later section, they will be briefly discussed now as they are almost always responsible for an acquired plantarflexed first ray deformity. In both of these situations, the plantar medial rearfoot is only able to make ground contact via excessive plantarflexion of the first ray (Figs. 3.74 and 3.75). Thus, an acquired plantarflexed first ray quickly develops. The uncompensated rearfoot varus deformity is notorious for producing an acquired plantarflexed first ray deformity, as the inverted rearfoot greatly increases the mechanical efficiency of peroneus longus as a first ray plantarflexor.

Weakness of the intrinsic muscles responsible for stabilizing the plantar proximal hallux (particularly abductor hallucis) and/or contracture or extensor hallucis longus. Both of these conditions allow the hallux to dorsiflex excessively, which places a retrograde plantarflectory force on the first metatarsal head. The extensor hallucis longus muscle will often produce a visible plantarflexion with the first ray during early swing phase.

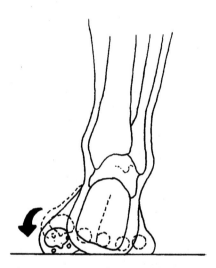

Figure 3.74. An acquired plantarflexed first ray secondary to an uncompensated rearfoot varus.

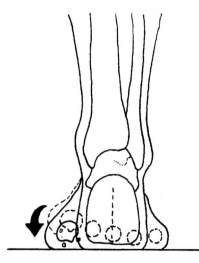

Figure 3.75. An acquired plantarflexed first ray secondary to an uncompensated forefoot varus.

The same poorly understood neuromuscular disorders associated with a pes cavus may also be responsible for an acquired plantarflexed first ray deformity. As mentioned, the pes cavus often presents with a rearfoot varus, forefoot valgus, and plantarflexed first ray. As with the forefoot valgus deformity, the extent of mechanical malfunction associated with a plantarflexed first ray is dependent on the size of the deformity and the rigidity of the midfoot (specifically, the availability of first ray dorsiflexion). Because of this, the plantarflexed first ray deformity is categorized as either flexible, semiflexible, or rigid, depending on the dorsiflectory range available to the first ray (Fig. 3.76).

Pathomechanics

Regardless of the range of motion available to the first ray, the downward projection of the first metatarsal shaft causes the first metatarsal head to strike the ground prematurely. When the plantarflexed first ray deformity is flexible, ground-reactive forces quickly shift the first metatarsal into a dorsiflexed and inverted position (Fig. 3.77).

During the contact period, the flexible plantarflexed first ray will dorsiflex and invert through a range of movement that is directly proportional to the range of subtalar pronation, i.e., the more the rearfoot everts, the more the first ray will dorsiflex and invert. Unfortunately, the flexible plantarflexed first ray deformity is almost always associated with a compensated rearfoot varus deformity which, as described earlier, requires sometimes large ranges of compensatory subtalar pronation. When the plantarflexed first ray and rearfoot varus deformities do occur together (as in Fig. 3.77), the second metatarsal head is particularly prone to injury, as the first ray is often forced to dorsiflex above the level of the lesser metatarsals, exposing the second metatarsal head to a greater percentage of ground-reactive forces.

This alteration in the distribution of ground-reactive forces typically produces a mild diffuse callus pattern under the first metatarsal head (associated with the premature loading of the first metatarsal head during the contact period) with a more localized and dense callus formation directly under the second metatarsal head (associated with the excessive loading of this metatarsal head during the propulsive period).

The flexible plantarflexed first ray may also be responsible for dorsomedial bunion pain and/or intermetatarsophalangeal bursitis, as the rapidly dorsiflexing and inverting first ray creates a shearing force between the first and second metatarsal heads (predisposing to bursitis) and between the dorsomedial first metatarsal head and the skin (which is held stationary by shoe gear), thereby shearing the adventitious bursa.

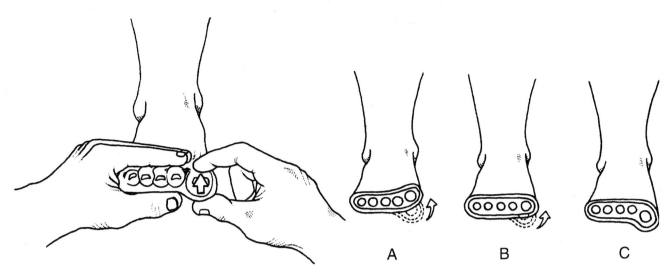

Figure 3.76. Categorization of the plantarflexed first rays. The first ray is maximally dorsiflexed as the lesser metatarsals are held stationary. If the first ray can dorsiflex above the common transverse plane of the lesser metatarsals (**A**), it is referred to as a flexible deformity. If it dorsiflexes to the same level as the lesser metatarsals (**B**), it is referred to as a semiflexible deformity, and if it is unable to reach the common transverse plane of the lesser metatarsals (**C**), it is referred to as a rigid deformity.

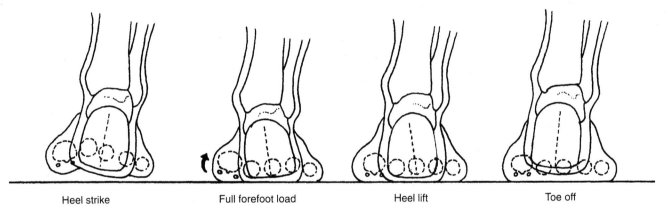

Heel strike   Full forefoot load   Heel lift   Toe off

Figure 3.77. Foot motions with a flexible plantarflexed first ray deformity. Note the sudden dorsiflexion and inversion of the first metatarsal head during the contact period. Normally, the first metatarsal does not move during early stance.

It is also quite common for the medial branch of the medial-dorsal cutaneous nerve (which passes over the dorsomedial aspect of the first metatarsal head) to become sheared between the rotating metatarsal head and the skin/shoe gear. The repeated compression of this sensory nerve often leads to a mononeuritis capable of producing pain and paresthesia along the dorsomedial aspect of the hallux. On occasion, this pain will be referred proximally towards the anterior aspect of the ankle (3) and should not be confused with radicular pain. The pain associated with this acute neuritis will typically subside quickly once the mechanical irritant has been removed, i.e., the range of subtalar pronation is controlled and/or the first ray is no longer forced to dorsiflex and invert through such an extreme arc.

When the first metatarsal is semiflexible, the first metatarsal head is unable to move above the common trans-verse plane of the lesser metatarsals, so the shearing forces associated with excessive first ray motion are minimized (which decreases the potential for bursitis/neuritis), and the second metatarsal head is protected from trauma. However, the sesamoids (particularly the tibial sesamoid) are now subjected to potential injury, as they are literally "driven" into the ground by forces everting the rearfoot (i.e., star in Fig. 3.78). Over time, a reactive hyperplasia of skin occurs along the plantar medial margin of the first metatarsophalangeal joint, which only acts to amplify pressure along the tibial sesamoid, as this hard callus is less yielding to ground-reactive forces.

In Figure 3.78 the midstance and propulsive period subtalar motions are not affected by the semiflexible plantarflexed first ray deformity. This would not be the case were the first ray rigid. When the first metatarsal head is un-

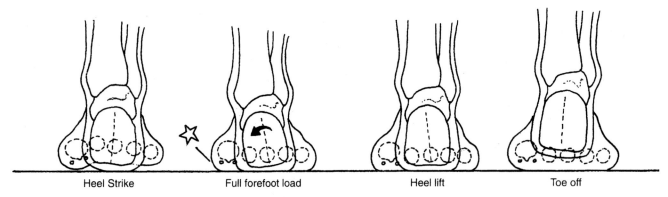

Figure 3.78. Foot motions with a semiflexible plantarflexed first ray deformity.

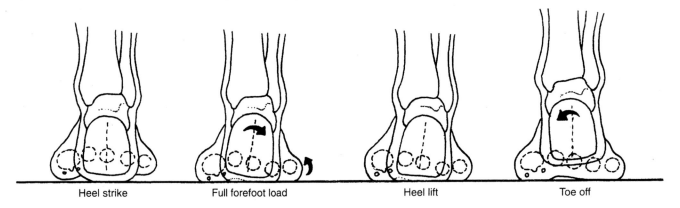

Figure 3.79. Stance phase motions with a rigid plantarflexed first ray deformity.

able to move to the common transverse plane of the lesser metatarsals, the entire lower extremity may be prone to injury, as subtalar pronation comes to an abrupt halt the moment the plantarflexed first metatarsal makes ground contact (Fig. 3.79). The entire foot actually tips laterally, thereby transferring ground-reactive forces from the first to the fifth metatarsal head. Because the fifth ray possesses its own independent axis of motion, the fifth metatarsal head is typically able to dorsiflex and evert into a safe position (Fig. 3.79, FFL). While this lessens the potential for injury to the fifth metatarsal head, it increases intermetatarsal shear (predisposing to intermetatarsophalangeal bursitis) and often results in the formation of an adventitous bursa along the dorsolateral fifth metatarsal head (i.e., tailor's bunion).

Of much greater clinical significance, the sudden contact period subtalar supination necessary to compensate for the rigid plantarflexed first ray creates asynchronous movement patterns between the talus and the shank (i.e., the talus is forced to abduct while the shank continues to internally rotate) and results in the rapid transfer of forces along the postaxial fibular border: this foot behaves identically to the rigid forefoot valgus foot type and is therefore subjected to some injuries, i.e., stress fractures in the foot, lateral ankle sprains, lateral knee pain, lateral achilles peritendinitis, etc.

As demonstrated in Figure 3.79, when it is able to, the subtalar joint will pronate during the propulsive period in an attempt to minimize the lateral instability. While this lessens the postaxial transfer of forces and decreases the risk of inversion sprain, it may predispose to other injuries, as it unlocks the midtarsal joint at a time when vertical forces are peaking. This may eventually lead to a pathological laxity of the supporting ligaments and joint capsules, as the tarsals will be allowed to shift with the application of propulsive period ground-reactive forces.

Classic Signs and Symptoms Associated with the Plantarflexed First Ray Deformity

The classic signs and symptoms associated with this deformity are dependent primarily on the range of motion available to the first ray. If the first ray is flexible, the following signs and symptoms should be expected:

1. A medium-to-high medial longitudinal arch height off-weight-bearing with a mild-to-moderate lowering of the arch upon weight-bearing.

2. Mild diffuse callus formation under the first metatarsal head with a denser more localized callus under the second metatarsal head. The mild callus centered beneath the first metatarsal head results from the premature loading of that metatarsal head during the contact period. This callus is also described as a "fullness," since the only sign of this mild hyperplasia may be a thickening of the skin lines under the first metatarsal head. Because the first metatarsal head often dorsiflexes above the common transverse plane of the lesser metatarsals, it is unable to bear weight effectively during the latter half of stance phase, and a greater percentage of ground-reactive forces are shifted to the second metatarsal head. Unless this individual learns to avoid the propulsive period by shortening length of stride, a dense localized callus will quickly develop under the second metatarsal head.

3. Dorsomedial bunion pain with intermetatarsophalangeal bursitis. Because the position of the first ray axis allows for almost equal amounts of frontal and sagittal movements, significant shearing forces will develop when the first metatarsal head is forced upward during the contact period. These shearing forces may traumatize any of the neighboring tissues, particularly the dorsomedial adventitious bursa and the first intermetatarsophalangeal bursa (which is sheared between the rotating first and stationary second metatarsal head). The dorsiflexing and inverting metatarsal head may also produce entrapment neuropathy (with associated paresthesias) of the cutaneous nerves located along the dorsomedial aspect of the metatarsophalangeal joint.

4. Dorsal base exostosis. In addition to shearing the neighboring tissues, the excessive contact period first ray motion may even lead to an osteoarthrosis of the first metatarsal-medial cuneiform articulation. This is often associated with decreased joint space, sclerosis of the articular margins and, if severe, exostoses along the dorsal margins of the joint (particularly along the base of the first metatarsal). A common sequela of such bony outgrowth is entrapment of the neurovascular bundle of the tibialis anterior artery and the deep peroneal nerve: because this bundle is located directly above the base of the first metatarsal, it is often entrapped between the rotating exostosis and the skin/shoe gear. The exact location of the neurovascular bundle is illustrated in Figure 3.174.

5. Medial plantar fascia strain and/or abductor hallucis myositis. As the first ray dorsiflexes and inverts during the contact period, the first metatarsal head traverses a forward and upward arc that greatly increases traction on the medial plantar fascia and abductor hallucis muscle (Fig. 3.80). This increase in tensile strain may produce chronic injury to these tissues.

6. Signs and symptoms associated with the rearfoot varus foot type. Because the flexible plantarflexed first ray is almost always associated with a rearfoot varus deformity (32), many of their signs and symptoms intermix.

If the plantarflexed first ray deformity is semiflexible, the following signs and symptoms should be expected:

1. A medium-to-high medial longitudinal arch off-weight-bearing with only a slight lowering of the arch on weight-bearing.

2. Moderate-to-marked callus formation under the plantar medial first metatarsal head with an occasional pinch callus under the distal medial aspect of the proximal phalanx. Because the first metatarsal can only dorsiflex back to the common transverse plane of the lesser metatarsals, any condition that allows the rearfoot to evert excessively will greatly load the plantar medial aspects of the first metatarsal head and hallux. The dense callus that forms under the metatarsophalangeal joint increases the potential of tibial sesamoiditis, as the hardened skin is less able to dampen ground-reactive forces.

Remember that as long as the range of rearfoot eversion does not exceed the range of midtarsal inversion (which is usually the case), the ability of the first metatarsal head to dorsiflex above the lesser metatarsals is of only limited concern since the longitudinal midtarsal joint axis is able to fully compensate for the range of subtalar pronation. Ideally, the first metatarsal head will never be forced to dorsiflex above the level of the lesser metatarsals. Therefore, when associated with a properly functioning subtalar and midtarsal joint, the semiflexible plantarflexed first ray deformity will rarely produce injury other than directly below the plantarflexed metatarsal head.

If the plantarflexed first ray deformity has been rigid, the following signs and symptoms should be expected.

1. A high medial longitudinal arch, both on and off-weight-bearing, with the heels inverted during static stance. The inverted heels are often responsible for lateral achilles peritendinitis (secondary to the increased tensile strain placed on the lateral achilles tendon), retrocalcaneal bursitis (this is particularly true when Haglund's deformity is present) and/or periostitis of the dorsolateral calcaneus

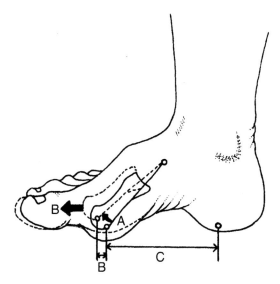

Figure 3.80. As the forefoot becomes fully weight-bearing, the first metatarsal head shifts forward and upward from its plantarflexed position (A). The forward motion **(B)** tractions the plantar fascia and abductor hallucis muscle **(C).**

(which is repeatedly compressed against the lateral heel counter).

2. Moderate-to-marked callus formation under the first, fifth, and sometimes fourth metatarsal head. As demonstrated by Cavanagh et al. (107), peak pressures beneath the forefoot during static stance are normally greatest directly below the second or third metatarsal heads (see Fig. 3.81A). However, when a rigid plantarflexed first ray is present, the foot absorbs ground-reactive forces like a tripod, with weight-bearing points centered beneath the first and fifth metatarsal heads and beneath the posterolateral plantar calcaneus (Fig. 3.81B).

This drastically altered distribution of ground-reactive forces may severely traumatize the first and fifth metatarsal heads. The tibial sesamoid is particularly prone to injury, as the first ray is usually everted as well as plantarflexed, which allows ground contact for the medial forefoot to occur directly below this sesamoid. The skin beneath the first and fifth metatarsal heads will typically respond to the marked increase in ground-reactive forces with a reactive hyperplasia that eventually leads to the formation of the characteristically dense, often nucleated callus pattern. If the fifth metatarsal is flexible, ground-reactive forces will also be distributed to the fourth metatarsal head, where a less localized hyperkeratotic lesion may form.

3. Tailor's bunion or bunionette. While fifth ray dorsiflexion and eversion will decrease the potential for injury to the fifth metatarsal head, it will increase the potential for tailor's bunion as the dorsolateral bursa is sheared between the rotating metatarsal head and the skin.

4. Interdigital neuroma and/or intermetatarsophalangeal bursitis. In addition to irritating the first and fifth metatarsal heads, the tripod arrangement for dissipating ground-reactive forces will allow for a superior displacement of the fourth and fifth metatarsals relative to the second and third metatarsals (Fig. 3.82). This results in a chronic shearing of the intermetatarsophalangeal bursa located between the third and fourth metatarsal heads. In addition, because the rigid plantarflexed first ray deformity maintains the foot in a low gear push-off throughout propulsion, the interdigital nerve (which may already be irritated by a swollen bursa) is often tethered against the transverse ligament by the dorsiflexing lesser toes.

5. Metatarsus adductus with digital contractures. When a large rigid plantarflexed first ray deformity is present, the exaggerated range of compensatory rearfoot inversion often forces the oblique midtarsal joint axis into a more vertical position. The vertical displacement of this axis allows the forefoot to adduct (which, over time, leads to a metatarsus adductus deformity) and causes the toes to claw (refer back to Fig. 3.71).

Also, because the medial longitudinal arch height increases as the forefoot supinates about the oblique midtarsal joint axis, the metatarsal shafts become progressively more plantarflexed, which in turn allows ground-reactive forces to dorsiflex the proximal phalanx. This sets the stage for even greater digital contracture, as the interossei and lumbricale tendons are displaced superiorly, and flexor digitorum longus is allowed to act unopposed in clawing the interphalangeal joints.

The hallux is particularly prone to clawing because the often severely plantarflexed position of the first metatarsal shaft forces the proximal phalanx into a position of extreme dorsiflexion (Fig. 3.83). In fact, it is not uncommon for a large dorsal bursa to overlay the first interphalangeal joint.

6. Signs and symptoms associated with the rigid forefoot valgus deformity. Because these two deformities behave almost identically, they share many of the same signs and symptoms, e.g., lateral knee and ankle pain, inversion sprains, lateral compartment syndrome, low back pain, etc.

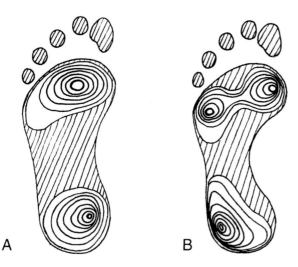

Figure 3.81. Plantar pressure distribution during static stance. (A) Weight-bearing points in a normal foot. (B) Weight-bearing points when a rigid plantarflexed first ray is present. Note that pressures beneath the heel are 2–6 times greater than forefoot pressures.

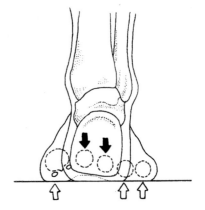

Figure 3.82. Ground-reactive forces *(white arrows)* **create a superior displacement of the fourth and fifth metatarsal heads while the unsupported second and third metatarsal heads are allowed to drop** *(black arrows).*

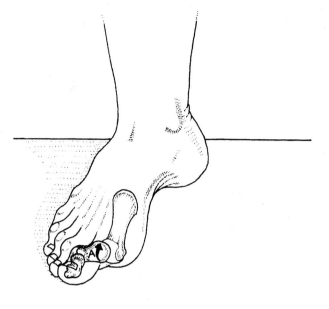

Figure 3.83. The rigid plantarflexed first ray deformity forces the proximal phalanx into a dorsiflexed position (A), which often results in an extreme clawing of the first digit.

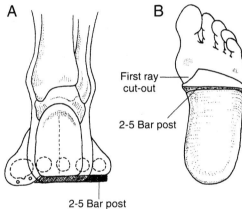
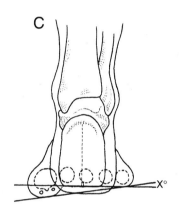

Figure 3.84. The 2-5 bar post. A forefoot bar post (a bar post represents an unangled forefoot post) is situated beneath the distal shafts of the second through fifth metatarsals. The portion of the bar post that would normally extend beneath the distal first metatarsal shaft is "cut-out" in order to allow the first metatarsal head to rest in its plantar position (hence the name 2-5 bar post). The thickness of the bar post is determined by the distance between the first metatarsal head and the common transverse plane of the lesser metatarsals; the post is of sufficient height so that the first metatarsal head makes ground contact, and the sagittal bisection of the rearfoot is vertical. As with all forefoot posts, shoe fit is the limiting factor, and a bar post greater than 10 mm is often difficult to tolerate. It should be noted that different laboratories use different terms to describe the 2-5 bar post. Because the plantarflexed first ray deformity behaves almost identically to the forefoot valgus deformity (particularly when the plantarflexed first ray is rigid), many laboratories prefer that you refer to the 2-5 bar post as a forefoot valgus post with a first ray cut-out. The degree of posting necessary to accommodate the first metatarsal head is determined by measuring the degree of forefoot valgus between the first and fifth metatarsal heads and the plantar calcaneus (angle X in **C**). (The foot should be maintained in its neutral position during this measurement.) While it is more accurate to refer to this addition as a 2-5 bar post (as long as the second through fifth metatarsals are neither in valgus or varus), either approach is fine, and it is really just a matter of semantics.

Orthotic Management for the Plantarflexed First Ray Deformity

Regardless of whether the plantarflexed first ray deformity is congenital or acquired, flexible or rigid, the initial goal of orthotic therapy is to accommodate the plantar position of the first metatarsal head. The first step in this process is to take an impression that accurately captures the degree of first ray plantarflexion while the foot is in its neu-tral position. (In flexible deformities, this requires neutral position casting while rigid deformities may tolerate semi-weight-bearing step-in techniques). A shell is then molded to the positive model, which has been slightly altered to allow for soft tissue displacement, and a 2-5 bar post is placed beneath the distal shafts of the lesser metatarsals (Fig. 3.84A and B).

The 2-5 bar post allows the forefoot to load smoothly from the lateral to the medial metatarsal heads, as the plantar first metatarsal head no longer strikes the ground prematurely. The 2-5 bar post is invaluable when treating the rigid plantarflexed first ray deformities as, during the contact period, it allows for the continued range of subtalar pronation necessary for adequate shock absorption. When treating a rigid deformity, Langer (108) recommends adding a 0° rearfoot post to stabilize the heel (Fig. 3.85) and incorporating shock-absorbing material into or under the orthotic.

The 2-5 bar post also serves an important function in the treatment of semiflexible and flexible plantarflexed first ray deformities, as it prevents the excessive dorsiflexion and inversion of the first ray that is so often responsible for injury, e.g., abductor hallucis myositis, intermetatarsophalangeal bursitis, bunion pain, etc. If the plantarflexed deformity is particularly large, orthotic control can be extended into the propulsive period by extending a compressible 2-5 bar post to the sulcus with a balance for lesion beneath the first metatarsal head (Fig. 3.86).

This balance is a custom-made pocket that supports the lesser metatarsals and allows the first metatarsal to drop into a cushioned well. (This is particularly effective when treating sesamoid pain.) When used in the treatment of semiflexible and flexible first ray deformities, this addition prevents the sudden first ray dorsiflexion and inversion that would otherwise have occurred during the early propulsive period. This in turn protects the second metatarsal head from trauma and decreases the shearing of tissues neighboring the first metatarsal. When used in the treatment of rigid plantarflexed first ray deformities, this addition prevents the compensatory propulsive period subtalar supination that normally forces the foot into a low gear push-off. This drastically reduces the risk of inversion ankle sprains, lateral ankle and knee pain, lateral achilles peritendinitis, and interdigital neuritis, as the heel is maintained in a more vertical position and the toes are no longer hyperdorsiflexed.

Unfortunately, the size of the deformity may occasionally exceed the accommodative capabilities of the orthotic. Sgarlato (74) notes that when a rigid plantarflexed first ray exceeds 10° (as measured by degrees of forefoot

valgus), surgical referral for a dorsal base closing wedge osteotomy may be necessary to correct the mechanical malfunction. Root et al. (3) noted that when performed during adolescence or early childhood, this operation often produces a spontaneous reduction of the cavus deformity (Fig. 3.87).

In conjunction with orthotic therapy, various manipulative techniques should be used to break down any soft tissue adhesions that may be limiting joint motion. Occasionally, particularly in uncompensated forefoot and rearfoot varus deformities resulting from trauma or prolonged immobilization, it is possible to restore subtalar/midtarsal motion to a point at which the acquired plantarflexed first ray deformity reduces. If this does occur, the 2-5 bar post and sub 1 balance should be removed. However, reduction of uncompensated foot types rarely occurs, as they are most often associated with fixed osseous deformity (particularly in older individuals). Because of this, the goal of manipulation is not to force the plantarflexed first metatarsal head back to the common transverse plane of the lesser metatarsals, but rather, to improve flexibility by breaking down potentially painful soft tissue adhesions (even slight improvements in flexibility can result in dramatic reductions in symptomatology). If aggres-

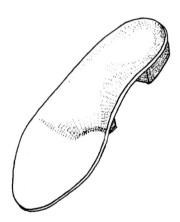

Figure 3.86. The sub 1 balance for lesion.

Figure 3.85. (A) Plantar view of a shell with a 2-5 bar post; (B) plantar view of a shell with a 2-5 bar post and a 0° rearfoot post, i.e., the post stabilizes the heel in a vertical position (C).

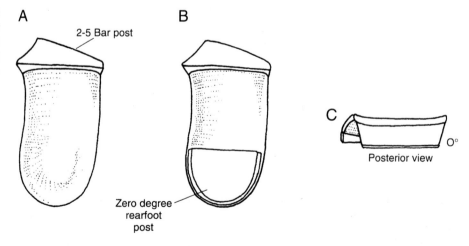

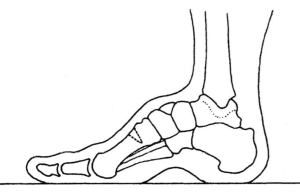 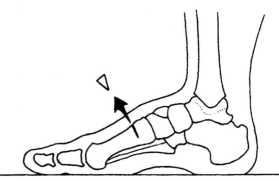

Figure 3.87. Dorsal base closing wedge osteotomy associated with a rigid plantarflexed first ray. By changing the decline angle of the first metatarsal, the cavus deformity is reduced. If a calcaneal osteotomy had been used to realign the inverted heel, the cavus deformity would most likely return as the cause of the deformity, in this case a rigid plantarflexed first ray, had not been corrected. This emphasizes the importance of a thorough biomechanical evaluation prior to surgical referral.

sive manipulation were used to return a congenital plantarflexed first ray to the level of the lesser metatarsals, a pathological laxity of the plantar tarsometatarsal and/or midtarsal joint restraining ligaments would result.

Keep in mind that the congenital plantarflexed first ray is in its most stable position functionally when it is plantarflexed (i.e., it possesses equal ranges of motion both dorsally and plantarly), and the goal of conservative treatment should be to accommodate, not alter, this deformity.

Treatment of the Plantarflexed Lesser Metatarsal

Thus far, the described methods of orthotic management have been limited to treatment of the plantarflexed first ray only. However, the same biomechanical principles used in treating the plantarflexed first ray can also be applied when one of the lesser rays is plantarflexed. For example, if the fifth metatarsal were plantarflexed, a bar post should be extended beneath the distal first through fourth metatarsal shafts (or, phrased differently, a forefoot varus post with a fifth ray cut-out should be used). If necessary, a sub 5 balance for lesion can be added to control propulsive period motions. Use of this post with a flexible plantarflexed fifth ray will decrease the pain associated with a tailor's bunion, as the fifth metatarsal head no longer dorsiflexes and everts during the contact period.

When used in the treatment of a rigid plantarflexed fifth ray, the bar post prevents compensatory subtalar pronation (and all of the potential injuries associated with this motion) as it supports the medial forefoot and accommodates the plantar position of the fifth metatarsal head. If it had been the third instead of the fifth metatarsal that was plantarflexed, treatment would be as simple as adding a balance for lesion (or a soft accommodating material) beneath the plantarflexed metatarsal head.

Although not discussed, it is possible to have a deformity in which all of the metatarsals are plantarflexed. This deformity is referred to as a plantarflexed forefoot, and Root et al. (3) claim it is the result of congenital malformation of the tarsometatarsal joints or midtarsal joint (although it seems likely that it may also result from acquired upper motor neuron dysfunction). The plantarflexed forefoot typically produces a marked clawing of the digits secondary to the increased metatarsal decline angle and is often responsible for injury to the anterior talocrural articulation and/or posterior knee, as the ankle is unable to provide the dorsiflectory range necessary to compensate for the plantarflexed metatarsals (Fig. 3.88).

Conservative treatment of this deformity requires a heel lift of sufficient height to allow the tibia to tilt a minimum of 10° forward from vertical. Rarely, the forefoot may be so severely plantarflexed that surgical intervention is necessary to realign the metatarsals.

Treatment of the Dorsiflexed Metatarsal

Lastly, although uncommon, it is also possible to have a deformity in which one or more of the metatarsals is dorsiflexed relative to the common transverse plane. As with plantarflexed metatarsals, the dorsiflexed metatarsals may be congenital or acquired and can be differentiated by checking the available ranges of dorsi and plantar motion, i.e., the congenital deformity (which is usually larger) possesses equal ranges of upward and downward movement (Fig. 3.89A) while the acquired deformity presents with asymmetrical dorsiplantar movement patterns that vary between the two feet (Fig. 3.89B).

When the first metatarsal is dorsiflexed relative to the lesser metatarsals, it is also referred to as a metatarsus primus elevatus. While the acquired form of this deformity may occasionally result from a tonic spasm of tibialis anterior, it is most often the result of a chronically everted heel that requires compensatory first ray pronation. Over time, bony and soft tissue changes occur that maintain the

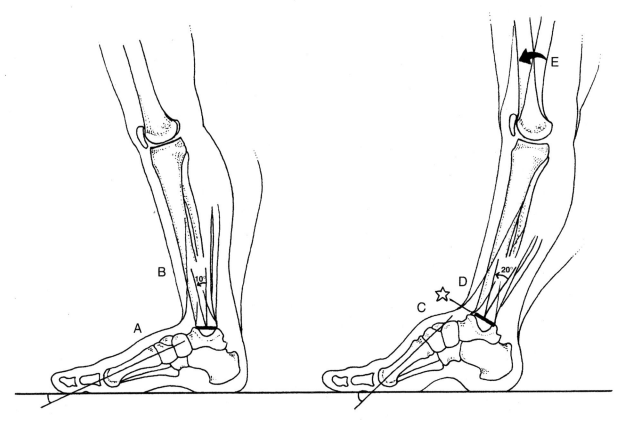

Figure 3.88. Mechanical dysfunction associated with a plantarflexed forefoot. When a normal metatarsal decline angle is present **(A)**, the ankle will readily supply the range of dorsiflexion necessary for noncompensated function during late midstance **(B)**. However, when a plantarflexed forefoot is present **(C)**, the entire rearfoot is tilted posteriorly, and the ankle, which typically possesses a maximum of 20° dorsiflexion, is often unable to allow the leg to reach vertical **(D)**. This forces the knee into hyperextension and predisposes to impingement exostosis, as the anterior tip of the lower articular surface of the tibia repeatedly collides with the neck of the talus *(star)*. The plantarflexed forefoot deformity may be so great that even with compensatory hyperextension of the knee **(E)**, the heel is unable to make ground contact, and the individual may walk and stand with weight supported entirely by the plantar forefoot.

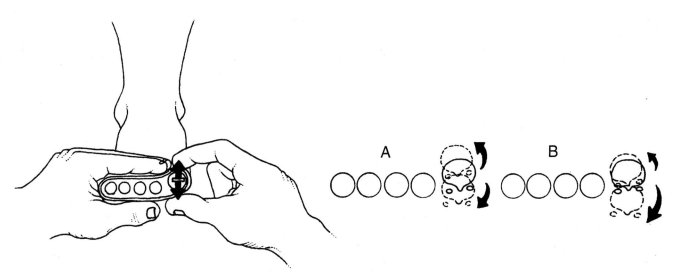

Figure 3.89. When stressed superiorly and inferiorly, the congenital dorsiflexed first metatarsal will display equal ranges of dorsi and plantar movement **(A)** while the acquired deformity will possess asymmetrical movement patterns **(B).**

dorsiflexed position of the first metatarsal. (A dorsal base exostosis is often present.) Assuming the dorsiflexed first ray is associated with an everted heel that is able to return to a more vertical position, treatment should include a functional orthotic that minimizes the degree of rearfoot eversion (by inverting the calcaneus, the orthotic will improve the mechanical efficiency of peroneus longus as a first ray plantarflexor and may potentially correct the deformity), along with the incorporation of various manipulative techniques necessary to break any soft tissue adhesions that may be limiting first ray motion.

If the heel had been fixed in a permanently everted position (as in many rigid flat foot deformities), orthotic therapy would be ineffective in reducing the metatarsus primus elevatus since dorsiflexion of the first ray is necessary to accommodate the everted calcaneus.

Conservative treatment may also be ineffective when dealing with a large congenital dorsiflexed first ray since the first metatarsal is often so elevated that it is unable to plantarflex into the position necessary for a normal propulsion. Therefore, the dorsal-posterior shift of the first metatarsophalangeal joint's transverse axis does not occur, and the hallux is unable to dorsiflex beyond 35°: hallux limitus/rigidus with compensatory hyperextension of the interphalangeal joint may quickly follow.

Successful management of a large congenital dorsiflexed first ray may necessitate a plantar base closing wedge osteotomy to realign the first metatarsal with the lesser metatarsals. Unfortunately, all too often the surgeon ignores or simply does not recognize the dorsiflexed first ray deformity and operates only on the deformed metatarsophalangeal joint. Should this occur, the first metatarsal joint deformity will quickly return since the biomechanical cause for deformity remains unchanged (3). If it had been one of the lesser metatarsals that were dorsiflexed, surgical realignment is typically not necessary, since a dorsiflexed lesser metatarsal does not predispose its metatarsophalangeal joint to deformity and conservative treatment with manipulation to maintain the full range of metatarsal plantarflexion, coupled with recommendations for shoes with a spacious toe box, will usually result in a complete resolution of any symptomatology.

The exception is when the dorsiflexed metatarsal is unable to effectively participate in the distribution of ground-reactive forces, thereby exposing the neighboring metatarsal heads to trauma. Conservative treatment in this situation simply requires placing a small metatarsal pad proximal to the dorsiflexed metatarsal head, thereby shifting ground-reactive forces away from the neighboring metatarsal heads and onto the shaft of the involved metatarsal.

ORTHOTIC MANAGEMENT FOR VARIOUS COMBINATIONS OF REARFOOT AND FOREFOOT DEFORMITIES

Because 98.3% of the population possesses some degree of tibiofibular varum (1), it should be expected that the coexistence of various combinations of forefoot and rearfoot deformities would be the rule, rather than the exception. This idea was consistent with the foot survey by McPoil et al. (1) in that nearly 85% of those individuals possessing subtalar and/or tibiofibular varum also possessed some type of forefoot deformity (either forefoot varus, forefoot valgus, or plantarflexed first ray). While the combination of a rearfoot varus with a forefoot valgus was the most commonly seen coupled malformation (which should not be surprising, considering the mutually dependent nature of these deformities), virtually any combination of forefoot and/or rearfoot deformity may coexist together, i.e., a forefoot varus with a plantarflexed first ray, a rearfoot varus with a forefoot varus, a rearfoot varus with a forefoot valgus and a plantarflexed first ray, etc.

As a general rule, orthotic management in these situations requires putting the foot in its neutral position and filling in the space between the foot and horizontal (109). Although the simplicity of this rule gives the impression that orthotic management for combinations of defects is a relatively uncomplicated procedure, in actuality it can be a confusing process of trying to decide which deformity to post and what post angles to use. The following section will review the pathomechanics and orthotic management associated with the more commonly seen combinations of defects.

The rearfoot varus/forefoot varus deformity. The individual with this combination of deformities is prone to injury throughout the entire stance phase because the rearfoot varus deformity requires rapid compensatory subtalar pronation during the early portions of stance while the forefoot varus deformity requires compensatory subtalar pronation during the latter portions of stance (Fig. 3.90).

Treatment in this situation requires taking a neutral position impression that accurately captures the forefoot deformity, then fabricating an orthotic that can control both the rearfoot and forefoot deformities. This can be accomplished in either of two ways. The first and most common approach is to post the forefoot so as to bring the rearfoot to vertical (Fig. 3.91A), then add a separate rearfoot post (referred to as an extrinsic rearfoot post) to tilt the entire orthotic laterally (Fig. 3.91B).

The only flaw with this approach is that because the rearfoot and forefoot posts rest on different planes (dotted lines in Fig. 3.91B), the orthotic, when placed on a flat surface (or more importantly, when placed in a shoe) will have a "rock line," where the entire orthotic will tip from being supported solely by the rearfoot post to being supported solely by the forefoot post, depending on which side of the line pressure is being placed (Fig. 3.92).

If you compare the location of the average rock line on an orthotic with separate rearfoot and forefoot posts with the normal progression of vertical forces (Fig. 3.93), it becomes clear that the rearfoot post becomes nonfunctional after early midstance since the entire orthotic will have tilted medially (everted) onto the forefoot post. Clinically,

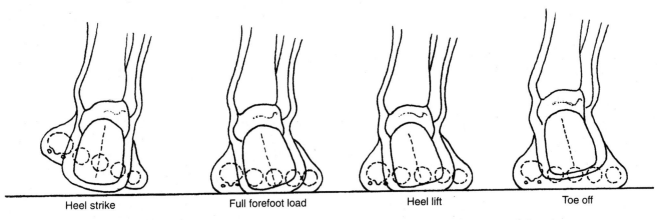

| Heel strike | Full forefoot load | Heel lift | Toe off |

Figure 3.90. Stance phase motions with a combination rearfoot varus/forefoot varus deformity.

Figure 3.91. (A and B) Use of independent forefoot and rearfoot posts.

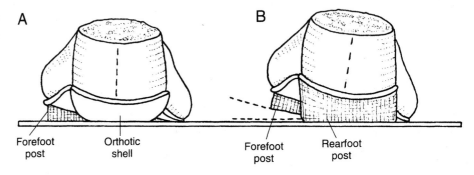

A — Forefoot post, Orthotic shell

B — Forefoot post, Rearfoot post

Figure 3.92. The rock line on an orthotic with independent forefoot and rearfoot posts. If pressure is applied posterior to the rock line (**A**), the entire orthotic will rest on the rearfoot post. Conversely, if pressure is applied anterior to the rock line (**B**), the orthotic will rock medially onto the forefoot post.

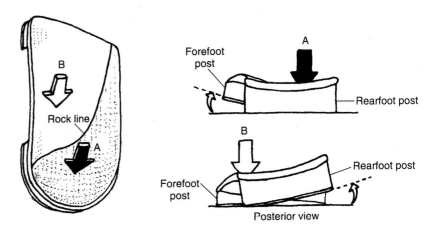

Rock line

Forefoot post — Rearfoot post

Forefoot post — Rearfoot post

Posterior view

Figure 3.93. (A) Location of average rock line; (B) normal progression of forces during stance phase. *TO* = toe-off; *HL* = heel lift; *FFL* = full forefoot load; *HS* = heel strike.

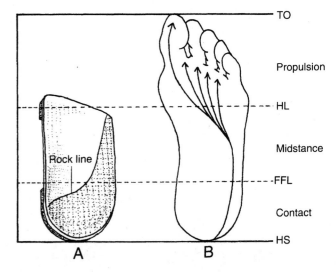

TO

Propulsion

HL

Midstance

FFL

Contact

HS

Rock line

A   B

this can create problems since the rearfoot post in this situation can control subtalar motions only during the contact and early midstance periods. After that, the control afforded by the rearfoot post is lost, and the subtalar joint is forced to suddenly pronate in compensation for the rearfoot deformity.

For example, if an individual with a 4° forefoot varus and a 12° rearfoot varus were treated with an orthotic with a 4° forefoot varus post and a 6° rearfoot varus post (the 6° rearfoot post would allow the subtalar joint to pronate 6° prior to contacting the shell), the orthotic would work well in controlling subtalar joint motions during the contact period, but the moment the body's center of mass passed anterior to the rock line, the subtalar joint would suddenly pronate an additional 6° (the amount equalling the rearfoot post) as the orthotic everts onto the forefoot post. While this additional range of subtalar pronation may not be a problem for many individuals since the motion occurs relatively slowly and may be controlled by the supporting muscles, it may be potentially injurious to others since it allows for an unlocking of the midtarsal joint (with the associated shifting of the tarsals and metatarsals) as vertical forces peak.

Rather than using separate rearfoot and forefoot posts, a better approach for treating combinations of rearfoot and forefoot varus deformities is to add the desired rearfoot and forefoot post angles together, then place a post of this size under the medial forefoot. Although this gives the impression that the forefoot is being overposted (which would produce iatrogenic injury), it should be kept in mind that the degree of forefoot deformity is captured in the orthotic shell, not by the location of the posts. For example, if an 8° forefoot varus post were used on an individual who would normally be treated with separate 4° forefoot and rearfoot varus posts, the larger forefoot varus post would actually achieve the same results as the combined smaller posts, as the rearfoot would continue to be inverted 4° from vertical (Fig. 3.94) while the plantar forefoot remains inverted 4° relative to the plantar rearfoot.

This example demonstrates an important principle in that an orthotic shell made from a neutral position impression has a specific forefoot-to-rearfoot relationship that is unaltered by either the forefoot or rearfoot post. If a flat rearfoot post is added to stabilize the heel (the post is flat in that it does not change the angle of the orthotic shell), the orthotic in Figure 3.94 with the larger forefoot varus post would allow for the same degree of subtalar control during the contact period as the orthotic posted with separate 4° forefoot and rearfoot varus posts. However, because the plantar surface of the orthotic with the large forefoot varus post and flat rearfoot post is perfectly level, the orthotic will not rock medially during midstance, and the subtalar joint will maintain a more aligned position throughout the remainder of stance phase.

Because this is an uncommon method for posting (usually separate rearfoot and forefoot varus posts are used), the orthotic laboratory should be informed that the goal with the large forefoot varus post is to invert the rearfoot a specific number of degrees and that the rearfoot should be posted flat to maintain the heel in this inverted position. If the laboratory has not been informed that inverting the rearfoot was done deliberately with an oversized forefoot post, it will assume that there was an error in either casting or measurements, and they will most likely use a forefoot post that brings the rearfoot only to vertical.

The rearfoot varus/forefoot valgus deformity. As noted earlier, this is the most commonly found combination of deformities. Orthotic management associated with this combination is dependent on the relative size of each deformity and the specific patterns of compensation present. If, for example, there is a large rearfoot varus deformity coupled with a small forefoot valgus deformity, and gait evaluation reveals that the subtalar joint compensates for the rearfoot deformity only, i.e., rapid pronation during the contact period with no signs of lateral instability during midstance or propulsion, then the goal of orthotic therapy will be to control the contact period subtalar motions with a rearfoot post and to leave the forefoot deformity alone. In fact, a slight degree of forefoot valgus in this situation is actually beneficial and may represent a developmental accommodation for the rearfoot deformity since it allows the subtalar joint to move closer to its neutral position prior to heel lift. If the forefoot deformity had been inadvertently

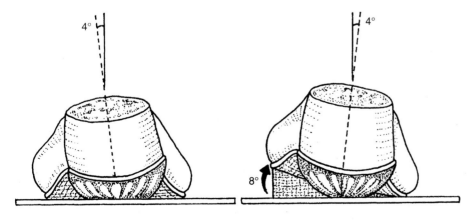

Figure 3.94. Use of an 8° forefoot varus post on an individual with a 4° forefoot varus has the same effect as separate 4° forefoot and rearfoot varus posts.

posted, the forefoot post would force the subtalar joint into a pronated position the moment the individual's progression of forces passed the rock line on the orthotic.

Clearly, this is not the goal of orthotic therapy. A common misconception that has become standard practice in the fabrication of orthotics is the belief that the practitioner should fully post both the forefoot and rearfoot deformity.

In the presence of a combined rearfoot varus and forefoot valgus, this practice is particularly dangerous and is responsible for many iatrogenic injuries since during late midstance and early propulsion the position of the subtalar joint is determined solely by the forefoot post. If an individual with a 5° rearfoot varus and a 5° forefoot valgus were fully posted on the forefoot, the 5° post would maintain the subtalar joint in a pronated position during heel lift, which would, of course, be detrimental (Fig. 3.95A).

In the presence of equal forefoot and rearfoot deformities, the forefoot deformity is necessary to allow the subtalar joint to reach its neutral position (Fig. 3.95B) and should accordingly be left alone. It should be mentioned that there are certain exceptions to this rule, as it is occasionally necessary to overpost the forefoot beyond subtalar joint neutrality in order to successfully resolve symptoms associated with a chronically inverted heel, e.g., recurrent inversion instability or a recalcitrant tarsal tunnel syndrome. In fact, Valmassy (110) advocates routinely posting combined rearfoot varus/forefoot valgus deformities with sufficient forefoot valgus posting to bring the rearfoot to a vertical position. He emphasized that when this is not possible because of a limited range of subtalar joint motion, the forefoot valgus post should be of sufficient height to maintain the subtalar joint in its maximally pronated position.

Because of the potential for iatrogenic injuries associated with this technique (specifically, plantar fasciitis, spring ligament sprain, soleus strain, and decreased stabilization associated with talonavicular incongruity), the large forefoot posts should be used with caution.

When treating combinations of rearfoot varus and forefoot valgus deformities, a forefoot post is used primarily when the size of the forefoot deformity exceeds the size of the rearfoot deformity. The exact degree of the forefoot post should then be determined by subtracting the rearfoot angle from the forefoot angle.

For example, an individual with a 4° rearfoot varus and a 9° forefoot valgus would receive a 5° forefoot valgus post to protect against lateral instability and maintain the subtalar joint in a neutral position during heel lift. In situations requiring both rearfoot and forefoot posting (e.g., an 8° rearfoot varus with a 12° forefoot valgus), the forefoot post is still determined by subtracting the rearfoot angle from the forefoot angle (in this case, 4°), only now a separate extrinsic rearfoot post can be added to control subtalar joint motions during the contact period, i.e., a 2° rearfoot post would allow 6° of subtalar pronation. The separate rearfoot and forefoot posts work well in this situation since the rearfoot post controls subtalar joint motions during the contact period and, once the rock line is passed, the forefoot post protects against lateral instability and maintains subtalar neutrality during heel lift.

The only drawback with the technique of subtracting the rearfoot angle from the forefoot angle in order to determine the size of the forefoot post is that it requires taking an impression of the foot in a non-neutral position: the forefoot angle captured in the cast should reflect the size of the desired post, not the size of the actual deformity.

To demonstrate this point, picture an individual with a 4° rearfoot varus and a 9° forefoot valgus. The negative cast in this situation should capture 5°, not 9° of forefoot valgus. This is accomplished by using less pressure when loading the lateral column during the casting procedure. If the full 9° of forefoot valgus had been captured in the impression, use of a 5° forefoot valgus post would maintain the rearfoot in position of 4° inversion, which would completely block the range of subtalar pronation necessary for

Figure 3.95. The combination of a 5° rearfoot varus with a 5° forefoot valgus. Use of a forefoot post in this case would force the subtalar joint *(STJ)* into a pronated position the moment the individual's progression of forces passed anterior to the rock line **(A)**. If left unposted, the 5° forefoot valgus will allow the 5° rearfoot varus to reach a neutral position by heel lift **(B)**.

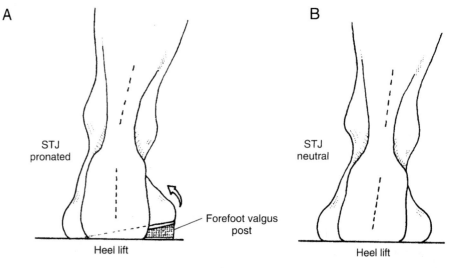

A

STJ pronated

Forefoot valgus post

Heel lift

B

STJ neutral

Heel lift

shock absorption (which would eventually result in iatrogenic injury).

Because a non-neutral impression has been used in this situation, it is the orthotic post, not the shell, that plays the primary role in controlling joint motions during stance phase. In all situations in which the forefoot post is not intended to bring the rearfoot to vertical, the laboratory should be informed of your treatment plans.

The rearfoot varus/flexible plantarflexed first ray deformity (Fig. 3.96). Since subtalar compensation for the rearfoot varus deformity often forces the first ray above the common transverse plane of the lesser metatarsals, orthotic management for this combination requires both the use of a 2-5 bar post to accommodate the plantarflexed first metatarsal head and a rearfoot varus post to prevent excessive contact period subtalar pronation.

The rearfoot varus post is invaluable in treating the combined rearfoot varus/flexible plantarflexed first ray deformity because, in addition to preventing excessive subtalar joint pronation, it also acts to increase the mechanical efficiency of peroneus longus as a first ray plantarflexor, which enables this muscle to protect more effectively against dorsiflexion and inversion of the first metatarsal.

If subtalar joint pronation during late midstance/early propulsion is a concern, an alternate posting technique would be to place the desired rearfoot post beneath the forefoot and have the rearfoot posted flat to stabilize the inverted orthotic shell. Also, a first ray cut-out and sub 1 balance for lesion should be added to accommodate the plantarflexed first metatarsal. This orthotic could control subtalar and first ray motions during the entire stance phase.

The rearfoot varus/rigid plantarflexed first ray deformity (Fig. 3.97). Because the rigid plantarflexed first ray deformity maintains the rearfoot in an inverted position and prevents the subtalar joint from pronating during most of stance phase, orthotic management requires the addition of a 2-5 bar post with a sub 1 balance for lesion to accommodate the first metatarsal head and to allow for a continued range of subtalar pronation. Rearfoot posts typically are not needed since controlling excessive subtalar joint pronation is rarely a concern.

The forefoot varus or forefoot valgus with a plantarflexed first ray deformity. Treatment of this combination requires use of the appropriate forefoot post (as measured with the second through fifth metatarsal heads as the reference) with a first ray cut-out added to accommo-

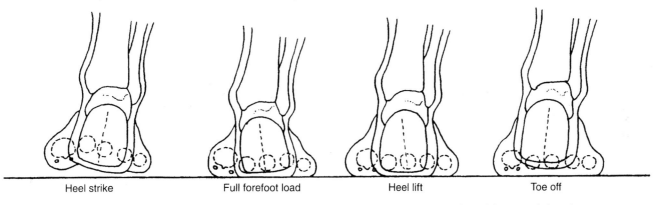

| Heel strike | Full forefoot load | Heel lift | Toe off |

Figure 3.96. Foot motions with a combination rearfoot varus/flexible plantarflexed first ray deformity.

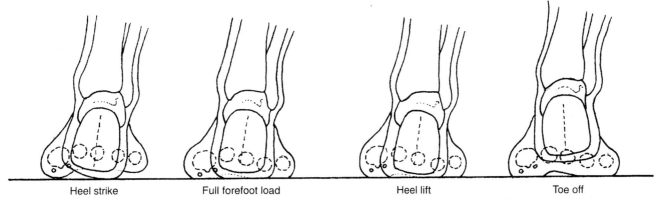

| Heel strike | Full forefoot load | Heel lift | Toe off |

Figure 3.97. Foot motions with a combination rearfoot varus/rigid plantarflexed first ray deformity.

date the plantarflexed first metatarsal. If the plantarflexed first metatarsal is semiflexible or rigid, a sub 1 balance should also be considered.

An outdated technique for treating a combination forefoot varus/flexible plantarflexed first ray requires dorsiflexing the plantarflexed first ray into a midline position (i.e., level with the lesser metatarsals) while the neutral position cast is being taken. Because this maneuver risks inadvertent supination of the forefoot about the longitudinal midtarsal joint axis, this technique has for the most part been abandoned (42).

VARIATION IN METATARSAL LENGTH

The relative lengths of the different metatarsals are readily evaluated by plantarflexing the digits and noting the positions of the dorsal metatarsal heads. Ideally, an imaginary line connecting the distal metatarsal heads should form a smooth parabolic curve (Fig. 3.98). In most feet, the relative lengths of the metatarsals can be expressed by the formula 2>1>3>4>5 or 2>1 = 3>4>5 (111). Because the second metatarsal is usually the longest, it is exposed to ground-reactive forces during both high and low gear push-off, with large amounts of pressure centered directly beneath the second metatarsal head as the transition from low gear to high gear push-off occurs.

Numerous investigators have demonstrated that plantar forefoot pressure values measured during walking are greatest beneath the second metatarsal head (112, 113). In fact, Gross and Bunch (114) took plantar force estimates and mathematically determined the bending strains, shear forces, and axial forces placed upon the individual metatarsal midshafts. Not surprisingly, bending strain and shear forces were greatest on the second metatarsal shaft (bending strain on the second metatarsal is nearly seven times greater than bending strain on the first metatarsal), while axial forces were greatest on the first metatarsal shaft

(presumably due to the larger forces on the hallux relative to the lesser digits).

Fortunately, even though the second metatarsal shaft appears slender and frail, its overall outline and composition of dense compact bone allows it to effectively manage propulsive forces. Furthermore, the second tarsometatarsal articulation seems to be specifically designed to handle these large forces, as the base of the second metatarsal is wedged into a relatively rigid socket between the medial and lateral cuneiforms (Fig. 3.99). This anatomical configuration serves as a locking mechanism for the entire tarsometatarsal complex (115).

Given the fact that the distribution of ground-reactive forces is dependent on the relative lengths of the metatarsals, it seems reasonable to assume that an excessively long or short metatarsal would subject its metatarsal head to a respective increase or decrease in pressure.

The Elongated Second Metatarsal

The most commonly seen variation in metatarsal length is an elongated second metatarsal, i.e., the second metatarsal is even longer than usual, with its metatarsal head projecting distal to the ideal parabolic curve (Fig. 3.100). If this metatarsal is even slightly elongated, its metatarsal head is subjected to tremendous forces as the

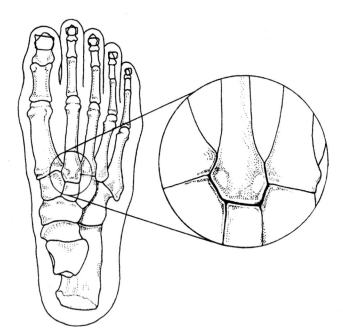

Figure 3.99. The second tarsometatarsal articulation (a.k.a. Lisfranc's joint). Note how the base of the second metatarsal is firmly stabilized against the neighboring metatarsals and cuneiforms. Because the plantar surface of the second tarsometatarsal joint is reinforced by the strong plantar ligament and an extension of the tibialis posterior tendon (106), it is particularly effective at resisting the dorsiflectory moments created by ground-reactive forces.

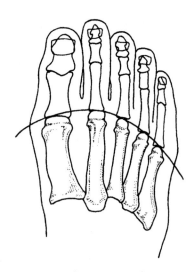

Figure 3.98. Ideal alignment of the metatarsal heads.

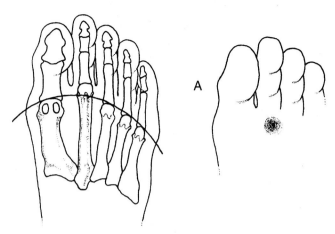

Figure 3.100. An elongated second metatarsal. (Modified from Gould JS (ed). The Foot Book. Baltimore: Williams & Wilkins, 1988:220.)

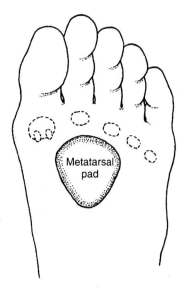

Figure 3.101. By distributing weight away from the central metatarsal heads, even a small metatarsal pad may decrease plantar metatarsal head pressures by as much as 60% (118).

foot pivots from low-gear to high-gear push-off. The resulting increase in pressure and friction produces a characteristic diffuse intractable plantar keratosis beneath the second metatarsal head (inset A, in Fig. 3.100) and may be a cause for primary metatarsalgia (64) and/or plantar warts, i.e., pressure stimulates growth of this virus (117).

Also, an elongated second metatarsal often produces a mallet toe deformity as compression from a tight toe box deforms the digit. (Because shoes are fit from heel to ball, an elongated second metatarsal is typically not taken into consideration.)

Treatment for an elongated second metatarsal may include the addition of cushioning materials placed directly beneath the painful metatarsal head (materials such as Spenco (Spenco Medical Corp., Waco, TX), poron, and/or plastazote may be invaluable in reducing shear forces), the use of metatarsal pads placed proximal to the metatarsal heads (Fig. 3.101) and, if necessary, an orthotic to accommodate any structural deformity that might be responsible for an increase in pressure beneath the second metatarsal head, e.g., a forefoot varus deformity. Recommendations should also be made for well-fitting shoes that do not compress the distal digit and, if symptoms warrant, a Thomas bar or rocker bottom may be added to the outer sole of the shoe to help reduce pressure beneath the metatarsal head. (These additions are discussed in a later section.) Of course, it is essential that the individual with an elongated second metatarsal avoid high-heeled shoes and have the hyperkeratotic lesions trimmed down regularly.

The Shortened First Metatarsal

Another cause for pain beneath the second metatarsal head is an excessively shortened first metatarsal. It has been theorized that this deformity, which was originally described by Dudley Morton in 1935 (119), allows for a redis-

tribution of pressure away from the shortened first metatarsal onto the neighboring second metatarsal.

Although the clinical significance of a shortened first metatarsal has been questioned (120), recent investigation (121) has corroborated Morton's theory in that peak pressure measurements taken beneath the second metatarsal head while the patient was walking were significantly greater in individuals possessing Morton's foot structure (i.e., the first metatarsal was 8 mm or more shorter than the second metatarsal) than they were in a control group. It should be clarified that a short first metatarsal by itself does not constitute Morton's foot structure. A true case of Morton's foot structure will present with a short first metatarsal, a thickened second metatarsal shaft, and a hypermobile first metatarsal with posteriorly displaced sesamoids (Fig. 3.102).

Because of its shorter length, the first metatarsal in this foot type is only able to participate in the propulsive period transfer of forces by excessively plantarflexing about the first ray axis (Fig. 3.103). It has been suggested that this increased range of first ray plantarflexion may predispose the individual with Morton's foot structure to degenerative changes at the junction of the first and second metatarsal bases (122).

In some individuals, the first metatarsal may be so severely shortened that the first ray is unable to plantarflex through the range necessary for the first metatarsal head to maintain ground contact during midpropulsion. (It should be remembered that first ray plantarflexion is usually less than 10°.) This being the case, the first metatarsal is unable to participate in the distribution of ground-reactive forces, and the neighboring second metatarsal head may be chronically traumatized. Furthermore, the subtalar joint will be al-

Figure 3.102. Morton's foot structure.

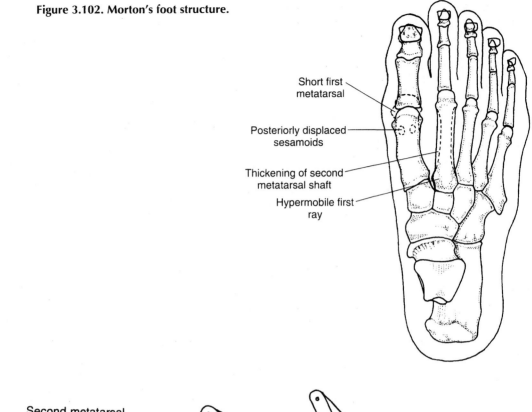

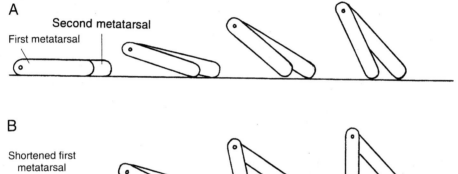

Figure 3.103. In order to demonstrate the effect of a shortened first metatarsal, this illustration uses an analogy in which ice cream sticks of various lengths are used to represent the first and second metatarsals. In series A, because the first metatarsal is only slightly shorter than the second metatarsal, the range of first ray plantarflexion necessary for the first and second metatarsal heads to maintain ground contact is minimal. However, when the first metatarsal is markedly shorter than the second (as in **B**), an extreme range of first ray plantarflexion is necessary for the first metatarsal head to maintain ground contact following heel lift.

lowed to pronate through larger ranges of motion during the propulsive period, as the medial forefoot is no longer stabilized by an effective peroneus longus muscle.

Treatment in this situation requires the addition of a platform (referred to as Morton's extension) placed beneath the first metatarsal head (Fig. 3.104). This extension allows the first metatarsal head to participate in the distribution of ground-reactive forces, which in turn allows for a lessening of pressure beneath the second metatarsal head, a decreased range of propulsive period subtalar pronation and, by allow-

ing the first metatarsal to assume more midline position, minimizes strain on the first tarsometatarsal articulation.

Travell and Simons (123) described a surprising relationship between Morton's foot structure and trigger points in the masseter and temporalis musculature. These investigators claimed that by correcting faulty biomechanics associated with this foot type, Morton's extension may allow for an immediate improvement of interincisor jaw opening by as much as 30%.

A word of warning regarding the use of Morton's ex-

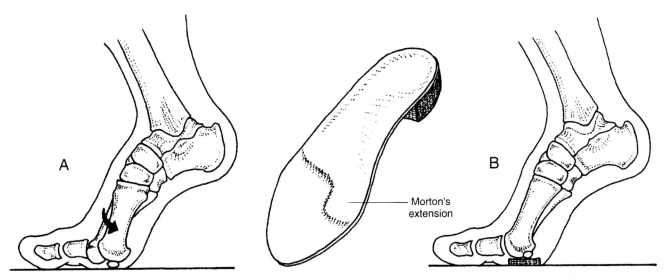

Figure 3.104. (A and B) Morton's extension. Compare first ray motions with and without this addition.

tension: While proper use of this platform may be essential to manage a true Morton's foot successfully, more often than not it is incorrectly used to treat a lengthened second metatarsal. (A true Morton's foot structure is actually quite rare.) The inappropriate use of a Morton's extension may result in sesamoiditis and, if continued, could eventually lead to degenerative changes at the dorsal first metatarsophalangeal joint secondary to impaired first ray plantarflexion. Because of this, Morton's extension should only be considered after careful static and dynamic evaluation. (Although this addition may be useful in treating recalcitrant pain beneath the second metatarsal head .)

The Elongated First Metatarsal

A final cause for potential injury occurs when the first metatarsal is the longest metatarsal. As the individual with this deformity moves into propulsion, there will be an increase in the amount of pressure centered beneath the first metatarsal head, and ground-reactive forces will prevent the range of first ray plantarflexion necessary for the dorsal-posterior shift of the first metatarsophalangeal joint's transverse axis (3). This often leads to subluxation of the first metatarsophalangeal joint, with the eventual development of a hallux limitus deformity.

Conservative treatment of the lengthened first metatarsal is always difficult and should include techniques that encourage the individual to maintain a low gear push-off throughout the propulsive period. This may be accomplished muscularly by having the patient consciously modify his or her gait pattern to maintain a low-gear push-off deliberately, by using an orthotic with an extended rearfoot varus post to maintain the subtalar joint in an inverted position during early propulsion and/or by cutting the sole of the shoe along an axis that parallels the bisection of the second and fifth metatarsal heads. All of these techniques

maintain the rearfoot in an inverted position during terminal stance phase, which allows a moderately lengthened first metatarsal to plantarflex during the propulsive period.

Another technique that is useful in treating a lengthened first metatarsal involves fabricating an orthotic with a large rearfoot varus post, then adding a kinetic wedge beneath the forefoot. This addition, which is described in more detail in a later section, requires placing a soft, triangularly shaped piece of foam beneath the first metatarsal head while the remaining metatarsal heads are supported by a dense rubber. According to Dananberg (124), the softer material placed beneath the first metatarsal head allows the first ray to plantarflex and evert during propulsion, thereby lessening the potential for first metatarsophalangeal joint deformity.

If these methods are ineffective and hallux limitus deformity continues to be painful, a rocker bottom may be added to the sole of the shoe (see Fig. 3.132). Unfortunately, Root et al. (3) claimed that when an elongated first metatarsal has resulted in a hallux limitus deformity, conservative attempts to restore hallux dorsiflexion are useless, and the deformity will continue to progress unless the first metatarsal is surgically shortened. They recommended surgically shortening the first metatarsal so that its distal tip lines up with the distal tip of the third metatarsal (assuming the third metatarsal is not excessively lengthened or shortened), while simultaneously altering the declination angle of the first metatarsal so that its metatarsal head rests on the common transverse plane of the lesser metatarsals. Failure to change the declination angle will result in the formation of a metatarsus primus elevatus.

It should be noted that this approach seems a bit extreme since the habitual use of a low gear push-off, coupled with a rocker bottom shoe, will successfully alleviate the symptoms in almost all situations.

Leg Length Discrepancy

Leg length discrepancy (LLD), which is divided into functional and structural categories, is a common cause of injury (19, 125). Messier and Pittala (19) demonstrated that structural leg length discrepancies greater than 0.64 cm (1/4 inch) predispose to plantar fasciitis while Rothbart and Estabrook (126) claimed that functional leg length discrepancy secondary to asymmetrical pronation is an etiological factor in the development of sciatica.

It is extremely important to differentiate a structural leg length discrepancy (which represents a fixed osseous malformation) from a functional leg length discrepancy (which is most often the result of asymmetrical pronation and/or soft tissue contracture in the pelvis/spine), since treatment for these two conditions is different. Unfortunately, differentiating these two deformities is not always easy. In many cases, structural and functional leg length discrepancy occur together, one masking the actual degree of the other (Fig. 3.105).

To help differentiate structural from functional leg length discrepancy, several examination techniques have been developed. The most accurate of these tests is the scanogram. This technique involves taking a series of x-rays with the central ray initially level with the femoral head, then with the tibial plateau, and finally with the ankle mortise. Information from these x-rays gives exact information regarding the length of the femurs and tibias.

An alternate method of x-ray evaluation involves po-

sitioning the standing patient with the feet directly beneath the femoral condyles, with the subtalar joint maintained in a neutral position (which should be maintained muscularly by the patient) and the A.S.I.S.'s equidistant from the buckey. An x-ray taken with the central ray parallel to the femoral heads will give fairly accurate information regarding the relative lengths of the lower extremities (although it is unable to give exact information regarding lengths of the femurs and tibias). Regardless of which x-ray procedure is used to detect leg length discrepancy, the subtalar joints should always be maintained in their neutral positions, and the femoral neck angles should always be measured and compared bilaterally since these are common causes for functional and structural leg length discrepancies, respectively (Fig. 3.106).

If exposure to x-ray is a concern or if cost is prohibitive, structural leg length discrepancy may be identified with manual examination techniques. The most common method of evaluation is to position the patient supine and measure the distances from the A.S.I.S. to the medial malleolus. Unfortunately, asymmetrical muscle tension may tilt the pelvis, thereby making accurate measurement difficult. To add to the problem, Rothbart and Estabrook (126) claim that supine measurements for determining leg length discrepancy should be avoided since pressure from the examining table flexes the sacrum while tension in the hip flexors simultaneously extends the innominates, thereby obliterating a structural leg length discrepancy. Because of inaccuracy with supine measurements, Ford and Goodman (127)

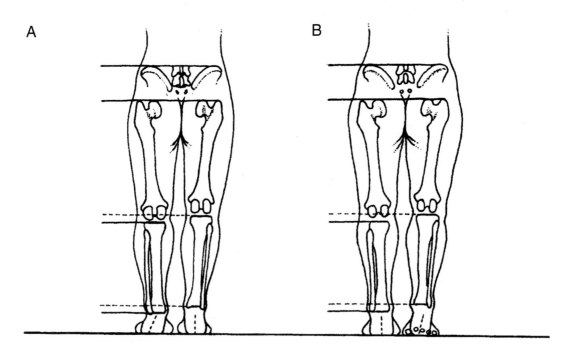

Figure 3.105. Masking of leg length discrepancies. In **A,** a functional leg length discrepancy on the left (which is secondary to asymmetrical pronation), coupled with a structural leg length discrepancy on the right (which is the result of a short femur), gives the appearance of symmetrical leg lengths. In **B,** the rigid plantarflexed first ray on the right produces a functional long leg on that side that hides the right short femur.

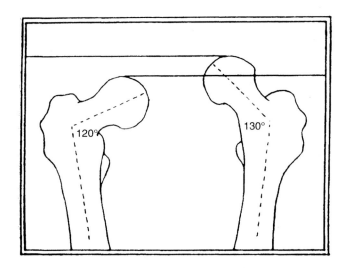

Figure 3.106. Asymmetrical femoral neck angles is a common cause for structural leg length discrepancy.

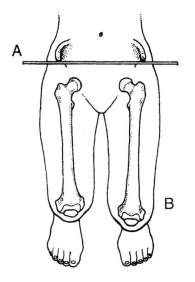

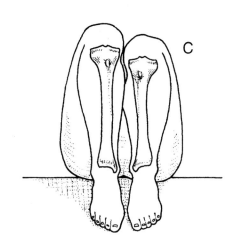

Figure 3.107. Allis' test. The examiner manually aligns the ASIS's so that they rest on the same frontal and transverse plane (**A**). The medial malleoli are then placed together, and femoral lengths are evaluated from above (**B**) while tibial lengths are determined by comparing the levels of the tibial plateaus (**C**).

suggest that leg length discrepancies less than 1/4 inch be ignored.

More accurate evaluation of structural leg length discrepancies requires that the examiner combine information from several different manual tests. To begin with, the relative lengths of the femurs and tibias can be evaluated with Allis' test (Fig. 3.107). Findings from this evaluation can then be compared with information from a weight-bearing evaluation, wherein the levels of the various bony landmarks can be observed from front and back (Fig. 3.108). Information from this evaluation, when coupled with information from off-weight-bearing and/or x-ray measurements, enables the practitioner to differentiate structural from functional leg length discrepancy accurately.

Pathomechanics

As related to its effect on gait, there are many ways that a patient may compensate for a leg length discrepancy. Because the short leg has a longer distance to fall during late swing phase (which results in an increase in vertical [128] and lateral [129] ground-reactive forces), many patients will attempt to modify impact forces by slowly lowering the shorter leg to the ground via eccentric contraction of the contralateral hip abductor musculature. This produces chronic strain on these muscles and may cause hypermobility of the L5-S1 articulation, as the body of L5 rotates towards the excessively lowered hip. (Normally, the pelvis drops only 4 or 5° during the middle portion of swing phase and returns to neutral by heel-strike.) Also, in an attempt to stabilize against the increased lateral shear forces at heel-strike, some individuals develop an out-toe gait pattern on the side of the short leg. Another common pattern of compensation for a leg length discrepancy occurs when the individual hyperextends the knee and inverts the subtalar joint on the side of the short leg. While both of these motions may be helpful in that they bring the heel closer to the ground during late swing phase, they may also be damaging in that hyperextension of the knee impairs the quadricep's ability to dampen vertical forces while inversion of the sub-

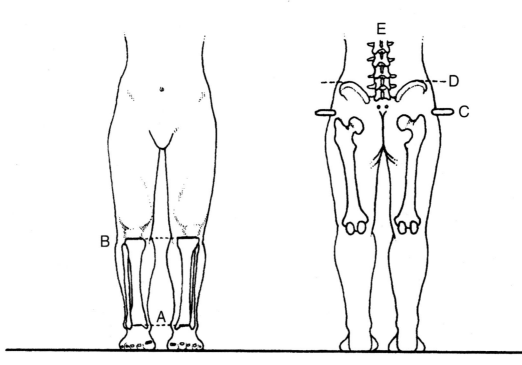

Figure 3.108. Weight-bearing evaluation for leg length discrepancies. The patient is carefully positioned with both feet directly beneath the greater trochanters. The level of the medial malleoli (**A**) can then be compared to determine whether asymmetrical subtalar pronation (or supination) is a cause of functional leg length discrepancy. Next, the tibial plateaus are compared (**B**) to determine the relative lengths of the tibias. To compare femoral lengths, the fingertips are placed on top of the greater trochanters (which can be found by having the patient flex and extend the hips), and their respective levels are noted (**C**). The levels of the posterior superior iliac spine (PSISs) are evaluated with the patient standing erect, then bent 90° at the hip. Finally, the levels of the iliac crests should be compared (**D**), and any deviation of the lumbar spine from vertical should be noted (**E**).

talar joint creates a functional rearfoot varus deformity that increases the range and speed of subtalar joint pronation present during the contact period.

It is also possible that compensation for a leg length discrepancy may produce injury on the side of the long leg. Because the long leg moves through a larger arc during swing phase (130), the individual often attempts to decrease the radius of this arc by flexing the knee. This motion may significantly increase compressive forces at the patellofemoral articulation. Furthermore, it is not uncommon for the individual to bring the long leg closer to the ground by maximally pronating the subtalar joint on that side. While Sanner et al. (131) noted an average vertical change of only 3 mm as the subtalar joint moves from a neutral position to a pronated position, it is possible for subtalar joint pronation to compensate fully for structural leg length discrepancies of 1/2 inch or more. In some cases, the head of the talus will actually make ground contact. Ironically, Hiss (132) claims that this makes the foot more stable, as plantar contact with the talar head serves as a point of support for the unstable medial column. So, even though it is a commonly held belief that the greater range of subtalar joint pronation occurs on the side of the structurally short leg, it is quite possible that an even greater range will occur on the side of the long leg if the individual attempts to level the pelvis.

Treatment in this situation requires placing a heel lift beneath the short leg and, if the range of subtalar joint pronation on the long leg side remains unchanged, an orthotic may be necessary to control the exaggerated motion. It is of particular interest that Novick and Kelley (133) noted that the addition of a 2-mm-thick functional orthotic produced a 4.8-mm elevation of the ankle joint's center of mass secondary to superior repositioning of the talus on the calcaneus. Because of this situation, treatment for combinations of structural and functional discrepancies requires careful pre- and postevaluation to ensure that proper correction has been attained.

Treatment of Structural vs. Functional Discrepancies. If a structural leg length discrepancy were present by itself, treatment should consist of placing the appropriately sized heel lift beneath the short leg. The actual height of the heel lift is best determined by placing lifts of various sizes beneath the short leg and reevaluating alignment. The ideal heel lift will level the iliac crest and, more importantly, bring the lumbar spine to vertical (123). This technique is surprisingly accurate for even subtle leg length discrepancies. If a heel lift is recommended based upon information from off-weight-bearing measurements (e.g., A.S.I.S. to medial malleolus), it is necessary to add approximately 33% to the measured discrepancy in order to attain full correction, i.e., because the talus is positioned one-third of the way between the calcaneus and metatarsal heads, a heel lift placed beneath the calcaneus will raise the talus only two-thirds of that distance. For example, a 3/8-inch heel lift will raise the talus 1/4 inch.

Most authorities recommend that heel lifts be used for structural leg length discrepancies greater than 1/4 inch (134, 135). However, Subotnick (136) claims that because of the threefold increase in ground-reactive forces associated with running, heel lifts should be used on running athletes that present with structural leg length discrepancies greater than 1/8 inch. It should be noted that Travell and Simons (123) are less concerned about the effects of relatively small leg length discrepancies. They recommended a 1/4-inch structural leg length discrepancy be treated only when it is suspected of being a perpetuating factor in myofascial pain syndromes. Otherwise, it is suggested that heel lifts be used preventively only in the treatment of structural leg length discrepancies exceeding 1/2 inch or more.

It is of interest that use of a heel lift to compensate for structural leg length discrepancies in children under the age of 15 is often associated with the complete disappearance of the leg length discrepancy (i.e., leg lengths become equal) after 3–7 months of wear (137). As a result, children should be evaluated at 6-month intervals to determine whether the heel lift is still necessary.

Because of problems with shoe fit, it is recommended that heel lifts greater than 3/8 inch be added to the midsole or heel and not placed inside the shoe. Heel lifts that run the full length of the midsole will prevent contracture of the posterior calf musculature. Also, to reduce the risk of injury to the contralateral hip flexors and adductors (which are stretched with heel lift), large structural leg length discrepancies should be treated by gradually increasing the size of the heel lift at a rate of approximately 1/4 inch every 4 weeks. During this break-in period, the rectus femoris, iliopsoas and adductor musculature should be gently stretched to reduce the potential for iatrogenic injury.

A primary contraindication for heel lift therapy occurs when the lumbar spine is not laterally flexed toward the structurally short leg. Use of a heel lift in this situation could result in recurrent injury to the lumbosacral spine.

Another contraindication is that a heel lift should never be used to treat a functional leg length discrepancy since it does not address the cause of the discrepancy and may even create a unilateral weakness of the involved lower extremity (138).

Treatment for a functional leg length discrepancy requires the appropriate manual therapies to address any soft tissue contractures that may be twisting the pelvis and, if necessary, an orthotic to correct any asymmetrical prona-

tion that may be causing the leg length discrepancy. In one study by Rothbart and Estabrook in which a combination of functional orthotics and manipulative techniques were used to correct functional leg length discrepancies secondary to asymmetrical pronation and its associated sacroiliac joint dysfunction, it was noted that 78 of the 81 patients treated exhibited a complete reduction in low back pain with 77% of these individuals remaining asymptomatic 6 months after their last manipulative treatment (126). They related the reduced chronicity to the fact that the orthotics (which were made from neutral position impressions) maintained a more functionally efficient posture, thereby allowing even short-term manipulation (i.e., 3 weeks) to have a more permanent effect.

Rothbart and Estabrook (126) also theorized that asymmetrical pronation (which was defined as side-to-side variations in stance phase pronation greater than 2°) forces the entire lower extremity to internally rotate and drop inferior, which allows the innominate on that side to extend, i.e., the posterior superior iliac spine (PSIS) moves antero-superior. This sets the stage for chronic sacroiliac joint dysfunction and may allow for entrapment of the sciatic nerve between the piriformis muscle and the sacrospinous ligament as the rotating innominate partially collapses the greater sciatic notch. They also claimed that prolonged asymmetrical pronation allows the normal amphiarthrodial sacroiliac joint to become diarthrodial as vertical forces on the repeatedly collapsing limb eventually produce ligamentous instability of the sacroiliac joint.

The list of possible injuries associated with asymmetrical pronation are detailed in Figure 3.109.

In ending this discussion of leg length inequalities, it should be clear that isolating the exact degree of structural vs. functional leg length discrepancy is not always easy and requires careful observation and examination. Before casually recommending a heel lift based upon information obtained from a single A.S.I.S. to medial malleolus measurement, the practitioner should have fully evaluated respective tibial and femoral lengths in a variety of positions, checked for soft tissue contracture that might be twisting the pelvis and/or lumbar spine, and carefully evaluated foot function, both statically and dynamically, to determine whether asymmetrical subtalar joint motion is contributing to a functional leg length discrepancy.

MINIMUM RANGES OF MOTION NECESSARY FOR A NONCOMPENSATED GAIT

An important prerequisite for normal function is that specific joints of the lower extremities and pelvis must move through certain minimum ranges of motion. This is complicated by the fact that these ranges are subject to change with different activities, i.e., the ankle must be able to dorsiflex 10° for walking and 25° for running. If for any reason a joint is unable to move through its required mini-

Figure 3.109. The effects of asymmetrical subtalar joint pronation. Excessive subtalar joint pronation (**A**) causes the lower extremity to internally rotate (**B**) and drop inferiorly (**C**). This, in turn, increases tensile strain on the iliopsoas and piriformis muscles (**D**) and leads to a narrowing of the greater sciatic notch (thereby predisposing the entrapment of the sciatic nerve). Also, as the lower extremity drops inferiorly, the ipsilateral innominate is lowered (**E**) and, as is consistent with Fryette's law, the body of L5 rotates toward the functionally shortened leg (**F**). As a result, the lumbar spine attempts to straighten itself by laterally flexing toward the long leg (**G**, on *inset*), which compresses the lateral aspects of the discs on that side and forces the facets on the concave side into a hyperextended or close-packed position *(stars)*. Over a period of years, these actions may lead to a variety of overuse injuries.

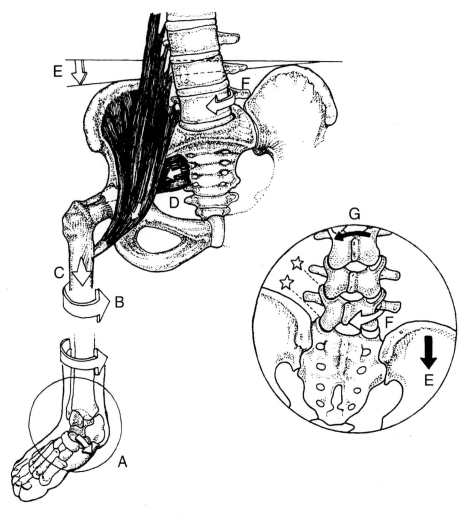

mum range of motion, potentially injurious compensation may occur elsewhere in the kinetic chain and/or the metabolic cost of locomotion would increase, as greater muscular effort would be required to produce a smooth translation of the body's center of mass.

While the loss of even subtle movements between the tarsals might be responsible for compensatory injuries, it is the larger more mobile joints that are more likely to produce pathological compensation. The following is a list of the minimal ranges of motion necessary for noncompensated function at the various lower extremity articulations.

The hip must rotate a minimum of 15–20°, flex 30°, and extend 10°. Conditions resulting in the loss of sagittal plane motions at the hip are most destructive since they may be readily compensated for by either flexion or extension of the lumbar spine (Fig. 3.110). An increased range of spinal flexion is particularly dangerous since numerous studies have demonstrated that repeated flexion of the lumbar spine can damage the annular wall of the intervertebral disc, allowing for a posterior migration of the nucleus (139, 140). Fortunately, while even slight limitation in hip flexion may damage the disc during sporting activities or actions

requiring frequent bending and lifting, the 30° range of hip flexion necessary for ideal locomotion is seldom lost, and compensatory spinal flexion during the gait cycle is rarely seen.

This is not the case with hip extension since osteoarthrosis and/or hip flexor contracture often limit the range of hip extension to 5° or less. This may lead to a chronic facet syndrome or even a dynamic lateral recess stenosis as the entire lumbar spine is often forced into a hyperextended position during late stance phase.

While decreases in transverse plane motions are less destructive than their sagittal plane counterparts, they still must be evaluated. At slower speeds of walking, compensation for decreased hip rotation may be associated with asymmetrical shoulder rotation and arm swing (141). As speeds increase, the asymmetrical arm motions become more exaggerated, and the effort required to move the pelvis with its rigidly attached femur becomes more noticeable. Also, there is an overall decrease in stride length, and an abductory twist of the rearfoot is often present during heel lift.

The knee must extend 180° and flex a minimum of

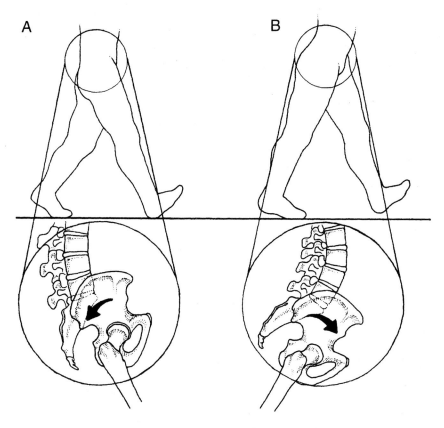

Figure 3.110. A limited range of hip flexion produces compensatory spinal flexion during late swing and early stance phase (A) while decreased range of hip extension produces compensatory spinal hyperextension during the propulsive period (B).

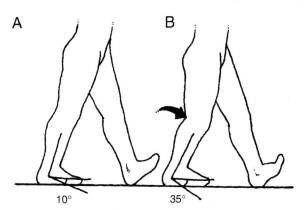

Figure 3.111. Just prior to heel lift, the range of ankle dorsiflexion is usually limited to 10° or less (A). However, when a limited range of knee extension is present **(B)**, the ankle is forced to dorsiflex excessively.

50°. If the knee is unable to fully extend, excessive tensile strains are placed on the posterior compartment muscles (particularly soleus and tibialis posterior) as the ankle joint is forced into an excessively dorsiflexed position during the late midstance period (Fig. 3.111). The individual with this deformity often avoids the latter half of stance phase by prematurely lifting the heel.

If the individual were to possess less than 50° of knee flexion (which is relatively uncommon), the metabolic cost of locomotion would be greatly increased as, in order to provide ample ground clearance during midswing, the individual is forced to circumduct the entire swing phase lower extremity. This is accomplished with great muscular effort via forceful contraction of the contralateral gastrocnemius and gluteus medius musculature (which function to elevate the center of mass and abduct the swing phase innominate), the ipsilateral quadratus lumborum (which lifts the swing phase innominate) and most importantly, vigorous contraction of the ipsilateral hip flexors (which pull the swing leg forward). Inman et al. (141) note that an adequate range of knee flexion is the single most important determinant of gait.

The ankle must dorsiflex a minimum of 10°. The ankle reaches its maximally dorsiflexed position just prior to heel lift. The greater the range of hip extension during late midstance (as with running and speed walking), the greater the range of ankle dorsiflexion necessary to compensate. If the ankle is unable to move through the full range necessary to compensate for hip extension, the foot will attempt to supply the remaining range by pronating the subtalar joint. This action tilts the oblique midtarsal joint axis into a more horizontal position that allows the forefoot to dorsiflex more effectively about this axis (Fig. 3.112).

While subtalar and midtarsal joint pronation allow for greater amounts of forefoot dorsiflexion, these movements may be destructive, as they unlock the tarsals as vertical forces peak, prevent locking of the calcaneocuboid joint, and prevent the approximation of the anterior and posterior

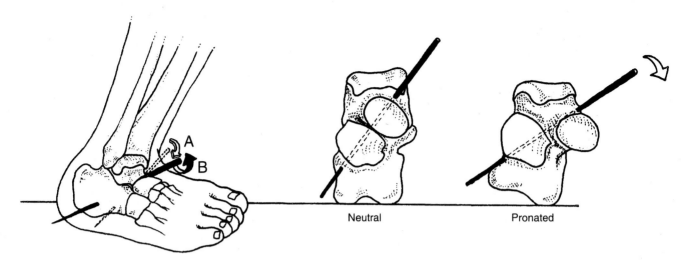

Figure 3.112. With the subtalar joint in its neutral position, the oblique midtarsal joint axis allows for much forefoot abduction (*arrow,* A). However, when the subtalar joint is pronated, the oblique midtarsal joint axis shifts into a more horizontal position, thereby allowing for greater amounts of forefoot dorsiflexion (*arrow,* **B**).

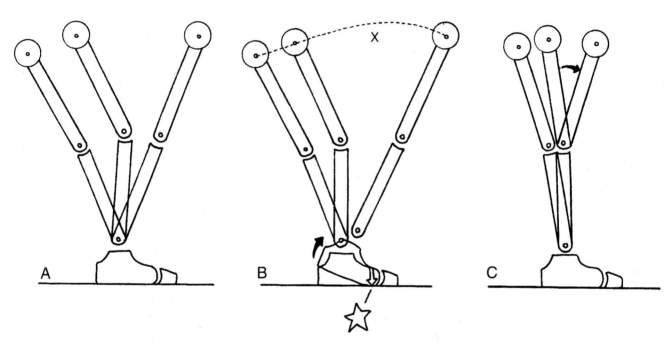

Figure 3.113. When an adequate range of ankle dorsiflexion is present (A), inertial forces associated with the forward progression of the center of mass act to prestretch the posterior calf musculature, thereby allowing for the eventual return of this energy during the propulsive period. If the ankle and foot are unable to supply the necessary range of dorsiflexion (**B**), the heel is prematurely lifted from the ground *(arrow)* and, as is consistent with Newton's third law, the forces associated with elevating the center of mass *(X)* will now drive the longer metatarsal heads into the ground *(star).* If the heel does not immediately lift from the ground (as with a weakened triceps surae), a recurvatum stress is applied to the posterior knee **(C),** which may eventually lead to a genu recurvatum deformity.

pillars normally associated with a functioning windlass mechanism.

If for any reason the subtalar and midtarsal joints are unable to fully compensate for the limited range of ankle dorsiflexion, the individual will be predisposed to a metatarsal stress syndrome (142), as inertial forces associated with forward progression of the body will forcefully drive the metatarsal heads into the ground (Fig. 3.113). Hughes (143) demonstrated that a decrease in ankle dorsiflexion greatly increases the potential for developing metatarsal stress fractures as soldiers with limited ranges of dorsiflexion were 4.6 times more likely to develop metatarsal stress fractures than their more flexible counterparts.

In addition to these problems, a restriction in ankle dorsiflexion (which is referred to as an equinus condition) may also damage the anterior talotibial articulation, as the leading edge of the anterior tibia often collides into the sulcus on the dorsal talar neck. If there is only a slight limitation in ankle dorsiflexion, the distal tibiofibular articulation will attempt to accommodate the talus by gapping anteriorly. (This articulation may gap by as much as 1.5 mm anteriorly [**144**].) However, the ability of the syndesmotic distal tibiofibular articulation to accommodate the dorsiflexing talus is at best limited.

Over time, repeated contact of the talar neck and the distal tibia results in a bony reaction with the eventual formation of an impingement exostoses (Fig. 3.114). O'Donoghue (145) stated that "this reaction has an adverse rather than a protective effect in that the more bone that is piled up, the more easily impingement occurs, and so a vicious cycle is formed, resulting in gradually increasing disability." He also stated that the pain associated with impingement exostoses is readily exacerbated by activities that increase the demands for ankle dorsiflexion, such as fast running, walking up hills, and prolonged squatting.

The subtalar joint must pronate 4° and supinate 12° from the neutral position. Because subtalar joint pronation is the body's primary shock absorbing system and because an adequate range of subtalar joint motion is necessary for the conversion of transverse plane shank motions into frontal plane heel motions, a properly functioning subtalar joint that possesses a minimum of 4° pronation is essential if the individual is to remain injury-free.

A range of less than 4° pronation greatly impairs the individual's ability to absorb shock since it inhibits both the cushioning effect associated with talar plantarflexion and the concurrent internal tibial rotation associated with talar adduction (which is necessary for knee flexion). The individual may attempt to compensate for the reduced shock-absorbing capabilities by dampening vertical forces via excessive ankle plantarflexion (which strains the anterior compartment musculature) or by avoiding heel-strike altogether, i.e., switching to a forefoot strike pattern allows the posterior compartment musculature more time to dampen impact forces.

If the individual has the misfortune of possessing an ankylosed subtalar joint (as occurs with triple arthrodesis and certain tarsal coalitions), in addition to a variety of high-impact symptoms associated with diminished shock absorption capabilities, the ankle joint often becomes a source of chronic pain since it is subjected to tremendous torsional strains as the subtalar joint is no longer able to convert the contact period internal rotation of the shank into rearfoot eversion. This results in large torsional strains being applied to the ankle mortise as the shank spins on top of the immobile talar trochlea.

Because shank motion occurs in a direction parallel to the ankle's axis of motion, it produces a shearing force capable of producing much damage. If ankylosis occurs in a child, nature, via the Heuter-Volkmann principle, has the ability to compensate by converting the ankle into a ball-and-socket joint that is better equipped to translate the transverse plane shank motions (141). In fact, a 10-year follow-up study of children subjected to triple arthrodesis found that 39% of the children showed evidence of a ball-and-socket ankle joint (146). Unfortunately, the adult is unable to accommodate the transverse plane shank motions with the formation of a new articulation, and severe osteoarthrosis of the ankle joint is often the final sequela of an ankylosed subtalar joint.

The ankle joint is not the only articulation predisposed to injury with an ankylosed subtalar joint. In a well-written article describing the pathomechanics associated with a peroneal spastic flatfoot, Outland and Murphy (147) described a series of joint interactions in which ankylosis of the subtalar joint produces an exostoses along the dorsal talar head. They referenced a personal communication regarding cinefluorographic films in which dorsiflexion of a foot with a normal subtalar joint is accompanied by an appreciable degree of forward gliding of calcaneus beneath the talus (Fig. 3.115A and B). This forward glide continues until near the end of ankle dorsiflexion when motion is checked, presumably by capsular ligaments. Then, as the final range of ankle dorsiflexion is reached, an upward gliding motion is seen both at the calcaneocuboid joint and the talonavicular joint as the upper portion of the navicular moves cephalad on the talar head (Fig. 3.115C). Throughout this process, the interspace between the head of the talus and the navicular acetabulum remains constant.

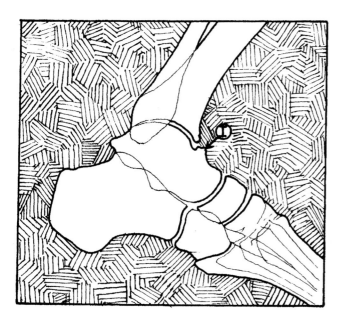

Figure 3.114. The impingement exostosis (I).

Figure 3.115. See text for explanation.

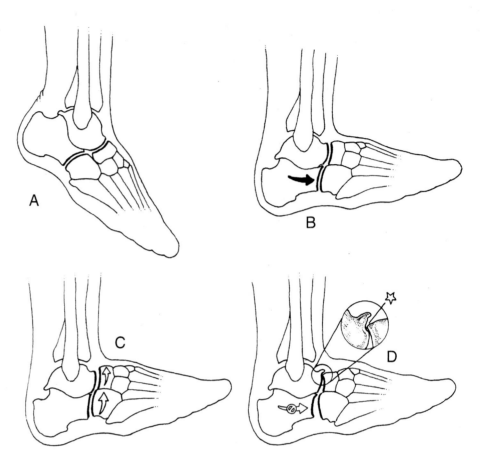

As pointed out by Outland and Murphy, these motions do not occur when the subtalar joint is ankylosed. In this situation, the normal gliding of the calcaneus beneath the talus does not occur, and the midtarsal joint functions as a hinge with ankle dorsiflexion accompanied by a narrowing of the dorsal talonavicular joint margins as the sharp upper edge of the navicular impinges upon the talar head (Fig. 3.115D). When the subtalar joint is completely ankylosed, talonavicular joint remodelling occurs, in which a characteristic exostoses forms along the talar head and neck (inset in Fig. 3.115D).

While a complete restriction in subtalar joint motion may result in dramatic bony changes in the ankle and neighboring tarsals, even a slight restriction in subtalar motion may lead to injury, as the foot is often unable to attain full plantigrade contact with the ground. As noted earlier, if the subtalar joint is unable to move through a range necessary to compensate for a specific foot type, it is referred to as an uncompensated version of that foot type. The most common examples are the uncompensated rearfoot and forefoot varus deformities (Fig. 3.116).

In addition to producing an acquired plantarflexed first ray deformity, the restricted subtalar motion might also be responsible for knee injury as, in an attempt to bring the medial plantar foot to the ground, the medial knee is gapped with a valgus stress while the lateral knee is compressed (Fig. 3.117).

Engsberg and Allinger (148) noted that individuals often attempt to compensate for limited subtalar motion by walking with a wider base of gait. While this may lessen the potential for knee injury, it produces a less effective gait pattern, as the body's center of mass is displaced further laterally over the stance phase leg (which strains the gluteus medius and the peroneal musculature), and the increased angular momentum present in the lower body is compensated for via excessive abduction of the arms.

Individuals with limited subtalar motions are also predisposed to interdigital neuritis and/or stress fracture of the lesser metatarsals, as the foot is maintained in a low gear push-off that tractions the interdigital nerves and increases the ground-reactive forces supported by the lesser metatarsal heads. Because of their aberrant distribution of plantar pressures, individuals with uncompensated foot types typically present with diffuse hyperkeratotic lesions beneath the lateral metatarsal heads.

Although it is possible to have an uncompensated forefoot valgus in which the subtalar joint lacks sufficient supination to bring the lateral forefoot to the ground, this situation is rarely seen since the range of subtalar joint supination is almost always sufficient to bring the lateral forefoot to the ground.

The midtarsal joint must allow for 6° of frontal plane motion. If the midtarsal joint is unable to invert a minimum of 6° (which occurs primarily about the longitudi-

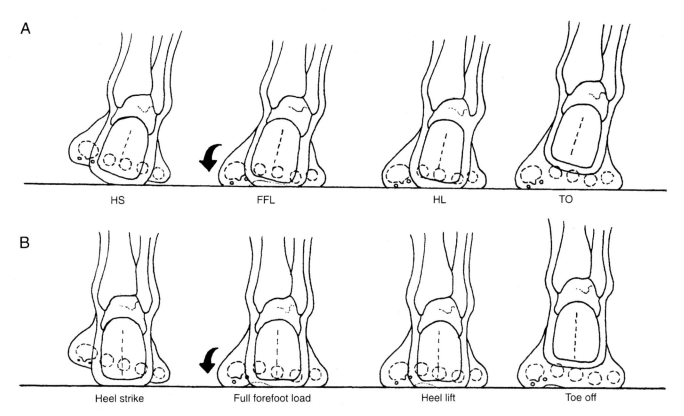

Figure 3.116. The uncompensated rearfoot varus deformity (A) and the uncompensated forefoot varus deformity (B). Note how compensatory first ray plantarflexion is necessary to bring the medial forefoot to the ground *(arrow)*. *HS* = heel strike; *FFL* = full forefoot load; *HL* = heel lift; *TO* = toe off.

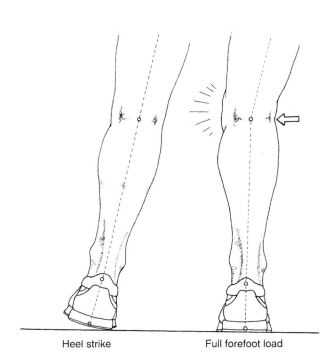

Figure 3.117. A limited range of subtalar joint motion creates a valgus stress at the knee. (Adapted from Engsberg JR, Allinger TL. A function of the talocalcaneal joint during running support. Foot Ankle 1990; 2:93–96.)

nal midtarsal joint axis), the subtalar joint is unable to move through an adequate range of pronation without compensatory dorsiflexion and inversion of the first ray (Fig. 3.118). When the first ray moves through its full range of motion and is no longer able to compensate, subtalar joint pronation comes to an abrupt halt.

The hallux must dorsiflex a minimum of 40°. Although 65° of hallux dorsiflexion is necessary for ideal propulsive period function, as little as 40° of hallux dorsiflexion will still allow the individual to move through the early stages of propulsion without injury. When the inflexible hallux achieves its fully dorsiflexed position, the individual often chooses to terminate the propulsive period by prematurely flexing the knee and hip.

Differentiating Causes of Restricted Motion

Once it has been determined that a joint with limited motion is a detrimentally affecting function, it is essential that the cause of the decreased motion be identified since this determines the proper treatment, i.e., a joint limited by muscular or capsular contracture will typically respond well to manual therapies while a joint limited by bony restriction should be treated with accommodative techniques. The nature of the restriction is determined by evaluating both the quality and quantity of the joint's passive and paraphysiological ranges of motion (Fig. 3.119).

Figure 3.118. When the midtarsal joint is unable to invert a minimum of 6°, continued subtalar pronation (A) can only occur if the first ray dorsiflexes and inverts (B).

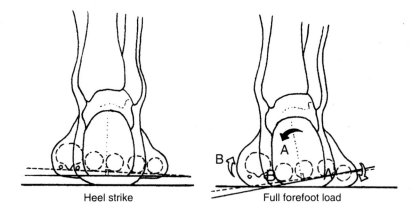

Heel strike   Full forefoot load

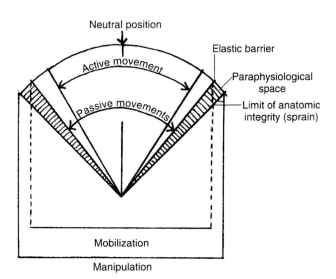

Figure 3.119. Range of motion available to a diarthrodial joint. If an examiner were to move a joint through its full range of motion, an elastic barrier would be felt at the end of its passive range of movement. This barrier normally possesses a springy end-feel that can be evaluated by gently stressing the joint. (A classic example of this end-feel is the springy resistance associated with long axis traction of a metacarpophalangeal joint) This end range rests within the limits of the joint's anatomical range of motion and can be accessed via careful manipulation. (Adapted from Sandoz R. Some physical mechanisms and effects of spinal adjustments. Ann Swiss Chirop Assoc 1976; 6: 91.)

When a joint's range of motion is limited by muscular contracture, the elastic barrier is difficult to access, and the end range is soft and constantly changing. The easiest way to identify a muscular restriction is to perform repeat hold-relax stretches: If the range of motion increases slightly with each successive stretch, the restriction is muscular.

In contrast to this situation, if the joint's range of motion is limited by a bony restriction, the end range is hard and abrupt and does not change with repeated hold-relax stretches. A classic example of a bony restriction can be felt by gently attempting to hyperextend the ulnohumeral joint.

A joint's range of motion may also be limited by joint dysfunction. In this situation, the normal elastic end play associated with accessing the paraphysiological space is replaced with a firm, tense end-play. As defined by Mennell (150), joint dysfunction represents a loss of the normal range of involuntary motion (joint play) of which all synovial joints are capable. He also notes that these involuntary movements are a necessary prerequisite for a full range of pain-free functional voluntary movement.

Although the exact nature of joint dysfunction remains controversial, the most plausible theory suggests that it is due to adhesions in the periarticular connective tissues that limit access to the joint's paraphysiological space (151). Because a joint's overall range of motion is dependent on the smaller accessory motions (152), loss of the paraphysiological range of motion may inhibit the normal rolling, spinning, and gliding motions necessary for the joint to move through its full range of movement. To compound the problem, because of discomfort associated with tensing the fibrous adhesions, the individual often learns to avoid using the dysfunctional joint, which only serves to perpetuate the restriction.

Another possible, albeit poorly understood cause for joint dysfunction relates to subluxation of a hypermobile articulation. Because the abnormal application of ground-reactive force in a mechanically malfunctioning foot often leads to a laxity of the restraining ligaments, subluxation of one or more of the tarsals is not uncommon.

Unfortunately, even slight subluxation may lead to a functional malalignment of axes that acts to limit further motion. This is analogous to how tilting one hinge on a door even 2 or 3° will drastically limit the range that the door will open. Because the articular surfaces are essentially frictionless, a subluxation could initially be reduced simply by moving the joint through its full range of motion: Pressure on opposing articular surfaces will cause the subluxation to reduce in order to allow for a parallelism of their shared axes. The same thing would happen if the door with the malaligned hinges were forced open, assuming the hinges were not secured too tightly.

As related to the body, however, ground-reactive forces are relentless in their maintenance of a subluxation, and the involved joint's range of motion remains limited due to the malaligned axes. If untreated, periarticular adhesions form that convert the one-time hypermobile joint into a hypomobile joint.

According to Hiss (132), these periarticular adhesions (which he refers to as "nature's cement") produce "joint tension that interferes with the synchrony of pivoting, balancing and the distribution of the moving load in walking." He notes that it is not uncommon for hypermobile pronated feet to have one or more of the tarsal bones become locked in an abnormal position. This is analogous to how a hypermobile glenohumeral joint may eventually become locked and frozen in the upper portion of the glenoid fossa.

Once the exact cause of limited motion has been determined, the appropriate treatment program can be initiated. The following sections will describe treatment for the various conditions limiting range of motion in the foot and ankle. For a more detailed description of manual techniques associated with knee and hip dysfunction, the interested reader is referred to other sources (150, 153–157).

Restricted Motion Resulting from Muscular Contracture

Resistance to a stretch results from tension on the active contractile components and the passive resistive (viscoelastic) components (158). The flexibility of these tissues can usually be improved through the use of various active and passive musculature relaxation techniques. The active muscular relaxation techniques (AMRTs), which are also referred to as PNF techniques, or muscle energy procedures, consist of various combinations of static stretches applied in conjunction with alternating combinations of antagonist and agonist contractions. A list of possible AMRTs is described as follows.

Maximum resistance hold-relax stretches. This technique requires that the examiner gently stretch the desired muscle to its fully lengthened position. The patient then isometrically tenses the muscle with maximum effort for approximately 10 seconds while the examiner provides resistance. On releasing tension, the muscle is gently stretched to its new end position, and the process is repeated until muscle length gains no longer occur.

Lewit technique. This stretching procedure is identical to the maximum resistance hold-relax stretch, with the exception that only gentle isometric contractions are used.

Rhythmic stabilization. This stretching technique involves alternate contractions of agonist and antagonist muscle groups while the examiner maintains the isometrically tensed muscle at the limit of its available range of motion.

CRAC technique (contract, relax, agonist contraction). As the name implies, this technique involves having the patient isometrically tense the desired muscle at the end of its fully stretched position (Fig. 3.120A). The muscle's antagonist is then contracted with full effort against resistance provided by the practitioner (Fig. 3.120B). (Note that the use of the term "agonist" in the title refers to agonists of the motion, not agonists of the stretched muscle.) The desired muscle is then stretched to its new end-position (Fig. 3.120C), and the process is repeated until muscle length gains no longer occur.

While the use of AMRTs is widely advocated because they more quickly increase range of motion (159–162) and improve the ability of the myotendinous junctions to resist tensile strains (163), more recent studies

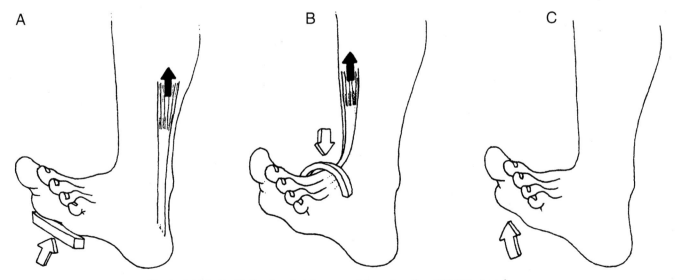

Figure 3.120. (A–C) Contract, relax, agonist contraction (CRAC) stretches.

suggest that the use of maximum resistance during these stretches should be avoided since forceful contractions produce a lingering after-discharge that can detrimentally affect muscle tension (164, 165).

While many authors believe that a maximum contraction is necessary to stimulate the Golgi tendon organ's reflexive relaxation of the agonist (166, 167), this has never been conclusively demonstrated. In fact, Holt (168) feels that the agonist relaxation following isometric contraction stems not from an increase in information from the Golgi tendon organ, but rather, from a decrease in information from the muscle spindle. Apparently, the isometric contraction somehow lessens the flow of impulses from the spindle complex. The exact mechanism for the lessened discharge remains to be proven.

It should also be mentioned that a study by Moore and Hutton (159) demonstrated that the CRAC stretches were associated with the highest level of EMG activity and that they were more likely to produce pain during the stretch. This prompted Stanish and Hubley-Kozey (169) to recommend that the stretched muscle's antagonist never be contracted during the stretching process for fear of producing an after-discharge that would eventually tighten the stretched muscle.

Because of the potential for delayed muscular tightening following the maximum resistance hold-relax stretches and the CRAC stretches, the resistance stretches described by Lewit are preferred over the more vigorous PNF stretches. Travell and Simons (123) claimed that the Lewit technique is remarkably effective at reducing painful trigger points as long as the fibers being stretched are precisely the fibers that have been tensed or shortened by trigger point activity. This is readily accomplished by alternating joint angles while performing repeat stretches until tension is felt in the area of the trigger point (e.g., a trigger point in the medial belly on the gastrocnemius muscle can be accessed by everting the subtalar joint while performing the gentle hold-relax stretches).

In addition to the use of AMRTs, the use of passive muscular relaxation techniques (PMRTs) should always be considered since a recent comparison of PNF vs. static stretches on hamstring flexibility demonstrated that static stretches produced significant reductions in oxygen consumption with corresponding improvements in gait economy (170). The decreased oxygen consumption was related to an improved antagonist response. Godges et al. (170) stated that the "static stretching procedure prepared the subject for more economical gait by applying the end range stretch in the same plane that the muscles are going to be used." The results of that study suggest that static stretching of the lower extremity musculature may be an effective way to improve endurance during locomotion.

Other advocates of PMRTs claim these techniques more effectively produce plastic deformity of connective tissues and allow for more permanent muscular elongation.

Sapega et al. (171) claim that the best way to permanently lengthen connective tissue structures is with prolonged, low-intensity stretches performed at elevated tissue temperatures (greater than 104°F), with the muscles cooled before releasing the tension. They imply that heating the muscle while stretching it allows for a destabilization of intermolecular bonding which, when cooled before release, allows the collagenous microstructure to restabilize in its new stretched length.

A list of the more commonly used in-office and home stretching procedures follows; the various perpetuating factors and the biomechanical effects of prolonged contracture are also noted (Figs. 3.121–3.125).

Restricted Motion Resulting from Osseous Block

The joints most likely to be affected by bony restrictions are the ankle joint, the subtalar joint, and the first metatarsophalangeal joint. The exact nature of these bony restrictions and the appropriate methods of treatment are discussed in the following sections.

The Ankle Joint. In addition to the relatively uncommon bony restriction associated with impingement exostoses (refer back to Fig. 3.114), ankle dorsiflexion may also be restricted by various congenital/developmental malformations. The most common deformity affecting ankle dorsiflexion is the flattened talar trochlea (Fig. 3.126). When present, the flattened talar trochlea allows for a premature bony contact between the anterior distal tibia and dorsal talus that limits ankle dorsiflexion.

Another bony anomaly that may restrict ankle dorsiflexion relates to a congenitally wide anterior talar dome. Normally, the wide portion of the anterior talus will fit snugly into the mortise formed by the distal tibia and fibula. If the talus possesses an unusually wide anterior dome or if the intermalleolar distance is narrowed secondary to fracture of the distal tibia or fibula, a bony restriction often develops that limits the available range of dorsiflexion (Fig. 3.127).

If a bony block sufficiently limits ankle dorsiflexion, the individual may attempt to compensate for the decreased range of motion by pronating the subtalar joint and, if necessary, the midtarsal joint. Since it is impossible to restore a decreased range of motion associated with a bony restriction, treatment must be geared toward accommodating the deformity.

For limited ankle dorsiflexion, this is accomplished simply by adding a lift beneath the heel (Fig. 3.128). A 1/4-inch heel lift will allow for an additional 3° of ankle dorsiflexion. Because of the relatively insignificant amount of ankle dorsiflexion restored with an in-shoe heel lift (which is typically no more than 1/4-inch high), it is suggested that large lifts be incorporated into the sole of the shoe or that the individual wear shoes with sufficient heel height (running shoes typically raise the heels 1/2 inch).

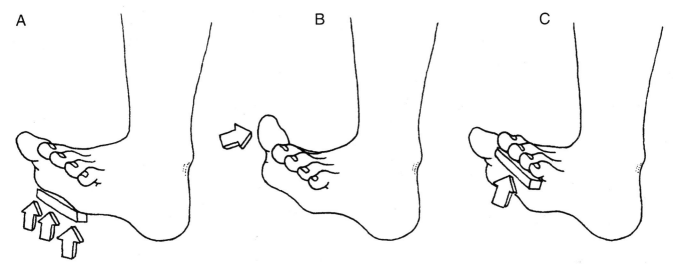

Figure 3.121. Posterior compartment stretches. The gastrocnemius muscle may be stretched by dorsiflexing the ankle with the knee fully extended. The medial, central, or lateral fibers of this muscle may be accessed by applying the dorsiflectory force beneath the lateral, central, or medial forefoot, respectively (i.e., applying pressure beneath the medial forefoot while dorsiflexing the ankle will invert the rearfoot, allowing for a better stretch of the lateral gastrocnemius muscle) **(A).** The same process is repeated to stretch the soleus muscle; only the knee is maintained in a flexed position. Tibialis posterior is also stretched by dorsiflexing the ankle with the knee flexed; only the lateral forefoot is loaded so as to maximally evert the heel. Flexor hallucis longus and flexor digitorum longus are stretched with the knee flexed, the ankle dorsiflexed, and the respective digits maximally dorsiflexed **(B and C). Effects of contracture:** Contracture in tibialis posterior and/or soleus is a common cause of functional rearfoot varus deformity. This often occurs in athletes involved in jumping sports (particularly basketball and volleyball), where exercise-induced hypertonicity of the posterior compartment musculature allows these muscles to overpower the antagonistic peroneals. As a result, the chronically tightened tibialis posterior/medial soleus muscles maintain the rearfoot in an inverted position during swing phase, and the foot behaves identically to the rearfoot varus deformity. Unlike the osseous rearfoot varus deformity, the functional rearfoot varus will reduce by stretching the contracted musculature and strengthening the antagonistic peroneals. Foot function will also be compromised by contracture in the triceps surae musculature as the subtalar and midtarsal joints attempt to compensate for a limited range of ankle dorsiflexion by pronating during the latter half of stance phase. When performing stretches on these muscles, the subtalar joint must be maintained in a neutral or supinated position to ensure locking of the midtarsal joint. Also, while contracture in flexor hallucis and flexor digitorum longus is fairly uncommon, it may result in flexion deformity of the involved distal phalanges (172). **Perpetuating factors:** Excessive subtalar joint pronation during the propulsive period is a major factor responsible for overloading the posterior compartment musculature. In addition, tibialis posterior may be chronically tightened in individuals possessing a rearfoot varus deformity. Activities that may perpetuate trigger point formation in these muscles include the frequent use of high-heeled shoes, sleeping in a prone position with the ankles plantarflexed, and sports requiring vigorous ankle plantarflexion. (Even swimming may aggravate these muscles.)

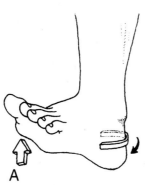
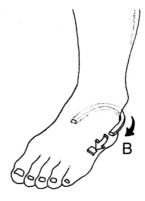

Figure 3.122. Lateral compartment stretches. Peroneus longus is stretched by inverting the heel, dorsiflexing the ankle, and applying a dorsiflectory force beneath the first metatarsal head **(A)**. Peroneus brevis is stretched by inverting the heel while plantarflexing and adducting the forefoot. This is accomplished by applying pressure over the dorsal base of the fifth metatarsal **(B)**. **Effects of contracture:** A tightened peroneus longus almost always results in a functional plantarflexed first ray. This is frequently seen in middle distance runners and classical ballet dancers, in whom the prolonged application of forces beneath the first metatarsal head produces a lingering after-discharge in peroneus longus that may eventually result in contracture. Although much less common, peroneus brevis may also present with contracture. This being the case, the subtalar joint is maintained in a pronated position throughout swing phase, and heel-strike usually occurs on the medial calcaneus. **Perpetuating factors:** The cavovarus foot type is the most common perpetuating factor for peroneus longus contracture. The improved mechanical advantage afforded peroneus longus by the inverted subtalar joint produces chronic strain on this muscle. Treatment for this condition should include manipulative techniques to improve foot function and, when necessary, a forefoot valgus post to lessen the degree of rearfoot inversion. Contracture in the lateral compartment musculature may also be perpetuated by overdeveloped posterior compartment musculature, various tarsal coalitions, and past history of trauma with resultant joint dysfunction in subtalar and/or calcaneocuboid joints.

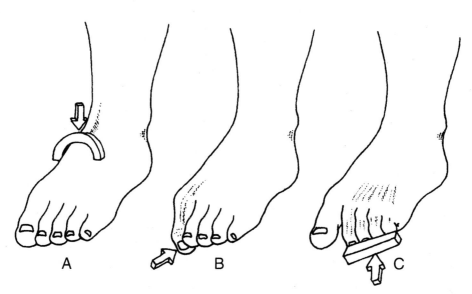

Figure 3.123. Anterior compartment stretches. Tibialis anterior is stretched by plantarflexing the ankle while contacting the base of the first metatarsal **(A)**. Extensor hallucis longus is stretched by plantarflexing the ankle and then maximally plantarflexing the hallux by pressing on the distal phalanx **(B)**. Extensor digitorum longus and peroneus tertius may be stretched by maintaining the ankle in a plantarflexed position and applying pressure to distal phalanges **(C)**. Note that the lateral fibers of extensor digitorum longus (including peroneus tertius) may be accessed by simultaneously inverting the rearfoot while plantarflexing and adducting the forefoot. **Effects of contracture:** Contracture in tibialis anterior may produce a functionally dorsiflexed first ray or even a functional forefoot varus if the contracture is severe enough. This may eventually result in hallux limitus or hallux abductovalgus, as first ray plantarflexion during the propulsive period may be blocked. It is also possible that contracture in extensor hallucis longus will produce a plantarflexed first ray deformity, as the compressive force generated at the hallux may produce a retrograde plantarflectory force at the first metatarsal head. Contracture in extensor digitorum longus is less damaging, although it may result in the development of digital contractures with hyperextension of the lesser metatarsophalangeal joints. **Perpetuating factors:** Tibialis anterior is chronically fatigued and tightened in individuals with excessive lowering of the medial longitudinal arch upon weight-bearing while the long digital flexors may be chronically contracted in individuals presenting with plantarflexed forefeet.

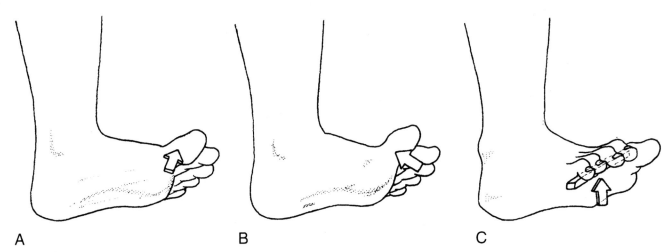

A   B   C

Figure 3.124. Intrinsic muscle stretches. Abductor hallucis is stretched by maintaining the ankle in neutral, slightly dorsiflexing the hallux, and applying an abductory force at the first interphalangeal joint **(A).** Flexor hallucis brevis and flexor digitorum brevis are stretched by applying a dorsiflectory force at the proximal phalanx of the hallux **(B)** and the middle phalanges of the lesser digits **(C),** respectively. The ankle should be maintained in its neutral position during all of these stretches to ensure that the stretch is generated in the short digital flexors. **Effects of contracture:** Kendall and McCreary (172) claimed that contracture in the abductor hallucis muscle will "pull the foot into forefoot varus," with the hallux being maintained in an adducted position. Severe contracture of the abductor hallucis muscle may be responsible for entrapment neuropathy of the medial and lateral plantar nerves (refer back to Fig. 3.20). Unlike their antagonists, the short digital flexors rarely produce digital deformity, although they may limit the overall range of digital dorsiflexion. **Perpetuating factors:** As with the lateral compartment musculature, abductor hallucis and the short digital flexors are almost always contracted in the presence of a cavovarus foot type. Also, the abductor hallucis muscle may be chronically contracted in individuals who sleep with their ankles plantarflexed. This may result in recalcitrant heel pain, particularly in the morning, as the contracted tissues are stretched upon weight-bearing. To treat this difficult-to-manage perpetuating factor, Wapner and Sharkey (83) suggested fitting the patient with a night brace that maintains the ankle in a position of 5° dorsiflexion. This form of treatment is remarkably effective for treating not only abductor hallucis myositis but also for treating recurrent achilles tendinitis and plantar fasciitis, which often result from faulty sleeping posture.

To prevent possible iatrogenic low back or knee injury, the individual with a unilaterally decreased range of ankle dorsiflexion must be treated with bilateral heel lifts.

It should be stressed that excessive subtalar or midtarsal joint pronation resulting from a decreased range of ankle dorsiflexion is not treated with a foot orthotic. If an orthotic were inadvertently prescribed to treat compensatory subtalar or midtarsal pronation and the decreased range of ankle dorsiflexion was not treated with a heel lift, iatrogenic injury would most likely result as the tissues beneath the medial longitudinal arch would collide into the orthotic shell as the foot continues to compensate for the limited ankle motion. This often results in neuropraxia of the medial plantar nerve and/or contusion of the abductor hallucis muscle.

In most situations, the addition of a heel lift allows for the restoration of proper subtalar and midtarsal motions. However, in certain situations, the subtalar and midtarsal joint continue to pronate excessively despite use of the heel lift. This most often occurs when the decreased ankle dorsiflexion is associated with other structural malformations (such as the forefoot varus deformity) or, when prolonged pronation associated with compensation for limited

ankle dorsiflexion has produced plastic deformity of the midtarsal restraining ligaments. In these situations, it may be necessary to use an orthotic in addition to the heel lift in order to control subtalar and midtarsal joint motions fully.

The Subtalar Joint.   Subtalar joint motion may be limited by bony restrictions that block pronation and/or supination. The most common cause of a bony restriction that limits supination occurs with the triarticulated subtalar joint. This anomaly occurs in approximately 36% of the population (173) and produces a restriction that prevents continued subtalar joint supination when the anterolateral facet of the calcaneus contacts the anterolateral facet of the talus.

Another example of a bony restriction that limits the range of subtalar joint supination is the rudimentary talocalcaneal bridge. As described by Harris (174), the rudimentary talocalcaneal bridge consists of an abnormal bony mass projecting from the sustentaculum tali that blocks supination when the tip of this mass impinges the medial side of the talar body (Fig. 3.129). This bony anomaly, which is very difficult to identify with conventional x-ray techniques, acts as an osseous block that maintains the heel in an everted position.

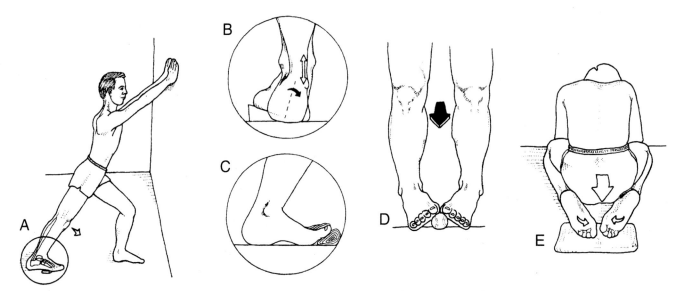

Figure 3.125. Home stretches. All of the posterior compartment muscles may be stretched with a standard calf stretch **(A).** By placing an angled piece of cork or a folded washcloth beneath the medial forefoot **(B),** the lateral fibers of the gastrocnemius muscle may be stretched. It is possible to stretch the medial fibers of the same muscle simply by placing the wedge under the lateral forefoot. The medial fibers of soleus and tibialis posterior should also be stretched with the wedge under the lateral forefoot; only the knee should be maintained in a slightly flexed position (the lateral fibers are stretched in **position B** with the knee flexed). The digital flexors can be stretched by placing a towel beneath the digits while performing bent knee calf stretches **(C).** Peroneus longus is best stretched by placing a tennis ball beneath the first metatarsal heads and then having the patient flex the knees **(D).** An alternate method of stretching peroneus longus is to have the patient abduct the hips 45°, internally rotate the lower

extremities, and slightly flex the knees: a gentle stretch should be felt along the outer leg. The anterior compartment and foot intrinsic muscles can be stretched by having the patient sit in a chair with the ankle crossed over the opposite knee. The different muscles may then be stretched as described in Figures 3.123 and 3.124. Another method of stretching the anterior compartment muscles is illustrated in **E.** By partially lowering body weight onto the plantarflexed ankles, the anterior compartment muscles are gradually lengthened. The lateral fibers of extensor digitorum longus and peroneus tertius may be accessed by adducting the forefeet *(arrows* in **E)** while placing a towel under the toes will increase the amount of stretch placed on all of the digital extensors. Of course, these are only a few of the potential home stretches, as a knowledge of each muscle's origin and insertion will allow the practitioner to prescribe any of a variety of stretches.

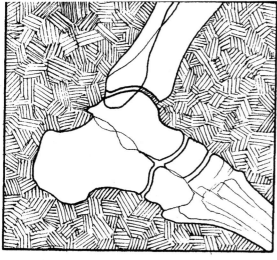

A

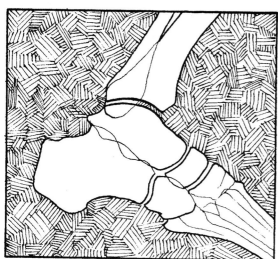

B

Figure 3.126. Comparison of the dorsal talus in a normal foot (A) and in a foot possessing a flattened talar trochlea (B). Note how the flattened talar dome is less curved, and the normal concave surface of the talar neck is absent. This deformity produces a bony block that limits ankle dorsiflexion as the thickened talar neck collides with the distal tibia. (Modified from photographs from Root MC, Orion WP, Weed JH. Normal and Abnormal Function of the Foot. Los Angeles: Clinical Biomechanics, 1977.)

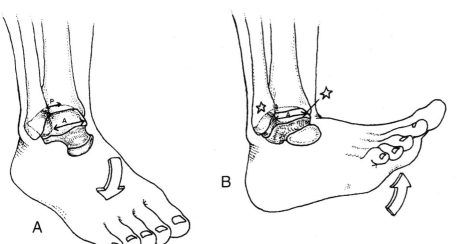

Figure 3.127. Although ankle plantarflexion is not affected (A), the foot with a wide anterior talus may dorsiflex only until the anterior talar dome engages the anterior surface of the distal talofibular articulation (*stars* in B). A = width of anterior talar dome; P = width of posterior talar dome.

Figure 3.128. The foot in A is unable to dorsiflex the ankle beyond the 90° mark, and the subtalar and midtarsal joints will most likely compensate for this deformity by pronating during late stance phase. Note how the addition of a heel lift allows this foot to move safely into its propulsive period (**B**).

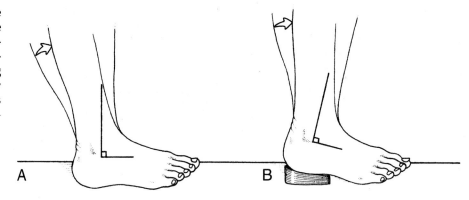

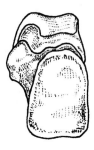 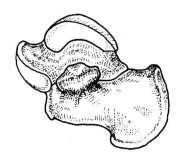

Figure 3.129. The rudimentary talocalcaneal bridge. The bony mass projecting from the sustentaculum tali acts as a bony block that limits subtalar joint supination. (Adapted from Harris RI. Rigid valgus foot due to talocalcaneal bridge. J Bone Joint Surg 1955; 37A(1): 169–183.)

In addition to anomalies that limit supination, there are also various bony blocks that limit the range of subtalar joint pronation. Because the use of triple subtalar arthrodesis is extensively used for various medical conditions, surgical fusion is the most common cause of restricted pronation.

Other causes include various tarsal coalitions (which are described in more detail in a later section) and a congenital anomaly in which the leading edge of the lateral process of the talus abuts the sinus tarsi (175). This particular malformation often results in an adhesive capsulitis of the subtalar joint (175).

Because the various bony restrictions often prevent the foot from making full plantigrade contact with the ground, treatment is to accommodate the bony restrictions by angling or posting the orthotic so as to bring the orthotic shell up to the high side of the foot (Fig. 3.130). Although the posted orthotic will not change the faulty biomechanics of the foot, it will reduce the risk of injury both to the medial knee and to the plantar lateral surface of the foot by distributing ground-reactive forces over a larger area.

First Metatarsophalangeal Joint. The characteristic degenerative changes associated with hallux limitus often produce a bony block that limits hallux dorsiflexion (Fig. 3.131). While manual techniques to restore hallux

dorsiflexion are indicated when bony changes are minimal, attempts to manipulate into a significant bony block would only accelerate the joint damage. Hiss (132) cautions against manipulating the first metatarsophalangeal joint when hallux limitus is present, stating that "every time the patient takes a step the metatarsophalangeal joint is manipulated (too much in fact) and it is this active motion of the joint that keeps the process going because of the excessive buildup of bone." Treatment in this situation requires the use of a steel shank or rocker bottom shoe to decrease the dorsiflectory moment on the first metatarsophalangeal joint (Fig. 3.132).

If the hallux limitus deformity is the result of mechanically malfunctioning foot (i.e., impaired first ray plantarflexion secondary to subtalar joint pronation), the appropriate orthotic must be prescribed in order to reestablish the propulsive period dorsal-posterior shift of the transverse metatarsophalangeal joint's axis. Surgical procedures to remove the exostoses from the dorsal first metatarsal heads should only be considered if comprehensive conservative care has failed.

Restricted Motion Resulting from Joint Dysfunction

The use of manipulation to improve function in the joints of the feet has a long and interesting history. Over 400 years ago, the early bone setters of England claimed to be particularly effective at reducing foot and hand pain by manipulating subluxations in the tarsals and carpals (176). In fact, these bonesetters singled out manipulation of the small bones of the hands and feet as one of six categories for which their treatments were particularly effective.

The importance of manipulating the foot was even acknowledged by D.D. Palmer (177) who, in his 1910 text, "The Science, Art and Philosophy of Chiropractic," stated that: "5% of all diseases are caused by displaced bones other than the vertebral column, more especially, those of the tarsus, metatarsus, and phalanges." While this may be somewhat of an overstatement, the clinical efficacy of adjustive techniques to improve function is readily apparent to anyone skilled in these procedures.

The various mobilizational and manipulative proce-

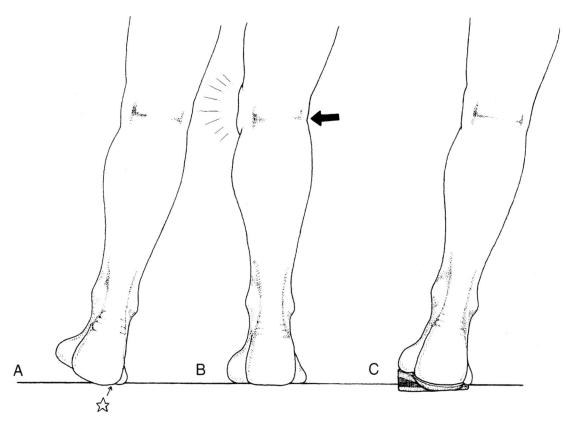

Figure 3.130. Lower extremity motion with limited subtalar joint pronation. The individual most often spends all of stance phase with weight supported beneath the lateral foot *(star in A)* or gaps the medial knee with a valgus stress **(B).** The varus post **(C)** prevents compensatory knee motions and distributes plantar pressures over a larger area.

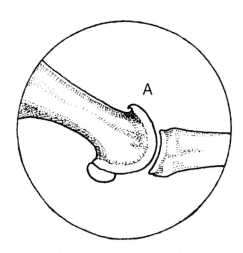

Figure 3.131. A dorsal exostosis on the first metatarsal head (A) often limits hallux dorsiflexion.

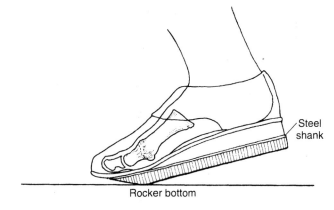

Figure 3.132. Addition of a steel shank or rocker bottom allows for a pain-free propulsion, even in the presence of ankylosis.

dures are used to break down the collagen fibral cross-linkages associated with prolonged disuse/immobilization and to restore the normal accessory motions necessary for a joint to move through its full range of motion. In a detailed study delineating histological changes associated with immobilization, Woo et al. (178) provided quantitative evidence that mobilization does, indeed, break down the collagen cross-fibers formed during immobilization.

In addition to being essential for nonrestricted range of motion, the restoration of a smooth end-play allows the articulations of the feet to dampen ground-reactive forces more effectively through the natural springiness or elasticity associated with stressing healthy connective tissue. Hiss (132), who has had the experience of adjusting several hundred thousand feet, stated that although it can takes months to restore motion to an old fibrotic foot ("it takes a lot of pounding to drive a nail into hard wood"), sometimes even the slightest increase movement can often spell the difference between pain and complete relief. Figures 3.134 through 3.157 illustrate the various manual techniques for joints of the foot and ankle.

Note that these procedures are not intended to represent a cookbook formula for manipulation. Rather, by coupling a thorough understanding of articular architecture with the experience gained by palpating motion barriers in thousands of feet, the practitioner is encouraged to modify the line of drives, contact points, and forces in ways that best suit each patient's individual needs. Maitland (179) describes five graded oscillations that may be used while performing these procedures (Fig. 3.133).

The decision of whether to mobilize or manipulate is dependent upon the practitioner's experience with these techniques. Because an improperly applied manipulation may potentially damage the joint, use of a high-velocity thrust should only be attempted by those experienced with such techniques. Although Good (180) claims that cavitation or cracking the dysfunctional joint is necessary for treatment to be completely successful, this claim is unfounded.

The only difference between mobilization and manipulation is that manipulation occurs so rapidly that it generates a negative pressure capable of pulling gases out of the synovial fluid. (Cavitation refers to the process of creating a cavity, in this case, a vacuum.) Because mobilization occurs more slowly, the vacuum never becomes strong enough to pull gases out of the synovial fluid. However, it is not the cavitation that produces the favorable response, but rather, the breaking of collagen cross-fibrils associated with the separation of joint surfaces.

The fact that mobilization effectively breaks these cross-links was demonstrated in the study by Woo et al. (178) in which the fibrotic joints were mobilized at the rate of 1 cycle of flexion/extension every 5 seconds (three cycles were performed, with the majority of changes occurring during the first cycle).

Although clinical experience suggests that manipulation more quickly restores motion, this has never been conclusively demonstrated. In fact, in many situations, the joints of the feet are so tightly articulated that even the high- velocity thrust of manipulation cannot create a sufficient separation of the articular surfaces to cavitate the joint. This is particularly true for the intercuneiform and the navicular-cuneiform articulations. In these situations, it is best to take the advice of Paris (181), who suggests mobilizing the very stiff joints and manipulating the slightly stiff joints. Using this approach, it is not uncommon for an extremely fibrotic joint to become so flexible that, over time, the joints can be effectively manipulated with a minimal amount of force.

It should be noted that the most common cause for injury associated with manual techniques is failure of the practitioner to evaluate motion barriers properly, thereby identifying a hypermobile joint prior to manipulation. This is especially important with the talocrural joint, where many practitioners routinely incorporate long axis manipulation as part of a postinversion sprain treatment regimen. (This is most likely because the popping noise associated with this manipulation gives both the practitioner and the patient a sense that something that was "out of place" is now "in place.")

Because repeated manipulation damages the already weakened restraining ligaments, it may be responsible for chronic pain pattern and/or recurrent injury. Treatment in this situation should include strengthening exercises, proprioceptive exercises, and manipulation of the neighboring hypomobile joints, not manipulation of the hypermobile talocrural joint. In addition to the dangers associated with manipulating hypermobile joints, manipulation is also contraindicated during the acute stages of inflammation, in the presence of active inflammatory disease, and when motion is restricted by a bony block.

Keeping these contraindications in mind, the following section will review the various manipulative/mobilizational techniques for each joint of the foot and ankle.

Manipulative Techniques

The Metatarsophalangeal and Interphalangeal Joints. All of these joints should possess an appreciable elastic spring when stressed in long axis extension. To perform this maneuver on a metatarsophalangeal joint, the ex-

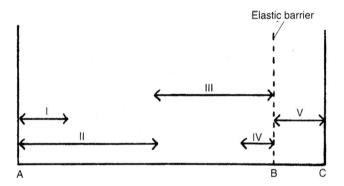

Figure 3.133. (A–C) The five graded oscillations used during manual therapy. *I* = small amplitude movement near the starting position; *II* = large amplitude movement near the starting position; *III* = large amplitude movement ending at the elastic barrier; *IV* = small amplitude movement bordering the elastic barrier; *V* = manipulation: a small-amplitude, high-velocity thrust accessing the paraphysiological space but not exceeding the anatomical limit of movement.

aminer should firmly grasp the proximal phalanx and gradually traction the joint in long axis extension (Fig. 3.134). If joint dysfunction is present, a short fast thrust is delivered once the end-range is reached.

These joints should also be evaluated by rotating the proximal phalanx on the fixed metatarsal. If a hard end feel is noted on rotating the phalanx, a manipulation may be performed by simultaneously rotating the phalanx while applying a dynamic thrust in long axis extension. Note that it is not uncommon for the toes in a chronically pronated foot to require rotational manipulations to reduce the varus position of the proximal phalanges. This test position is also used when evaluating medial and lateral side tilt.

As illustrated in Figure 3.135, lateral tilt at the second metatarsophalangeal joint is checked by tractioning the proximal phalanx with the right hand while simultaneously abducting it on the stabilized metatarsal head, which is being contacted on its dorsal and plantar surface by the thumb and index finger of the left hand. If joint dysfunction is present, a manipulation is performed with the left hand, driving through the metatarsal head while the right hand continues to traction and abduct the phalanx. To evaluate these joints in medial tilt, the hands are switched, and the process is repeated.

The metatarsophalangeal and interphalangeal joints should also be evaluated for superior-inferior glide. On reaching its full range of plantarflexion, each of these joints should possess an appreciable amount of inferior glide of the distal articulation on the proximal articulation. Conversely, the end-range of dorsiflexion should include a slight superior glide of the distal articulation on the proximal articulation. Unfortunately, digital deformity often results in contracture in the dorsal metatarsophalangeal joint capsule that limits the range of inferior glide. This is particularly true with claw toe deformity.

If this gliding motion is limited, the manipulation illustrated in Figure 3.136 may be performed in which the proximal phalanx is plantarflexed by the thumb while the index finger drives the metatarsal head superiorly. This manipulation, which is accomplished with a gentle squeezing motion, may be facilitated by tractioning the proximal phalanx in long axis extension and by performing several hold-relax stretches prior to delivering the adjustment in order to relax the digital extensor musculature. Note that superior glide at the metatarsophalangeal joints is rarely lost and when restriction in this motion is noted at the interphalangeal joints, it may be restored with simple long axis manipulation performed while stabilizing the more proximal phalanx.

It should also be noted that an invaluable form of treatment for metatarsophalangeal joint pain is to add a compressive component when evaluating the joints. As described by Maitland (182), this process involves positioning the digit in a midrange position and adding a compressive

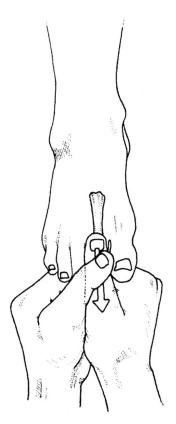

Figure 3.134. Long axis extension at the second metatarsophalangeal joint.

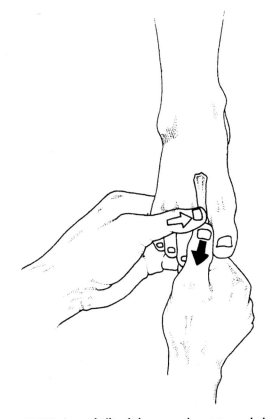

Figure 3.135. Lateral tilt of the second metatarsophalangeal joint.

Figure 3.136. Inferior glide of proximal phalanx on metatarsal head.

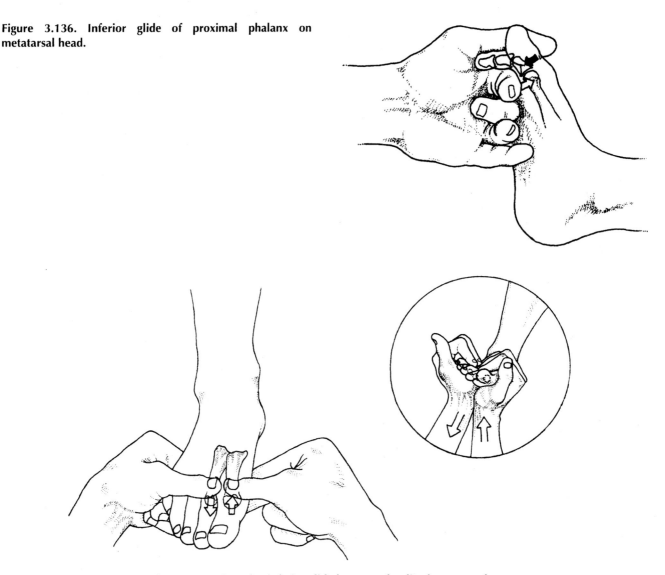

Figure 3.137. Superior-inferior glide between the distal metatarsals.

force while simultaneously applying a small-amplitude abduction-adduction and/or rotational motion. (These movements are applied in an oscillatory manner with a range of motion not to exceed 10°.) Because this procedure is performed with the digit in a midline position, neither the joint capsule nor the stabilizing ligaments are stretched in any way, thereby giving the practitioner information that could not have been attained with noncompressive tests.

The classic example of when this procedure should be used is on the individual presenting with a stubbed toe. Normally, such a patient will report no pain on passive testing, but the addition of a compressive force will often produce excruciating pain. This being the case, treatment would consist of small-amplitude oscillatory motions performed while gently compressing the joint. As patient tolerance improves, the compressive force is gradually increased until the symptoms are gone. Repeated treatments, which are readily performed by the patient at home, are remarkably effective at reducing pain associated with this type of injury.

Although the exact mechanism for the surprising success rate of this treatment is unclear, it is possible that stimulation of mechanoreceptors in the subjacent bone blocks a pain cycle associated with reflex sympathetic impairment. Maitland (152) stated that the joints most often requiring treatment with compression are the first metatarsophalangeal joints, the hip joint, the glenohumeral joint, the patellofemoral joint, and the carpometacarpal joint of the thumb.

The Distal Intermetatarsal Joints. Normally, a superior-inferior gliding motion is present between all of the metatarsal heads. Because the central metatarsal heads are stabilized by the strongest ligaments, intermetatarsal motion is least between the second and third metatarsals, slightly greater between the neighboring metatarsals, and greatest between the fourth and fifth metatarsals. The range of movement may be evaluated by grasping the heads of adjacent metatarsals between the thumbs and index fingers and alternately shearing up and down (Fig. 3.137).

Another method of contacting the metatarsals is illustrated in the inset in Figure 3.137. If motion is restricted between any of the metatarsals, a Grade 4 mobilization is performed to patient tolerance. It is of clinical interest that restricted superior-inferior glide between the second and third metatarsals is a common cause for intermetatarsophalangeal bursitis between the third and fourth metatarsals.

The Tarsometatarsal Joints. These joints may be evaluated with any of several different maneuvers. First, superior-inferior glide is checked by stabilizing each metatarsal's proximal tarsal and alternately dorsiflexing and plantarflexing the desired metatarsal.

For example, in Figure 3.138, the cuboid-fourth metatarsal articulation is stabilized with the left hand while the shaft of the fourth metatarsal is stressed in dorsiflexion/plantarflexion. A restricted end-range in superior glide between the fourth or fifth tarsometatarsal articulation may be manipulated by stabilizing the dorsal cuboid while applying a dynamic thrust through the plantar base of the involved metatarsal. (A pisiform contact may also used on the plantar metatarsal; see Fig. 3.139.) Conversely, inferior glide at the fourth and fifth tarsometatarsal joints may be restored by stabilizing the plantar cuboid with the center finger while thrusting downward upon the dorsal metatarsal base (thenar eminence contact; see Fig. 3.140).

Because the central metatarsals are so firmly attached to the cuneiforms, superior-inferior gliding motions at these tarsometatarsal articulations are best restored by vigorously mobilizing the proximal metatarsals with the grip illustrated in the inset of Figure 3.137. It is also possible to mobilize these articulations with a grip similar to the one illustrated in Figure 3.138 in which the left hand securely stabilizes the proximal cuneiform while the right hand vigorously inverts and everts the forefoot, thereby dorsiflexing and plantarflexing the desired tarsometatarsal articulation.

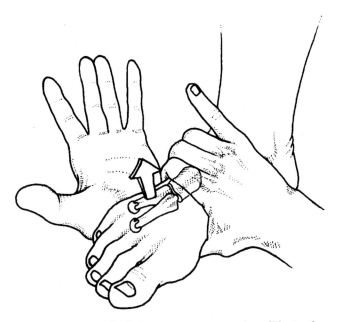

Figure 3.139. Manipulation to restore superior glide to the fifth tarsometatarsal articulation.

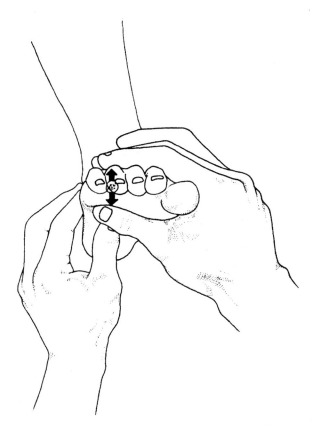

Figure 3.138. Evaluation of superior-inferior glide at the cuboid-fourth metatarsal articulation.

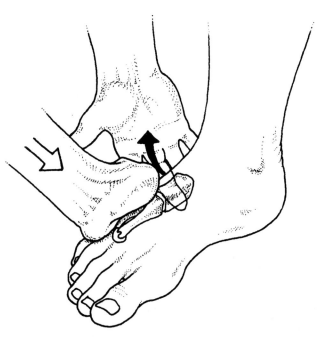

Figure 3.140. Manipulation to restore inferior glide to the fifth tarsometatarsal articulation.

With regards to the first tarsometatarsal articulation, a very effective method of restoring inferior glide is with the manipulation illustrated in Figure 3.141. In this manipulation, the patient is supine as the practitioner's right hand contacts the first metatarsal between the middle phalanx of the index finger and the thenar eminence. The left hand then "hooks" the medial cuneiform with the third finger and tractions upwardly (black arrow) as the right hand begins to plantarflex the first metatarsal. As the joint reaches its endrange, the palm of the left hand wraps securely over the dorsal midfoot.

The manipulation is given with the left wrist extending (thereby providing tractioning on the medial cuneiform upwardly via contact with the third finger) and the right wrist radially deviating (which allows the thenar eminence to plantarflex the first metatarsal). The practitioner's chest is directly over the patient's foot so that a long axis traction may be applied during the manipulation. Interestingly, Hiss (132) noted that joint dysfunction in the first tarsometatarsal articulation, which is almost always present in a chronically pronated foot, is a common cause of decreased proprioception.

An alternate method of restoring inferior glide at the first tarsometatarsal articulation is to contact the dorsal first metatarsal with the center finger while the palmar aspect of the opposite hand contacts the plantar surface of the second metatarsal (Fig. 3.142). By gradually increasing the shearing force between the first and second metatarsals, the practitioner can build up to a dynamic thrust with which the first metatarsal is plantarflexed and everted while the second metatarsal is stabilized against the palm of the left hand. This process may be repeated to restore inferior glide at all of the tarsometatarsal articulations simply by moving the contact points laterally, i.e., contacting the plantar third metatarsal while shearing the dorsal second metatarsal inferiorly, etc. Note that this manipulation is invaluable when attempting to reduce a functional forefoot varus deformity.

Superior glide at the tarsometatarsal articulations may be evaluated and treated by positioning the hands as in Figure 3.143A. By placing the pisiform of the right hand against the plantar first metatarsal shaft with the palmar surface of the left hand contacting the dorsal second metatarsal shaft, a shearing force is developed by contracting the pectoralis musculature (the practitioner's chest is positioned directly over the patient's foot) that drives the first metatarsal superiorly and the second metatarsal inferiorly (Fig. 3.143B).

This manipulation may be repeated at any of the tarsometatarsal articulations and is particularly useful when attempting to reduce a functional plantarflexed first ray and/or functional forefoot valgus deformity. It should also be noted that it is possible to restore a restricted range of

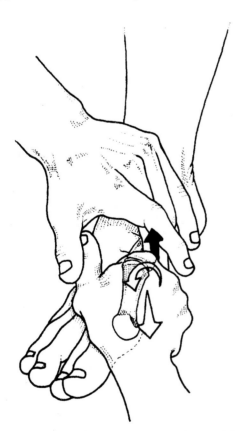

Figure 3.141. Manipulation to restore inferior glide to first tarsometatarsal articulation.

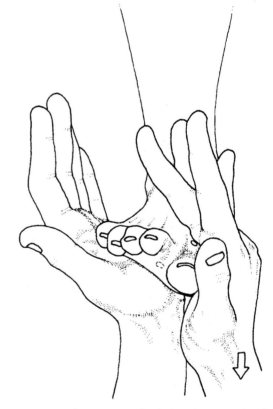

Figure 3.142. Alternate manipulation for restoring inferior glide at tarsometatarsal articulations.

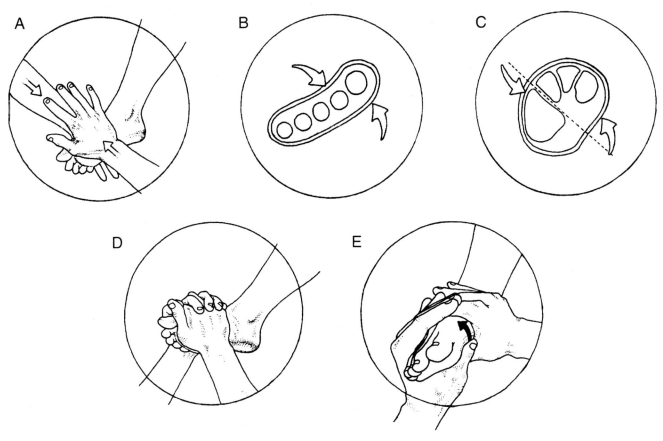

Figure 3.143. (A–E) Superior glide at tarsometatarsal and intertarsal joints.

forefoot inversion with this manipulation by moving the hands proximally over the midfoot and generating a force that drives the cuneiforms upward and the cuboid downward (Fig. 3.143C). Note that many practitioners prefer to use the grips illustrated in Figures 3.143D and E when performing these manipulations.

Perhaps the most effective treatment for restoring superior glide at the tarsometatarsal and intertarsal joints is with the manipulation illustrated in Figure 3.144. In this manipulation, the left hand dorsiflexes and inverts the proximal first metatarsal while the right hand is shearing the medial cuneiform inferiorly. To manipulate the intertarsal and midtarsal articulations, the hands are moved proximally so as to contact the cuneiform-navicular articulations and the talonavicular articulation, respectively. It is also possible to restore inferior glide at these articulations simply by reversing hand positions and actions.

The Midtarsal Joints. Like the tarsometatarsal and intertarsal joints, the midtarsal joints should also possess superior-inferior gliding motions. In addition to the shearing manipulation illustrated in Figure 3.144, superior-inferior gliding motions may also be restored with the manipulation illustrated in Figure 3.145.

In this procedure, the left hand stabilizes the heel by making firm contact proximal to the midtarsal articulations

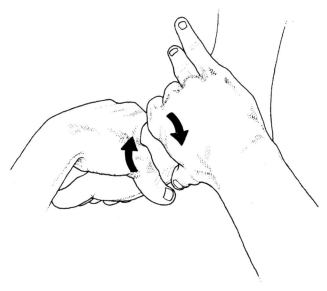

Figure 3.144. Superior-inferior glide at tarsometatarsal articulations.

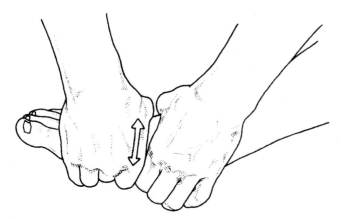

Figure 3.145. Superior-inferior glide at the midtarsal joints.

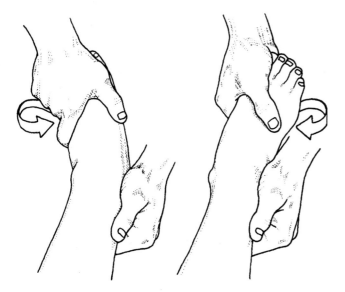

Figure 3.146. Figure eight mobilization of the midtarsal joint.

while the right hand creates a strong superior-inferior shearing force on the fixated rearfoot. Mennell (150) emphasizes that the thumb and index finger of the left hand must be carefully positioned over the navicular and cuboid to ensure that the shearing motion is produced at the proper joints. He goes on to state that the "resilience of the foot to take up the stresses and strains of function" largely depends on the superior-inferior gliding motions of the cuneiform bones on the navicular and the navicular on the talus.

A generalized manipulation that is very effective at restoring superior-inferior glide at the midtarsal joint is illustrated in Figure 3.146. To perform this manipulation, the left hand securely stabilizes the calcaneus while the right hand grasps the forefoot. The right hand then moves the forefoot through a figure-eight pattern while the left hand continues to stabilize the fixated rearfoot. This manipulation is very effective at restoring the limited range of midtarsal motion that often results from cast immobilization.

A more specific adjustment for restoring inferior glide

at the midtarsal joint is illustrated in Figure 3.147. While the thumb of the right hand stabilizes the distal calcaneus, the thenar eminence of the left hand drives through the dorsolateral forefoot (black arrow) while simultaneously inverting the forefoot (white arrow). By varying contact points, this adjustment may be used on any of the tarsals and is particularly effective for restoring inferior glide at the central tarsometatarsal joints.

In addition to superior-inferior glide, different foot types will present with a loss of other gliding motions. For example, the navicular in an individual with a rigid cavovarus foot will often be maintained in an adducted position that results in the loss of lateral glide of the navicular upon the talar head. This motion may be restored by stabilizing the talar head with the tip of the thumb while the opposite hand abducts the forefoot (thereby gliding the navicular laterally across the talus; see Fig. 3.148). This procedure may also be used to glide the cuboid laterally over the stabilized calcaneus (Fig. 3.149).

It is also not uncommon for an individual with a severely pronated foot to present with an inability of the cuboid to supinate on the calcaneus. (This is because the cuboid in a pronated foot is maintained in an abducted and dorsiflexed position for so long that capsular contracture prevents plantar-medial gliding of the cuboid on the calcaneus.) This being the case, calcaneocuboid supination may be restored via the manipulation illustrated in Figure 3.150, in which the right hand everts the calcaneus (pisiform contact on medial calcaneus) while the left hand plantarflexes and inverts the cuboid (pisiform contact on lateral cuboid). This motion is performed gently, as if one is squeezing clay. It is noteworthy that Hiss (132) claimed that calca-

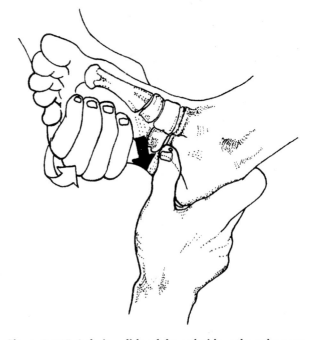

Figure 3.147. Inferior glide of the cuboid on the calcaneus.

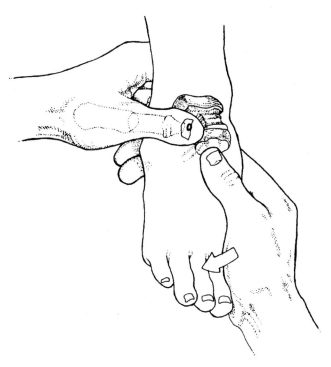

Figure 3.148. Lateral glide of the navicular on the talus.

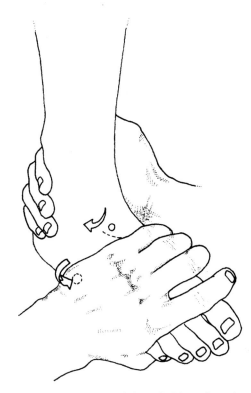

Figure 3.150. Supination of the cuboid on the calcaneus.

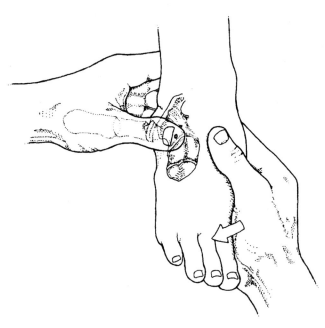

Figure 3.149. Lateral glide of the cuboid on the calcaneus.

neocuboid joint dysfunction is a common cause of recurrent inversion ankle sprain.

In addition to the gliding motions already described, Mennell (150) noted that there is a wide range of intertarsal movements (usually superior-inferior in direction) that "cannot be appreciated clinically unless there has been traumatic subluxation of one of the bones upon another." Hiss

(132) noted that these subluxations, which are usually in a plantar direction and produce pain with dorsal compression, may be corrected with the adjustment illustrated in Figure 3.151.

This manipulation involves positioning the standing patient so that the sole of the foot is presented to the practitioner. Contact points are then taken by crossing the thumbs beneath the subluxated tarsal. The adjustment is then given by driving the thumbs superiorly through the involved tarsal while slightly plantarflexing the forefoot. As the thrust is given, the foot is brought downward to help open the tarsals, and the wrists are relaxed so as not to injure the ankle mortise. Also, when performing this adjustment on a subluxated cuboid (which Newell and Woodle [183] claim is maintained in an everted position secondary to contracture of the peroneus longus muscle), the contact point with the thumbs should be made beneath the plantar-medial cuboid, and the line of drive should be in a superolateral direction in order to reduce the rotational component of subluxated cuboid.

It is of interest that Hiss (132) claimed that a subluxated cuboid may cause interdigital neuritis as it compresses the lateral plantar nerve and may also result in chronic pain beneath the lateral plantar foot, as the quadratus plantae muscle may be repeatedly contused.

The Subtalar Joint.   While John McM. Mennell repeatedly demonstrated a knowledge of functional anatomy that was far ahead of his time, perhaps his greatest contribu-

Figure 3.151. Reduction of plantar subluxations.

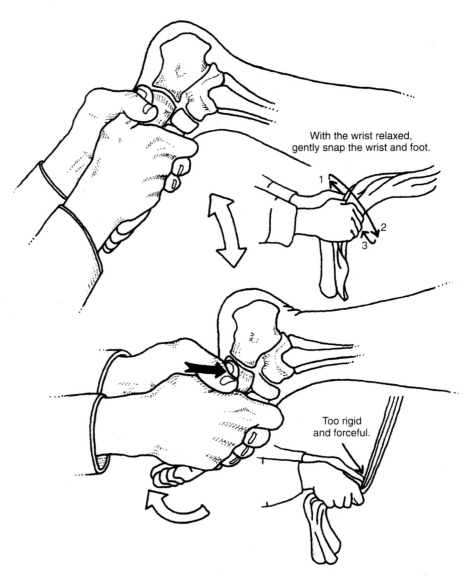

With the wrist relaxed, gently snap the wrist and foot.

Too rigid and forceful.

tion to the field of manipulative rehabilitation was his description of subtalar joint function. While other anatomists in the 1950s and 1960s discussed subtalar joint motion only as it related to passive ranges of inversion and eversion, Mennell was describing subtle rocking motions between the talus and calcaneus that absorb shear forces at heel strike and toe off and act to prevent injury about the ankle complex when the foot/ankle is sprained or stubbed (150). In fact, Mennell (150) states that if it were not for these involuntary rocking and gliding motions, "fracture dislocations around the ankle would be commonplace."

These joint play movements, which consist of long axis extension, forward and backward glide, and medial and lateral side tilt, may be elicited in the following manner. The supine patient is positioned with the hip abducted and externally rotated, with the knee flexed 90°, and with the ankle in its neutral position. While sitting on the edge of the examining table, the practitioner places his or her back

against the patient's distal thigh while firmly grabbing the foot just below the ankle (Fig. 3.152). The examiner then leans back against the patient's distal femur (A) while maintaining a counterforce along the long axis of the tibia (B). This long axis force is transferred equally through the webs of both hands, where it opens the talocrural and subtalar joints in long axis extension. If joint dysfunction is present, a dynamic thrust is applied at the end-range of this movement.

This position also allows for evaluation of forward glide of the calcaneus beneath the talus (which was previously illustrated in Fig. 3.115). By stabilizing the anterior talus with the right hand, the examiner's left hand gently glides the calcaneus forward beneath the talus (C) while maintaining a long axis traction on the joint. Backward glide can be evaluated by reversing hand actions so the left hand serves as the stabilizer while the right hand glides the calcaneus posteriorly (D). It is possible to evaluate lateral

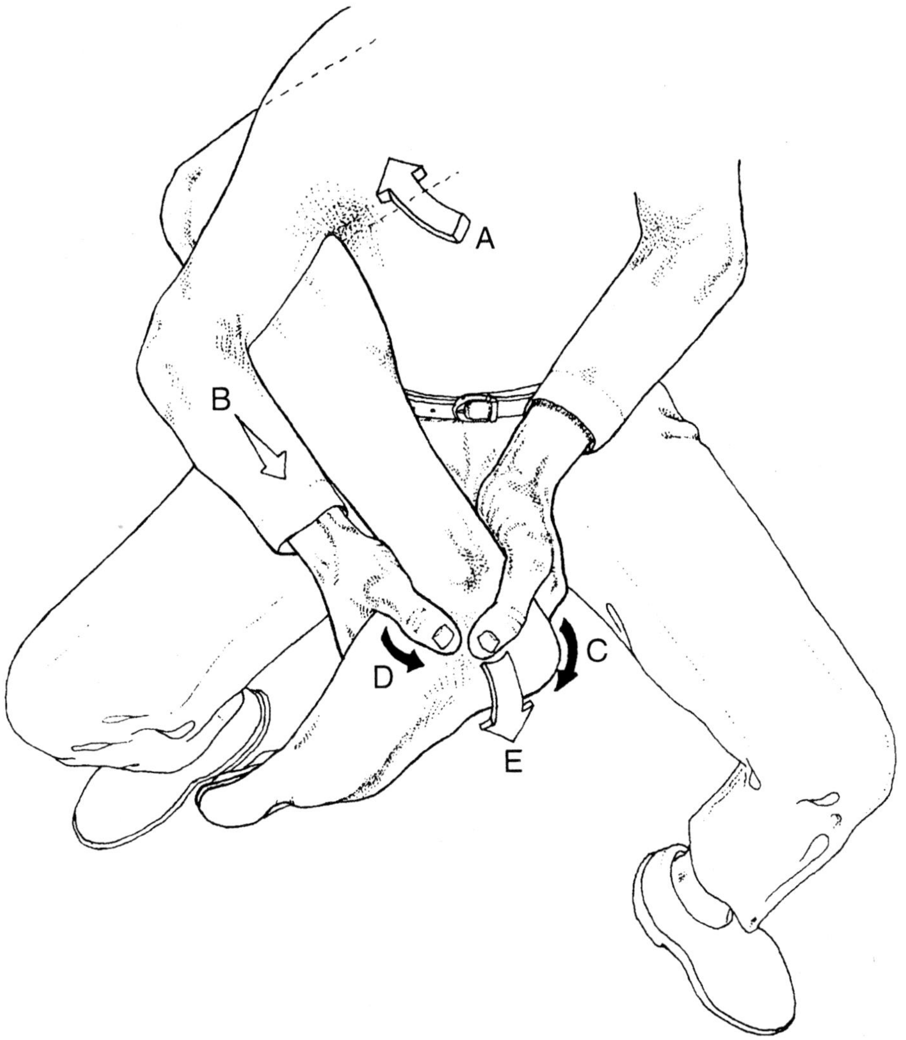

Figure 3.152. (A–E) Evaluation of subtalar joint motions.

tilt by maintaining the long axis traction while everting the calcaneus (E). Medial tilt, which is frequently lost following inversion sprain of the ankle, is evaluated by inverting the calcaneus with the tips of the lesser digits. If joint dysfunction is noted in any of these testing positions, a gentle manipulation may be performed by continuing the test movement while simultaneously tractioning on the subtalar joint. Care must be taken when performing these procedures, as the practitioner can generate a surprising amount of long axis traction by leaning back into the patient's thigh.

An alternate method for adjusting the subtalar joint in medial or lateral side tilt is illustrated in Figure 3.153. While maintaining the subtalar joint in long axis traction, lateral tilt may be restored by having the palm of the right hand evert the calcaneus while the left hand drives through the talus (thereby shearing the calcaneus laterally beneath the talus). To manipulate the subtalar joint in medial tilt, the hand positions and movements are reversed.

Another manipulation for restoring forward glide of calcaneus beneath the talus is illustrated in Figure 3.154. In

this adjustment, the plantar heel is stabilized by friction from the examining table while the crossed thumbs apply a posterior shear force through the talus. Initially, a force is applied gently, causing the talus to glide posteriorly on the fixated calcaneus. When performed properly, a smooth gliding motion should be felt, and the forefoot should lift slightly off the examining table. At the joint's end-range, a springy end-play should be noted as the crossed thumbs push into the elastic barrier. If joint dysfunction is present, several short dynamic thrusts may be applied at this end-range.

The Talocrural Joint. This joint should possess both long axis extension and anterior-posterior glide. Long axis extension may be evaluated with the same testing procedure used in Figure 3.152 or, more commonly, by hooking the talar neck with crossed fingers and tractioning inferiorly (Fig. 3.155). If joint dysfunction is noted, a dynamic thrust is applied by tractioning the joint in long axis extension while slightly radially deviating the wrists (black arrow). Anterior-posterior glide of the talocrural joint may be evaluated as illustrated in Figure 3.156. A loss of either

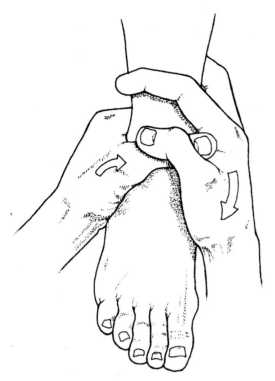

Figure 3.153. Manipulation to restore lateral tilt to the subtalar joint.

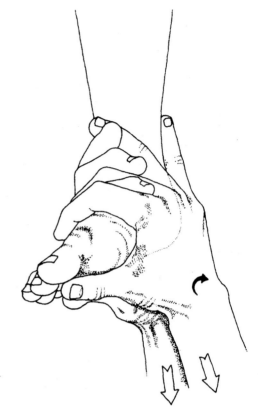

Figure 3.155. Long axis extension of the talocrural joint.

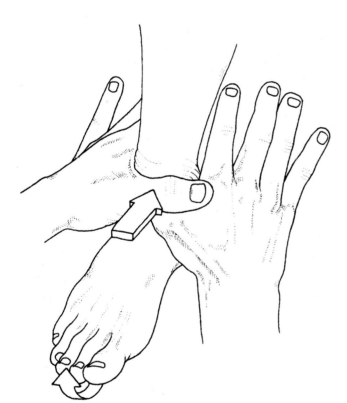

Figure 3.154. Manipulation to restore forward glide of the calcaneus beneath the talus.

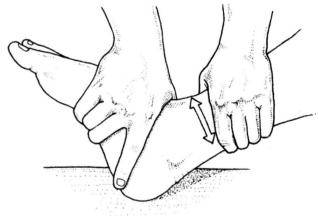

Figure 3.156. Evaluation of anterior-posterior glide at the talocrural joint.

of these motions may usually be restored by vigorously mobilizing the joint in this test position.

Distal Tibiofibular Joint. Although this is a fibrous syndesmotic joint, it should still possess a clinically appreciable range of anterior-posterior glide (Fig. 3.157). Dysfunction in this joint may be addressed by gradually increasing a Grade 4 mobilization until the desired motion has been restored. Note that motion in the distal tibiofibular

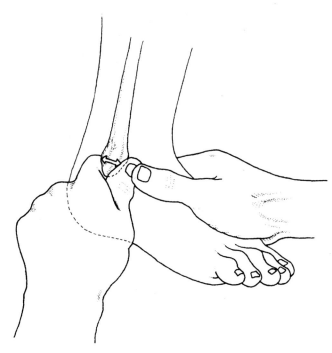

Figure 3.157. Evaluation of anterior-posterior glide at the distal tibiofibular joint.

joints should always be compared bilaterally to get a reference for norm.

NEUROMOTOR COORDINATION AND PROPRIOCEPTION

This is one of the more important criteria for normal function since a well-coordinated patient may be able to tolerate even large structural malformations without injury, while the uncoordinated patient may be constantly injured as he or she responds to even minor changes in terrain with uncontrolled, potentially injurious movement patterns. An extreme example of this is the destructive joint changes associated with the neurotrophic arthropathies, i.e., Charcot's joint.

While neuromotor coordination may be impaired secondary to upper or lower motor neuron lesions, a much more likely cause for dysfunction occurs when either disuse or injury damages the sensory receptors so that they are no longer able to provide enough position sense information to initiate the desired motor response. Position sense or proprioceptive information is supplied by neural input originating from receptors located in the muscles, tendons, joint capsules, and other associated deep tissues. These proprioceptors are categorized into three different groups: muscle proprioceptors, proprioceptors of the joints and skin, and labyrinthine and neck proprioceptors. As a group, proprioceptors relay constant information regarding static and dynamic joint positions, i.e., some of these receptors are slow to adapt and discharge only when the joint is held at a

specific angle, while others are rapidly adapting and discharge in bursts to signal changes in acceleration or tension.

The muscle proprioceptors consist of the muscle spindle and the Golgi tendon organs (GTOs). Spindles, which are presently considered to be the most important receptor for kinesthetic awareness (184), are located in parallel series with contractile muscle fibers and consist of fluid-filled capsules 2 to 20 mm long, enclosing 5–12 small specialized muscle fibers referred to as nuclear chain and nuclear bag fibers. Collectively, they are referred to as intrafusal fibers (see Fig. 3.158).

The nuclear bag fibers are very sensitive to stretch and, via primary afferents, relay information regarding dynamic changes in muscle length, i.e., phasic responses. Conversely, the nuclear chain, which is innervated by both annulospiral and flower spray nerve endings, relays information regarding the static position of muscle fibers, i.e., tonic responses. The sensitivity in which these receptors will discharge can be preset by activating the gamma-motor neurons: by producing contraction at the polar ends of the intrafusal fibers, the gamma-motor neurons increase tension on the central portions of the chain and bag (particularly the bag), producing a heightened sensitivity to a change in length (Fig. 3.159). The process of setting spindle sensitivity via gamma-motor neuron activity is referred to as gamma-bias.

The gamma-motor neurons may also produce voluntary movement via an indirect pathway known as the gamma-loop. In this pathway, signals from the pyramidal tract, which in a more direct pathway would travel directly to the α-motor neurons to produce movement, activate the gamma-motor neurons to tense polar portions of intrafusal fibers to the point of stimulating their afferents. This in turn sends a signal back to the cord, which traverses a monosynaptic pathway to activate the appropriate α-motor neuron. Although this obviously occurs at a much slower rate, stimulation of the gamma-loop system is associated with a greater control of muscular actions. In most situations, voluntary movements are accomplished by a combination of direct and indirect (via gamma-loop) activation of the α-motor neurons referred to as alpha-gamma coactivation.

While activation of spindle afferents will result in reflex contraction of the neighboring muscle fibers, activation of the Golgi tendon organs (which are located in the tendon fibers near the muscle tendon junctions) will produce autogenic inhibition or relaxation of the involved muscle. Because muscles are capable of producing greater contractile forces than their own structural makeup can withstand, the Golgi tendon organs play a protective role by inhibiting contraction (and facilitating the antagonist), should the contractile force become too great.

Although these receptors have relatively low thresholds (i.e., the GTOs located in a cat's soleus muscle will discharge with an applied force of less than 0.1 g [215]) their inhibitory effect may be offset by the annulospiral ac-

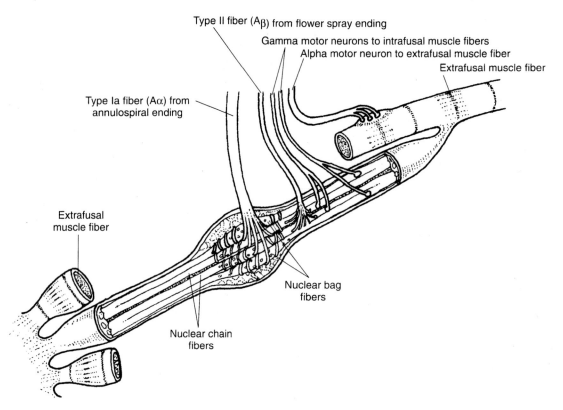

Figure 3.158. The intrafusal fiber and its innervation. (Modified from Netter F. The Nervous System. Part One, Anatomy and Physiology. West Caldwell, NJ: The CIBA Collection of Medical Illustrations, 1983: 1985.)

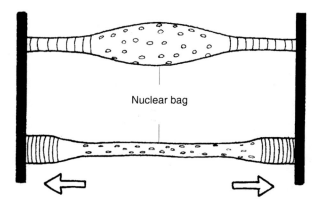

Figure 3.159. Stimulation of the gamma motor neurons produces contraction at the polar ends of the intrafusal fibers (arrows), which creates a heightened sensitivity in these fibers, as the nuclear region is now tensed. (Modified from Gowitzke BA, Milner M. Scientific Bases of Human Movement. Ed 3. Baltimore: Williams & Wilkins, 1988.)

tivity associated with voluntary movement. In fact, success with strength training depends upon the ability of the athlete to learn how to inhibit information from Golgi tendon organs successfully.

In a study delineating interactions between annulospiral and GTO fibers, Hufschmidt (187) found that a stimulus sufficient to excite both the annulospiral and Golgi tendon organs produces only facilitation, indicating that the inhibiting effect of the Golgi tendon organ can somehow be cancelled. It seems that although the GTOs supply the cord with constant feedback regarding the forces acting on the muscle, they may produce inhibition only when dangerously high tension levels are reached.

Unlike the muscle proprioceptors (GTOs and spindles), joint and skin proprioceptors travel all the way to the cortex and, because their receptors connect with so many interneurons, they are able to favorably modify activity in all limbs, not just in the stimulated limb. In addition, joint and skin receptors also have a facilitatory effect upon the vestibular apparatus which, by enhancing activity in specific motor neurons, acts to stabilize the extremities during the gait cycle by stimulating the requisite muscles to contract with more force.

When properly functioning, the various joint, skin, and muscle proprioceptors work together to supply the central nervous system with a constant barrage of sensory information regarding body position and movements. In ways that are still poorly understood, the central nervous system analyzes this information by comparing it to a desired pattern (which nature, conditioning, and past experiences have established) and produces an appropriate motor response. The cycle is then immediately repeated, wherein each response is analyzed and the movements are fine-tuned.

A perfect example of how proprioceptors interact to produce a desired movement occurs during the positive supporting reaction. In this reflex, the weight of the body pressing upon the foot spreads the metatarsophalangeal and interphalangeal joints and stretches the interossei muscles. In turn, information from the stimulated muscle and joint proprioceptors produces immediate reflex contraction of the extensor musculature, thereby converting the entire lower extremity into a firm but compliant pillar.

The importance of the foot proprioceptors is clear to anyone who has ever had his or her foot fall asleep after sitting cross-legged; upon standing, it is not uncommon for the knee to buckle as the temporary anesthesia associated with circulatory impairment inhibits the positive supporting reaction. O'Connell and Gardner (188) verified the significance of the foot proprioceptors by performing an experiment in which a blind-folded individual was suddenly dropped from an elevated chair onto a gymnasium floor mat. (By randomly raising and lowering the chair various amounts prior to the release, the subject lost accurate sense of distance to the mat.) In the first two trials, when the foot proprioceptors were left intact, the individual readily regained balance upon contacting the floor. However, in the third trial, the foot proprioceptors were anesthetized by submerging them in ice water for 20 minutes. Upon contacting the floor during this trial, the individual immediately crumbled to the mat as reflexive extension of the lower extremity did not occur. It is of clinical significance that shoe gear that inhibits abduction of the digits (such as pointed dress shoes) may also inhibit the positive supporting reaction (186).

In addition to the stability afforded by the muscle and joint proprioceptors, the importance of skin proprioceptors (particularly Meissner's corpuscles) was recently demonstrated in a particularly interesting study by Robbins et al. (189).

These researchers demonstrated that reflex response to noxious stimulation of the plantar cutaneous receptors varies in relation to the location of the stimuli, i.e., stimulation of the skin under the metatarsophalangeal joint produces reflex contraction of the digital plantarflexors (which allows for a redistribution of ground-reactive forces away from the metatarsal heads toward the distal digits) while stimulation of the skin under the medial longitudinal arch has the opposite effect in that it causes the digits to reflexively dorsiflex (which concentrates pressure beneath the metatarsal heads as ground-reactive forces are no longer distributed equally between the metatarsal heads and the distal digits).

Robbins et al. (189) contend that inappropriate use of arch supports may result in stimulation of the skin beneath the medial longitudinal arch, thereby exposing the metatarsal heads to trauma, as the digits are no longer able to plantarflex with full force. They also contend that excessive cushioning placed beneath the metatarsal heads may

reduce the proprioceptive information supplied by skin receptors, thereby lessening the plantarflectory force developed by the digits. Because of their research findings, Robbins et al. (189) claim that inappropriate stimulation of the skin receptors beneath the arch and/or excessive cushioning beneath the metatarsal heads may result in a "pseudo-neurotrophic arthropathy" of the metatarsophalangeal joints. They support this hypothesis by noting that shod populations have a greater incidence of osteoarthrosis at the metatarsophalangeal joints, while unshod populations have a greater incidence of osteoarthrosis at the distal interphalangeal joints (190).

Given the delicate balance between afferent and efferent discharges, it should be clear that even slight impairment of the proprioceptive system will detrimentally affect the appropriate motor response. This situation may result in injury, as the muscular reaction to a given stimuli may occur too late to protect the joint. In fact, Lentell et al. (191) demonstrated that individuals with recurrent ankle sprains usually present with proprioceptive deficits, not strength deficits, as is most commonly reported. Impaired proprioception may also be responsible for more subtle symptoms, as recent investigation (192) suggested that muscle activity during the gait cycle is maintained by a centrally generated neural locomotor pattern (which exists primarily at local spinal levels) that is dependent upon the proprioceptive input associated with rhythmic limb movements.

In describing this relationship, Rowinski (193) stated that aberrations of joint proprioceptors may "disrupt the phasic relationships between feedback and the central pattern" and produce symptoms such as the inability to develop high velocities and accelerations during the gait cycle, an increased sense of effort in the control of gait, and an increased amount of total conscious involvement in the function of ambulation. While this may not be as serious or obvious a problem as recurrent ankle sprains secondary to impaired proprioception, the significance of this information cannot be overstated.

Defects in the proprioceptive system are readily determined by what Freeman (194) refers to as a modified Romberg's test. The patient is instructed to stand on one leg with eyes open and closed. If after several attempts the patient is unable to balance for 10 seconds, then it can be assumed that the proprioceptive system is malfunctioning. (The average length of time an asymptomatic individual can balance on one leg before losing balance is 22 seconds [195].)

While damage to the proprioceptive system may be the result of peripheral neuropathy or posterior column disease, a much more common cause is previous trauma (such as inversion sprains) or repeated microtrauma (as occurs in a mechanically malfunctioning foot). These injuries theoretically destroy proprioceptive afferents and may produce injury due to impaired muscular stabilization. Cyriax (196) claimed that if the proprioceptive system is malfunctioning because of a previous sprain, the extensibility and function of the dystrophic tissue may be restored with cross-frictional massage. This technique, which involves stroking massage in a direction perpendicular to the sprained ligament's natural fiber orientation, will theoretically lengthen the fibrotic scar tissue that is impairing function.

When done properly, cross-fictional massage favorably stimulates proprioceptors and may produce a temporary anesthesia that is helpful in identifying the involved tissue. When done improperly, cross-frictional massage may produce an inflammatory reaction (with resulting fibrosis) and may even damage the Golgi tendon organs located in the muscle tendon junctions (197).

If the proprioceptive system is malfunctioning because of repeated microtrauma associated with a mechanically malfunctioning foot, an orthotic should be considered in an attempt to improve the mechanical efficiency of the supporting muscles (which lessens the irritation of the abnormally stressed joints) and to reestablish the normal progression of forces along the plantar foot. By improving the progression of forces, the orthotic acts to reeducate the central nervous system as to the ideal patterns for muscle recruitment. The efficacy of orthotics in favorably stimulating proprioception was demonstrated by Novick and Kelley (133), as they noted orthotics that are able to decrease calcaneal eversion by 2.4° during static stance will decrease calcaneal eversion by 4.2° during the gait cycle. They suggested that the decreased range of calcaneal eversion during locomotion results from "improved tactile and proprioceptive feedback" during dynamic function.

Though rarely mentioned, it is also possible that the proprioceptive system may be damaged secondary to decreased output from periarticular proprioceptors surrounding hypomobile joints. The importance of subtle intertarsal motions in maintaining balance is evidenced by the fact that individuals with certain tarsal coalitions are unable to effectively balance on one foot. While this represents an extreme situation in which the joint is ankylosed, it emphasizes that proprioceptive function cannot be considered fully restored until each joint can move through its full available range of motion.

In addition to limiting proprioceptive information, Hiss (132) claimed that a hypomobile joint produces a certain degree of "tissue tension" that forces the individual to alter the progression of forces through the plantar foot. This situation, according to Hiss, interferes with the synchrony of pivoting and balancing movements and, over time, results in an abnormal pattern of motor recruitment that is eventually reprogrammed into the central nervous system. Hiss (132) claimed that the only effective treatment in this situation is to restore flexibility to the dysfunctional joints with the appropriate manipulative procedures.

It appears that not only do manual techniques decrease potentially destructive compensatory movement patterns but they also serve to increase the quality and quantity of sensory information supplied to the central nervous system. This result, in turn, has a facilitatory effect on the vestibular apparatus (which improves motor activity) and may even block a chronic pain pattern that may be perpetuating an injury, i.e., stimulation of the faster Aβ fibers responsible for transmitting information from joint proprioceptors will "close the gate" to the slower Aδ and C type fibers responsible for pain transmission.

A perfect example of how pain and decreased proprioception may produce a chronic pain pattern occurs with reflex sympathetic dystrophy. Although the exact mechanism remains poorly understood, it is believed that nociceptive input associated with a relatively mild injury excites the internuncial neurons in the gray matter of the cord. These neurons then initiate a reverberating cycle that excites the anterior horn cells (producing muscle spasm) and lateral horn cells (producing sympathetic vasomotor and sudomotor responses). The increased sympathetic discharge may perpetuate the dystrophy, as it leads to trophic changes in the involved bone and connective tissues that further stimulate the nociceptive afferents, thereby irritating the already hyperexcited internuncials. As explained by Korr (198), the peripheral afferents and aberrant sympathetic discharge become "reflexively coupled to their mutual detriment." By stimulating the faster position sense joint proprioceptors immediately after an injury, manipulation is often able to break this dangerous cycle, thereby preventing the characteristic trophic changes.

In addition to the use of cross-frictional massage, foot orthoses, and manipulation to improve proprioception, Voss et al. (199) recommended various proprioceptive neuromuscular facilitation exercises that incorporate specific spiral and diagonal motions (Fig. 3.160). Because these techniques require a trained assistant to perform them, they are of somewhat limited value. Perhaps the simplest and most effective method for redeveloping the proprioceptive system is with home balance board exercises (Fig. 3.161). These exercises, which may be made progressively more difficult by performing them with one leg, and finally, with eyes closed, restore kinesthetic awareness by stressing proprioceptive pathways. This type of exercise system has an advantage over conventional exercises that require conscious effort (e.g., isotonic, isokinetic, etc.) in that it activates the subcortical pathways which, once trained, will operate on an automatic basis (200).

Because compensation for even minor injury may trigger a new state of centrally generated motor control, the rehabilitation process should attempt to resolve the acute stage as quickly as possible with techniques that minimize scarring and maintain range of motion. Various gait training exercises should be incorporated to ensure the synchronous interaction of all body segments, thereby preventing damage to the proprioceptive system. This may be as simple as instructing the patient to walk with a normal progression of force, i.e., make initial heel contact along the lateral calca-

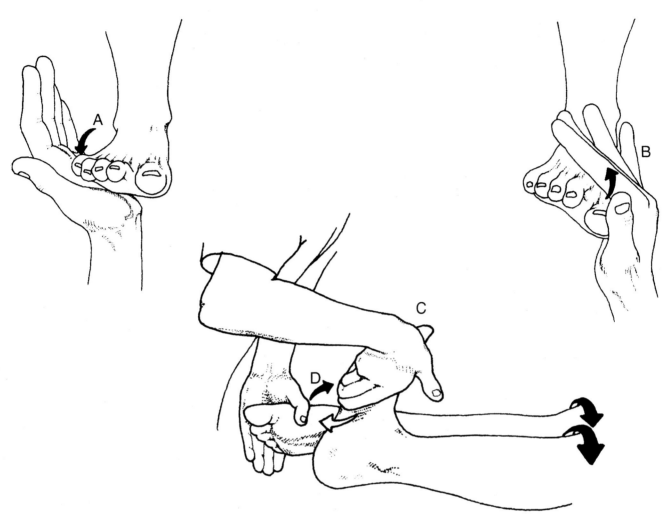

Figure 3.160. PNF patterns. *Insets* **A** and **B** demonstrate the simplest PNF pattern: the patient is instructed to alternately plantarflex and invert the forefoot (**A**) and dorsiflex and invert the forefoot against resistance provided by the practitioner. A more complicated series of movements requires that the patient alternate between plantarflexing and inverting one foot (**C**) while the opposite foot is dorsiflexing and everting (**D**).

Throughout the process, the foot that is plantarflexing is maintained with the lower extremity in an externally rotated position while the opposite lower extremity is internally rotated *(arrows)*. (For more information on these and other PNF patterns, the interested reader is referred to Voss DE, Ionta MK, Myers BJ. Proprioceptive Neuromuscular Facilitation. Ed 3. Philadelphia: Harper & Row, 1985.)

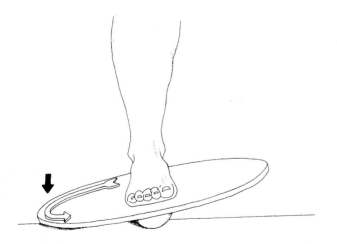

Figure 3.161. Balance board exercises. In the early stages of rehabilitation, the patient is instructed to sit next to the balance board with both feet contacting the outer edges of the board. The patient then rotates the board so that each section of the periphery contacts the ground. If this range of motion is too painful, the angle that the board tilts from horizontal (usually 16°) can be modified by placing magazines beneath the edges. (Medial and lateral placement will reduce the range of inversion/eversion while maintaining the full range of dorsiflexion/plantarflexion). As the patient improves, the magazines are removed, and the exercise is repeated with the patient standing, progressively bringing the feet towards the center of the board. Eventually, this exercise may be performed while the patient stands on one leg with eyes closed. For particularly large patients, it is possible to increase the angle that the board tilts by placing a magazine beneath the center sphere.

neus, progress along the lateral column during the midstance period and, finally traverse the metatarsal heads and roll off the hallux to terminate the propulsive period. If superimposed body weight makes early return to activity difficult, the patient should be encouraged to walk waist deep in a swimming pool.

Another alternative would be to have the patient march or gently bounce on a home minitrampoline: possible variations are limited only by the practitioner's imagination. In chronic cases, it may be necessary to have the patient permanently alter his or her gait pattern. For example, an individual with a rigid forefoot valgus deformity and hammer toes may have to develop a high gear push-off in order to avoid irritating a chronic interdigital neuritis. Also, individuals with recalcitrant calcaneal stress fractures may have to develop a forefoot strike pattern in order to lessen ground-reactive forces beneath the heel: Cavanagh and Lafortune (201) noted that shock scores are often halved when experimental subjects switch from a heel strike to a mid or forefoot strike pattern.

It should be noted that a forefoot strike pattern may markedly aggravate an achilles tendon and/or plantar fascia injury. With these injuries, it is best to have the patient maintain a rearfoot strike pattern and, if necessary, to shorten his or her length of stride in order to reduce forces during the propulsive period. While recommendations to either increase or decrease a patient's natural stride length is usually associated with a 1 or 2% increase in the metabolic cost of locomotion (202), the potential benefits associated with a reduced rate of injury usually greatly outweigh any metabolic penalties.

MUSCULAR STRENGTH, POWER, AND ENDURANCE

Perhaps no topic in the field of rehabilitative foot care has been the center of more controversy than the role of strengthening exercises in the maintenance and development of the medial longitudinal arch. Over 40 years ago, in an article describing the etiology and treatment of the hypermobile flatfoot, Harris and Beath (203) argued that muscular strength was not the most important factor in maintaining the shape of the medial arch (this was the most widely accepted view at that time) and that a poorly developed arch was the result of bony abnormalities in the tarsal bones (primarily in the subtalar joint) that makes them structurally unable to support body weight. They stated that the muscular mechanisms responsible for maintaining the arch are for occasional use only, since, unlike bony and ligamentous restraints, they are unable to function unremittingly. They supported this belief with the observation that feet that are completely paralyzed with poliomyelitis often have little deformity.

This is not to say that muscular support of the medial longitudinal arch is not important. On the contrary, a recent study by Hannah and Robbins (204) demonstrated that

barefoot running produced an increased tone in the intrinsic foot musculature (particularly flexor digitorum brevis) that resulted in an increased height of the medial arch as measured on lateral weight-bearing x-rays. Although the relative importance of muscular vs. osseous support in maintaining the medial longitudinal arch remains unclear, it is reasonable to state that the demands placed upon the muscular system vary inversely with the bony architecture, i.e., an individual with a single articulated subtalar joint is going to require greater muscular support than an individual with a triarticulated subtalar joint, where motion is stopped primarily by joint incongruity. It must be emphasized that there is a limit to the support afforded by the muscular system. As stated by Perry (205), "Even with maximal muscular participation, the capability to meet the valgus torques imposed on the foot is limited, providing a strong rationale for the careful selection of footwear and the addition of added support."

In most situations, when an individual with a mechanically malfunctioning foot presents with muscle weakness, strengthening exercises should initially be avoided, since the muscles are almost always overworked and weak from fatigue. The premature incorporation of a strengthening program will overload the already fatigued muscles and may perpetuate a faulty movement pattern in the individual who has learned to compensate for the chronically strained musculature. This being the case, the first stage of the rehabilitation process is to stretch the overworked muscles gently.

As noted by Janda (206), the postural muscles, such as tibialis posterior, soleus, and gastrocnemius, are particularly prone to tightening with fatigue. This is troublesome in that the fatigued and tightened postural muscle will often produce reflex inhibition of the antagonistic phasic muscles (particularly peroneus longus and tibialis anterior) which, needless to say, creates a confused state of motor control. Because of this, stretches for the fatigued and tightened postural muscles should be incorporated simultaneously with strengthening exercises for the weakened and lengthened phasic muscles.

The classic example of how postural and phasic muscles work together to produce foot deformity occurs with the hypermobile subtalar joint: the overly mobile subtalar joint often requires more muscular stabilization than the postural muscles can provide. As a result, these muscles fatigue and tighten, which in turn produces reciprocal inhibition of the antagonistic peroneals. Since even slight weakness of peroneus longus will allow for an increased range of subtalar pronation secondary to decreased stabilization of the first ray, the subtalar joint is allowed to move through an even greater range of pronation, which stresses the tibialis posterior, soleus, and gastrocnemius muscles to the point at which they can no longer stabilize the rearfoot. This places the forefoot into a constantly inverted position relative to the rearfoot, which may eventually become fixed by soft tissue contracture. This condition is referred to as a functional forefoot varus deformity.

Unlike the true forefoot varus, treatment of the functional forefoot varus deformity does not require a forefoot post (which would only maintain the deformity). Rather, treatment should consist of a well-designed program of manipulation to restore the range of first ray plantarflexion and midtarsal eversion, stretches for the posterior compartment musculature, exercises for the phasic muscles and an orthotic to minimize the range of subtalar joint eversion (which was the original cause of the deformity).

While weakness may be secondary to a mechanically malfunctioning foot, it may also be the end-result of prolonged immobilization. As demonstrated by LeBlanc et al. (207), immobilization has different effects on different muscle groups. After a 5-week period of horizontal bed rest, there was no change in muscle area or strength in the ankle dorsiflexors (as measured with MRI and Cybex 2 dynamometry) while the ankle plantarflexors, particularly the gastrocnemius and soleus, suffered a 12% reduction in mass and a 26% reduction in strength. This study emphasized the importance of strengthening the posterior compartment musculature after even brief periods of immobilization or inactivity.

Following is a series of illustrations (Figs. 3.162–3.165) that detail the various manual tests for muscles of the foot and leg. Also discussed are the possible side effects associated with prolonged weakness. It should be stressed that in addition to evaluating these muscles, the practitioner should also evaluate muscular strength along the entire kinetic chain since weakness of a more proximal muscle may detrimentally affect foot function, e.g., a weak piriformis muscle may allow for excessive talar adduction and produce a chronically pronated foot (172).

Once it has been determined that muscle weakness from fatigue is not a factor, strengthening exercises can be initiated. These exercises are readily performed by having the patient duplicate the manual muscle tests at home. These exercises may be done isometrically (changing joint angles approximately 15° after each contraction to allow for sufficient overflow) or isotonically (either eccentric or concentric contraction). Travell and Simons (123) recommend that muscles with trigger points should not be isometrically exercised and that initially only the eccentric portion of an isotonic contraction should be emphasized.

A popular method of isotonic exercise requires moving the muscle through a range of motion against resistance provided by different sized rubber bands or surgical tubing

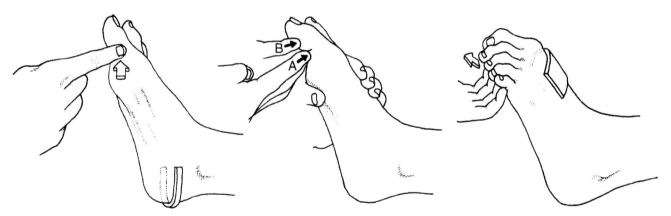

Figure 3.162. Abductor hallucis. Test: The examiner forcefully attempts to abduct the hallux against patient resistance *(left)*. (This direction is reversed to test adductor hallucis). Weakness: prolonged weakness of the abductor hallucis muscle may result in hallux abductovalgus deformity, plantarflexed first ray deformity, and/or an excessive lowering of the medial longitudinal arch. Weakness of adductor hallucis is rarely seen. **Flexor hallucis brevis and longus.** Tests: To test flexor hallucis brevis, the examiner attempts to dorsiflex the proximal phalanx against patient resistance *(center, A)*. Flexor hallucis longus is tested by applying the same force beneath the distal phalanx (B). Note that the interphalangeal joint is maintained in a flexed position when testing flexor hallucis longus. Weakness: A weak flexor hallucis brevis will allow for clawing of the great toe and lessened stability of the medial longitudinal arch (172) while a weak flexor hallucis longus may allow for injuries associated with inadequate sta- bilization of the medial forefoot during the latter half of the propulsive period (e.g., second metatarsal stress fracture, capsulitis, etc.) and for hyperextension of the first interphalangeal joint. Strangely enough, complete paralysis of flexor hallucis longus is occasionally found in long distance runners. Flexor digitorum brevis and longus. Tests: Strength in flexor digitorum brevis is evaluated by applying a dorsiflectory force beneath the middle phalanges of the patient's second through fifth digits *(right)*. The long digital flexor is evaluated by applying the same force beneath the distal phalanges while maintaining the interphalangeal joints in a flexed position. Weakness: As suggested by Robbins et al. (189), weakness in the digital flexors may allow for a lowering of the medial longitudinal arch and for chronic injury to the metatarsophalangeal joints, as the distal digits are unable to effectively distribute ground-reactive forces away from the metatarsal heads.

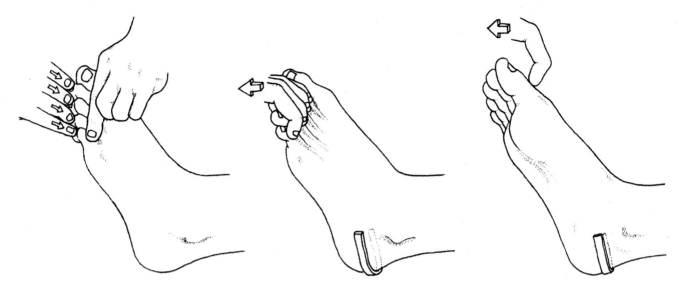

Figure 3.163. Lumbricales. Test: By contacting the dorsal distal surfaces of the distal phalanges, the examiner attempts to plantarflex the digits while stabilizing the foot at the metatarsophalangeal joints *(left)*. Weakness: Weakness of this muscle often results in digital deformity. **Extensor digitorum brevis and longus.** Test: These muscles are tested together (172) by positioning the foot in a slightly plantarflexed position with the examiner attempting to plantarflex the digits by applying pressure along the dorsal surface of the toes *(center)*. Weak-ness: The most common problem associated with weakness of these muscles is a clawing of the lesser digits. Extreme weakness may result in a mild drop-foot. **Extensor hallucis brevis and longus.** Tests: The patient resists a plantarflectory force applied at the proximal phalanx (testing brevis) and then the distal phalanx (testing longus) *(right)*. Weakness: Because extensor hallucis longus is an important ankle dorsiflexor, weakness in these muscles may result in a drop-foot.

(Fig. 3.166). Other common home exercises are illustrated in Figure 3.167. In all situations, an exercise program should attempt to duplicate the speed of contraction, joint angles, and types of contraction (i.e., eccentric vs. concentric) that the muscles are to be functionally stressed. The easiest way to do this is with barefoot walking. As the patient improves, the exercises can be made more difficult by having the patient perform repeat side-to-side running drills, progressively tighter "figure 8" drills, various plyometric exercises, along with Carioca maneuvers (Fig. 3.168). In addition to increasing strength, these movements produce the coordinated, synchronous muscular interactions that are essential for full recovery. In situations where large deformity and/or proprioceptive deficits are present, it may be necessary for the patient to wear orthotics and/or protective wrapping to prevent reinjury.

In certain cases, a given muscle may not respond to a strengthening program. Possible causes for this include the continued presence of active trigger points (which impair the muscle's ability to recruit fibers), joint dysfunction in the neighboring articulations (two separate studies (209, 210) demonstrated that mobilization of a hypomobile articulation may produce immediate strength gains in the supporting musculature), and/or nerve root entrapment.

As noted by Lee (211), one of the first signs of nerve root irritation is an accelerated fatigability of the involved muscle. This decreased endurance may not be apparent with a single full effort muscle contraction (as is used in most neurological assessments) and must be evaluated by stressing the involved muscle to the point of fatigue, then comparing the final number of repetitions to the uninvolved side. The neurologically induced fatigue may be a source of chronic foot injury and treatment must be directed toward restoring optimal spinal biomechanics: in order for an exercise program to be effective, one must first identify any and all factors that may be perpetuating the weakness.

EXCESSIVE/ABNORMAL MOTIONS

Because of the extremes in ground-reactive forces associated with locomotion, the most reliable protection against abnormal or excessive motion is a well-designed skeletal system. Ideally, the articulations of the foot are formed in such a way that they functionally interlock and remain stable even with the superimposed stresses of weight-bearing (215).

There are, however, numerous congenital anomalies that significantly impair the ability of bony restraining mechanisms to resist excessive motion.

The most significant of these congenital anomalies occurs in the subtalar joint. As described by Harris and Beath (215), an architecturally stable subtalar joint will form in such a way that the head of the talus is positioned directly over the anterior end of the calcaneus. In this posi-

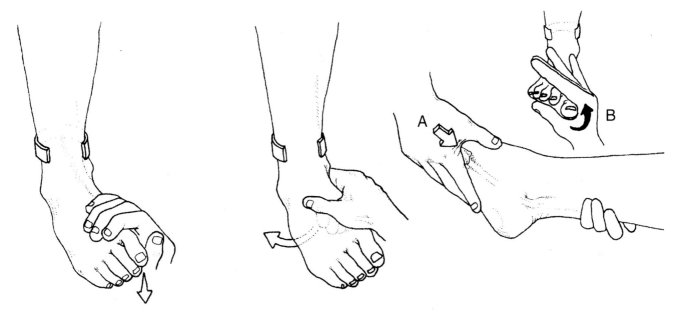

Figure 3.164. Tibialis anterior. Test: The examiner grasps the patient's medial forefoot (just distal to the insertion of tibialis anterior) and attempts to vigorously plantarflex the inverted foot against patient resistance *(left)*. Weakness: The most obvious problem associated with weakness of tibialis anterior is a drop-foot. Also, the forefoot often "slaps" the ground loudly during the contact period. Root et al. (3) noted that extreme weakness of tibialis anterior may allow the antagonistic peroneus longus to create a plantarflexed first ray deformity. **Tibialis posterior.** Test: The most common test position is to have the patient adduct and plantarflex the forefoot while the examiner, with a medial midfoot contact, attempts to dorsiflex and evert the foot *(center)*. Gould (208), who claimed that tibialis posterior is probably the most overlooked muscle in the body in terms of muscular strength, suggests testing this muscle by firmly grasping the heel and having the patient resist the examiner's eversion stress. If the heel is "broken" with less than 20 lbs of pressure, tibialis posterior should be considered weak. Weakness: Progressive lowering of the medial longitudinal arch with the possible development of a functional forefoot varus deformity and/or dorsiflexed first ray. **Peroneus longus and brevis.** Tests: As a group, the peroneals are tested by positioning the patient with the forefoot slightly supinated (adducted, plantarflexed, and inverted) *(right)*. Against resistance provided by the examiner (contact point on dorsal, proximal fifth metatarsal), the patient attempts to abduct, dorsiflex, and evert the forefoot **(A)**. It is possible to isolate

peroneus longus with the test position illustrated in **B**. In this test, the patient is positioned with the forefoot slightly plantarflexed and everted while the examiner grasps the medial forefoot. Against maximal resistance provided by the patient, the examiner attempts to dorsiflex and invert the forefoot. Weakness: A weak peroneus longus allows for the development of an acquired dorsiflexed first ray, as the medial forefoot is no longer stabilized during the propulsive period. This may eventually lead to deformity at the first metatarsophalangeal joint. Weakness in peroneus brevis is also troublesome, as it allows for the development of a functional rearfoot varus deformity as the muscles responsible for inverting the subtalar joint overwhelm the weakened peroneals during late swing phase, allowing heel-strike to occur with the rearfoot excessively inverted. (The foot will behave identically to one with an osseous rearfoot varus deformity until strength is restored to the lateral compartment muscles.) Also, weakness in the peroneals may result in chronic inversion ankle sprains, as peroneus brevis is unable to evert the lateral column, forcing the foot to roll through its propulsive period with the rearfoot excessively inverted as a low gear push-off is maintained. This movement pattern may eventually lead to interdigital neuritis, recurrent ankle sprain, and/or lateral hip pain as the gluteus medius muscle fires vigorously in an attempt to displace the center of mass medially towards the stance phase leg.

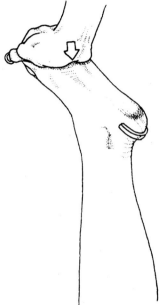

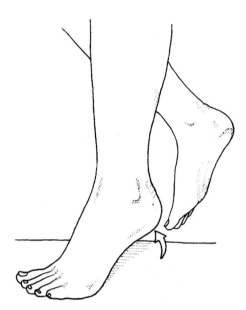

Figure 3.165. Soleus and gastrocnemius. Tests: Soleus is evaluated by positioning the patient in a prone position with the knee flexed 90°. (This position minimizes the ability of gastrocnemius to effectively assist in resisting the test motion.) The examiner then contacts the posterior calcaneus and plantar forefoot and attempts to dorsiflex the ankle against patient resistance *(left)*. Because the gastrocnemius is such a strong muscle, it is best evaluated by having the patient perform repeat single leg-heel raises while standing *(right)*. The number of repetitions necessary to produce mild fatigue should be compared bilaterally. Weakness: A weakness of these muscles is almost always associated with a marked delay in heel lift. This often results in the development of claw toe deformity and/or an acquired plantarflexed first ray deformity, as the long digital flexors and peroneus longus (which are all extremely weak ankle plantarflexors) attempt to initiate heel lift during late midstance (3). Because gastrocnemius crosses the knee joint, weakness in this muscle often results in genu recurvatum and/or recurrent knee injury.

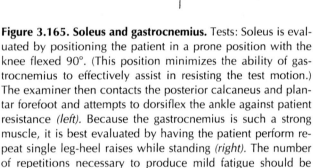

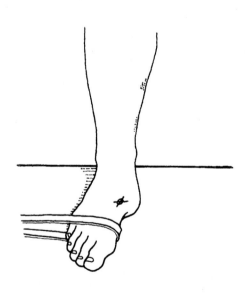

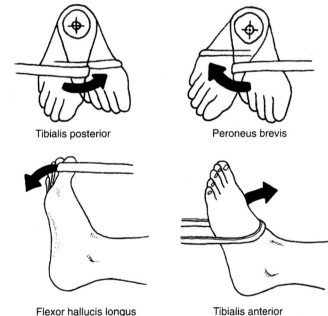

Tibialis posterior

Peroneus brevis

Flexor hallucis longus

Tibialis anterior

Figure 3.166. By anchoring the opposite end of an exercise band, it is possible to exercise virtually any muscle in the body.

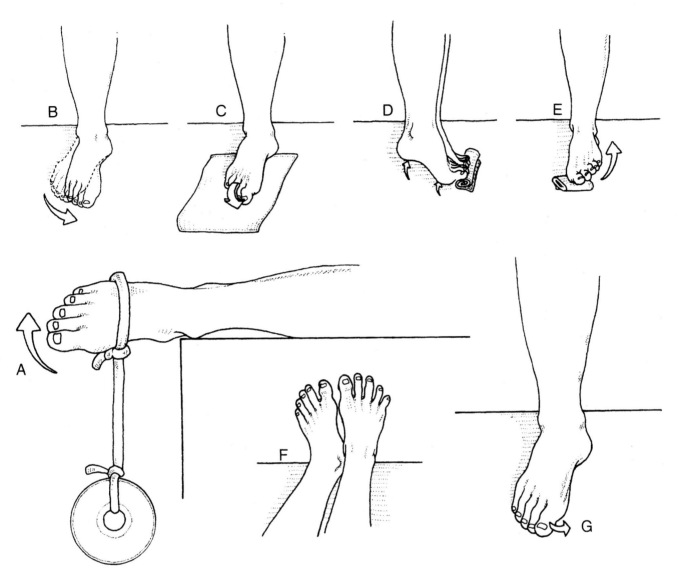

Figure 3.167. Home exercises. The peroneals may be exercised isotonically, as illustrated in **A.** Tibialis posterior may be exercised with what Alter (202) describes as a sand-scraping motion: the patient actively adducts and inverts the forefoot against resistance provided by friction beneath the lateral forefoot **(B).** The use of towel-curls has become a standard for strengthening the digital flexors and extensors. The patient first curls the towel into a ball (trapping the towel between the heel and the tips of the toes) and then attempts to straighten the towel by extending the toes **(C).** This exercise may be performed by using friction from the floor (or the inside of a shoe) instead of the towel. The posterior compartment muscles may be exercised with single leg-heel raises (weights may be added to the shoulders or hands) or by performing repeat single leg jumps (gradually increasing the height of the jump). Part **D** illustrates how placing a towel beneath the digits and instructing the patient to raise first the heel and then the plan-tar forefoot allows for an improved strengthening of the digital flexors. By placing the towel beneath the first metatarsal head and instructing the patient to plantarflex the ankle and evert the forefoot **(E)**, peroneus longus is effectively exercised. (This is a particularly useful exercise when trying to teach the patient how to initiate a high gear push-off) The interossei may be exercised by having the patient alternately adduct and abduct the digits with full effort **(F)** while abductor hallucis may be exercised by having the patient adduct the great toe against friction from the floor **(G).** It should be pointed out that while many practitioners claim that strengthening the foot musculature is an effective form of treatment for various overuse injuries, these claims seem to be exaggerated (46, 213). In fact, Awbrey et al. (213) found that patients treated with 3 months of foot exercises for plantar fascial injury showed no improvement, as compared to a control group.

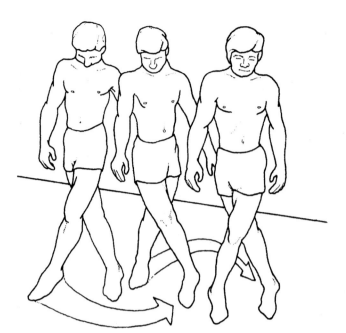

Figure 3.168. Carioca exercises. The patient performs repeat side-to-side drills while alternately crossing one leg in front of the other. (Adapted from Seto JL, Brewster CE, Lombardo ST, et al. Rehabilitation of the knee after anterior cruciate ligament reconstruction. J Orthop Sports Phys Ther 1989; 11 (1): 8–18.)

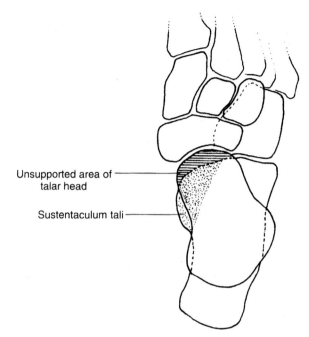

Figure 3.169. Ideal development of the sustentaculum tali.

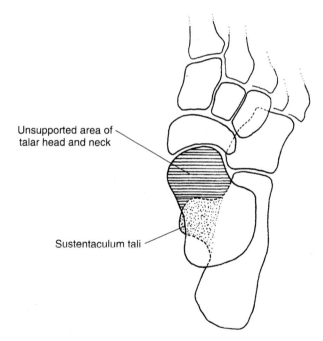

Figure 3.170. The poorly developed sustentaculum tali is unable to adequately support the talar head. (Adapted from tracings of x-rays as illustrated by Harris RI, Beath T. Hypermobile flatfoot with short tendo achilles. J Bone Joint Surg 1948; 30A(1): 116–138.)

tion, the talar head receives firm support from the sustentaculum tali, which is broad, rounded, and runs forward to the anterior margin of the calcaneus (see Fig. 3.169). This particular formation allows for much stability in that superimposed body weight compresses and locks the talus onto the calcaneus, thereby protecting against excessive motion with little or no stress placed on the restraining muscles and ligaments.

The Hypermobile Subtalar Joint

Unfortunately, a structurally stable subtalar joint is not always present, as ontogenic defects in subtalar development may allow for deformity in which the head of the talus lies anterior and medial to the end of the calcaneus, with the sustentaculum tali existing as a tongue-like process that projects proximally (Fig. 3.170). This being the case, the calcaneus is unable to support the head of the talus and superimposed body weight allows the talus to adduct and plantarflex as the calcaneus simultaneously everts. The excessive talar plantarflexion only serves to amplify the instability as the head of the talus acts as a wedge that further separates the incompetent sustentaculum tali from the navicular. This wedge-like action of the talus is a constant source of irritation, as it places the spring and long plantar ligaments on tension and may eventually lead to plastic deformity of these tissues.

Talar adduction also leads to instability, as the head of the talus may escape transversely from the navicular acetabulum. Vogler (216) noted that when the talar head escapes approximately 50% of the navicular acetabulum, it is functioning "out of control," and a retrograde compressive force develops at the proximal navicular that drives the talus further medially and downward, eventually leading to the complete collapse of the midtarsal joint. (Normally the compressive force from the navicular allows for greater stability in the modified ball-and-socket talonavicular joint; see Fig. 3.19.)

Furthermore, the adducted and plantarflexed talus impairs the windlass effect of the plantar fascia and allows ground-reactive force to create a jamming of the upper margins of the unstable tarsus as the undersurfaces of these articulations collapse (Fig. 3.171). Because the supporting muscles and ligaments are unable to resist the progressive collapse of the tarsals, the talar head often continues its plantar migration until it eventually makes ground contact. The final result is a hypermobile foot that presents with an inverted and abducted forefoot, an everted heel, and an unstable first ray.

Harris and Beath (203) claim that the architecturally unstable subtalar joint with its incompetent sustentaculum tali is the primary etiological factor responsible for the development of the hypermobile flatfoot deformity. This particular malformation, which may also be secondary to congenital ligamentous laxity, will always present with a normal medial longitudinal arch off-weight-bearing that completely collapses upon standing. The forefoot in this situation often moves through extreme ranges of inversion and abduction (the midtarsal joint may allow for as much as

50° of forefoot inversion) while contracture of the posterior calf musculature usually maintains the ankle in a plantarflexed position (e.g., negative 25° of ankle dorsiflexion, as measured with the subtalar joint in neutral, is not uncommon). Harris and Beath (203) emphasized that the decreased range of ankle dorsiflexion is not the cause of the hypermobile flatfoot deformity, but probably develops because "the structure of the foot and the laxity of the tarsal joints deprive the tendo Achilles of tension stresses, which normally would facilitate elongation of these tissues."

Because the stresses placed upon the muscular and ligamentous restraining mechanisms are so great, individuals with this deformity often learn to avoid strenuous sports or heavy activities. Although symptoms such as painful joints and/or fatigued muscles may be delayed indefinitely with a sedentary life-style, they most often begin by the early teens and may be evident as early as 5 years of age (203). Because there is a strong tendency for this subtalar anomaly to be inherited, the condition is often recognized by a parent afflicted with the same deformity. It cannot be overstated that early recognition of the hypermobile flatfoot deformity is essential since it is often possible to correct this deformity with the use of custom-molded orthotics that maintain bony alignment during growth years (217). (Note: treatment of the child's foot will be discussed in detail in a later section.)

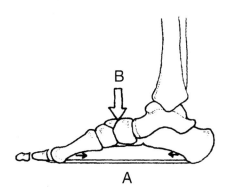
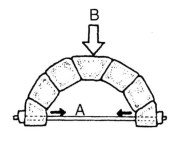
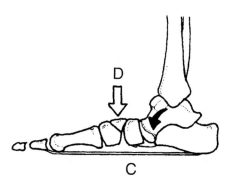
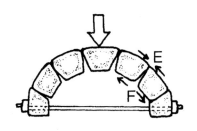

Figure 3.171. Normally, the plantar fascia has a tension banding effect (A) that allows imposed forces (B) to induce stability by interlocking the tarsals. When the tension banding effect of the plantar fascia is absent (C), imposed forces produce a collapse of the tarsals (D), with the dorsal surfaces being compressed (E) while the plantar surfaces are distracted (F). (Modified from Vogler H. Biomechanics of talipes equinovalgus. J Am Podiatr Med Assoc 1987; 77 (1): 21–28.)

The hypermobile flatfoot deformity can be identified by the extreme lowering of the medial longitudinal arch on weight-bearing, the chronically everted heel, the drastically increased range of forefoot inversion (with the concomitantly decreased range of ankle dorsiflexion) and, most importantly, by the medial displacement of the talus relative to the calcaneus during static stance. A superior/inferior x-ray serves as a useful index for determining the degree of deformity, as it demonstrates a shadow where the head of the talus is not supported by the anterior calcaneus (e.g., compare the shaded area in Fig. 3.170 to the shaded area in Fig. 3.169).

To be comprehensive, treatment of this subtalar anomaly should include various manual techniques to address any soft tissue contractures associated with this deformity, and an orthotic, which acts as a physical barrier to prevent excessive displacement of the talar head. Although the orthotic will not correct the deformity when used after osseous maturity, it can greatly reduce strain placed upon the supporting muscles and ligaments, as it basically acts as an extrinsic sustentaculum tali.

When applicable, a rearfoot varus post should be used to reposition the center of mass of the calcaneus beneath the center of mass of the talus. This post may be invaluable, as it lessens the length of the lever arm afforded body weight for pronating the subtalar joint, which in turn allows the muscular system to become more effective at controlling subtalar motions. The use of a forefoot varus post should be prescribed with caution, as prolonged subtalar pronation often results in the development of a functional forefoot varus where the forefoot deformity is maintained by soft tissue contracture. Use of a forefoot varus post in this situation would only maintain the forefoot deformity and may eventually lead to progressive deformity of the first metatarsophalangeal joint.

The most important clinical concern when dealing with a hypermobile flatfoot is how to accommodate the decreased range of ankle dorsiflexion. Because the limited range of ankle dorsiflexion is almost always associated with a pathological range of compensatory midtarsal joint pronation, it is important that the practitioner incorporate the appropriately sized heel lift and/or use only the softer orthotic shells, as use of a rigid shell without a heel lift almost always leads to iatrogenic injury as the pronating midfoot collides into the orthotic shell. Also, attempts should always be made to lengthen the achilles tendon (the subtalar joint must always be in a neutral or supinated position when performing calf stretches) and strengthen the supporting musculature (particularly tibialis posterior and abductor hallucis).

The Hypermobile First Ray

In addition to faulty foot function associated with an anomalous subtalar joint, another osseous malformation that allows for abnormal motion is obliquity of the first tarsometatarsal (Fig. 3.172). This particular deformity is a throwback to the primitive arboreal foot, where grasping skills, not mechanical stability, was the primary concern. Evolutionary remodeling of the foot necessitated a medial migration of the first ray in order to allow a more effective propulsive period (218).

If deformity of the first tarsometatarsal joint allows the first ray to be maintained in an adducted position, the first metatarsal head would be unable to bear weight effectively since, unlike the second metatarsal, it is not securely stabilized by an osseous locking mechanism. Note that when the first metatarsal is in a midline position, it can be effectively stabilized by the supporting musculature (the first metatarsal has stronger muscles attached to it than any of the other metatarsals [219]) and by ligamentous attachments to the secured second metatarsal base (the base of the

Figure 3.172. The ideal first tarsometatarsal articulation allows for a midline position of the first metatarsal (A). If obliquity of the first tarsometatarsal joint is present **(B)**, the first metatarsal shifts into an adducted position.

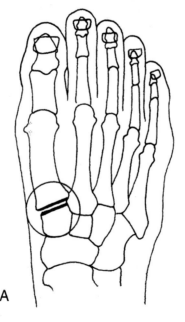
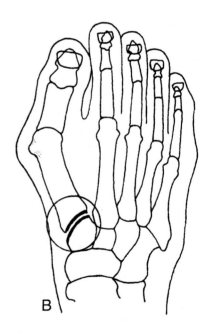

A   B

first metatarsal is loosely held to the base of the second metatarsal by the Lisfranc's ligament).

With the first ray situated in this biomechanically stable midline position, evaluation of the ranges of motion between the bases of the first through fifth metatarsals will show an average movement ratio of 2, 1, 2, 4, 5, respectively (132). In other words, the first metatarsal should move twice as much as the second metatarsal, just as much as the third metatarsal, half as much as the fourth metatarsal, and two-fifths as much as the fifth metatarsal. When obliquity of the first tarsometatarsal articulation is present, it is not uncommon for the adducted first ray to be so poorly stabilized that the intermetatarsal movement ratio becomes 5, 1, 2, 4, 5.

The extreme hypermobility of the first ray makes it unable to resist ground-reactive forces and allows for an exaggerated range of subtalar pronation. This is particularly damaging when it occurs with a rearfoot or forefoot varus deformity, as the exaggerated range of subtalar pronation is greatly increased, thereby forcing the first metatarsal into a dorsiflexed and inverted position. This allows for rapid development of a Grade 3 hallux abductovalgus as the forces of propulsion subluxate the proximal phalanx (Fig. 3.173).

The dorsiflexed and inverted first ray may also produce degenerative changes at the base of the first metatarsal, where a dorsal base exostosis often forms secondary to the compressive forces that develop along the dorsal tarsometatarsal articulation. This exostosis is particularly troublesome in that it often produces entrapment of the deep peroneal nerve and/or tenosynovitis of the extensor hallux longus/brevis tendons, as these tissues become sheared between the constantly shifting exostosis and shoe gear (Fig. 3.174).

Treatment of a hypermobile first ray requires a properly posted orthotic that prevents excessive subtalar pronation and improves the mechanical efficiency of the supporting musculature (particularly peroneus longus). Also, it is often necessary to include balance board exercises and manipulation of the intertarsal and tarsometatarsal articulations since the individual with a hypermobile first ray often presents with impaired proprioception and a decreased range of first ray plantarflexion.

Careful selection of shoe gear is a must since the adducted first ray almost always requires a roomy toe box to prevent compression of the metatarsal heads. It is often necessary to have a cobbler stretch the upper over the dorsomedial first metatarsal head to prevent the formation of a painful bunion. (Note: This treatment program can also be used when treating a splay foot deformity in which articular variation has allowed for an abnormal transverse plane spreading of the metatarsals, see Fig. 3.175.)

Malpositioned Subtalar Joint Axis

An important consideration in this discussion of articular anomalies is that, in addition to predisposing to injury

because they allow for excessive motion, articular anomalies may also produce injury because they allow for abnormal motion, i.e., because it is the articular surface geometry that determines where a joint will go upon mechanical or muscular demand (221), variation in articular shape may allow for a functional malposition of a joint's axis of motion. As previously described in the anatomy section, variation in subtalar joint anatomy may allow the joint's axis of motion to be positioned anywhere from 20 to 68.5° relative to the transverse plane (Fig. 1.24C and D).

The approximate position of the subtalar axis can be clinically determined by standing behind the patient and noting the relative amounts of calcaneal inversion/eversion, as compared to external/internal tibial rotation. If the axis lies near 70°, the amount of tibial rotation will greatly ex-

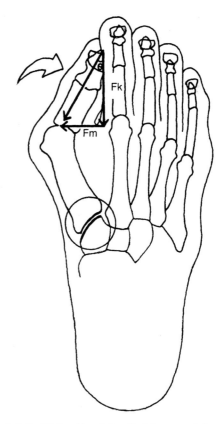

Figure 3.173. Obliquity of the first tarsometatarsal articulation *(inset)* results in an adducted first metatarsal that in turn results in abduction of the hallux (arrow). As the foot with this deformity moves into its propulsive period, ground-reactive forces centered beneath the hallux *(FK)* will have a medially directed component *(FM)*, which equals FK x tangent of angle θ. As a result, a hallux that is abducted 60° will push the head of the first metatarsal medially with a force that is 1.7 times greater than that of push-off. As stated by Bojsen-Moller (106), this spoils the stability and the mechanics of the forefoot and causes painful pressures between the metatarsal head and the shoe. These internal forces may eventually result in the "total collapse of the first ray." (Partially adapted from Bojsen-Moller F. Anatomy of the forefoot, normal and pathologic. Clin Orthop Related Res 1979; 142: 10.)

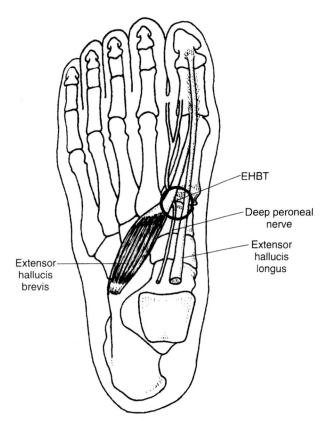

Figure 3.174. The dorsal base exotosis *(inset)* may produce tenosynovitis of extensor hallucis longus and/or brevis and may result in entrapment neuropathy of the deep peroneal nerve where it passes beneath the extensor hallucis brevis tendon (EHBT). This entrapment neuropathy may be clinically detected by a positive percussion sign (Tinel's test) performed at this junction and/or by a decreased vibratory sense/two-point discrimination at the first dorsal web space. (Adapted from Lee Dellon A: Deep peroneal nerve entrapment on the dorsum of the foot. Foot Ankle 1990; 11 (2): 73–78.)

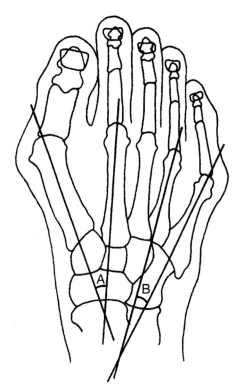

Figure 3.175. The splay foot deformity. This deformity is identified by the substantial increase in intermetatarsal angles, particularly between the first and second **(A)** and the fourth and fifth **(B)** metatarsals. (These angles are typically less than 10 and 5°, respectively.) Root et al. (3) claimed that this deformity results from either abnormal propulsive period pronation of the subtalar joint or loss of function in the transverse pedis muscle. They went on to state that attempts to halt the progression of this deformity by eliminating the abnormal pronation are destined to fail if the first metatarsal angle exceeds 14° and the fifth ray is in subluxation in a pronated position (as evidenced by a concave lateral border of the fifth metatarsal shaft on a dorsiplantar x-ray).

ceed rearfoot motion, i.e., 2° of rearfoot eversion will be accompanied by 8° of internal tibial rotation. Conversely, an axis situated 20° to the transverse plane will allow for large amounts of rearfoot motion with relatively small amounts of tibial rotation.

When a high axis of motion is present, the lower leg is predisposed to injury, as even small ranges of rearfoot inversion/eversion may result in potentially injurious amounts of torsional strains being placed upon the lower leg. The low axis motion has the opposite effect in that the lower leg is most often spared from injury, but the foot may be chronically injured, as it is forced to move through large ranges of frontal plane motion.

Treatment for both the high and low axis of motion requires a strong, well-coordinated muscular system to help control the aberrant frontal and transverse plane of motion of the heel and tibia. While orthotics may be invaluable in controlling motion associated with a low axis of motion, they are less helpful when a high axis of motion is present, since the rearfoot in this situation moves through such small ranges of motion that orthotic control is usually not indicated. In some cases, however, the high axis of motion is associated with a normal or even increased range of subtalar pronation, which makes orthotic control essential for minimizing torsional strains on the lower leg.

Vertically Displaced Oblique Midtarsal Joint Axis

In addition to variation in positioning of the subtalar joint axis, it is also possible that articular anomalies in the midtarsal joint may allow for a variation in positioning of the oblique midtarsal joint axis. Normally, the oblique midtarsal joint axis rests 52° to the transverse plane and 57° to the sagittal plane and allows for relatively equal amounts of abduction/adduction and dorsiflexion/plantarflexion (Fig. 3.176). However, variation in articular geometry may allow for a more vertical displacement of the oblique midtarsal joint axis. The high oblique midtarsal joint axis allows for a marked increase in transverse plane motion of the forefoot (abduction/adduction) with a corresponding decreased range of sagittal plane motion (dorsiflexion/plantarflexion). The position of the oblique midtarsal joint axis can be determined clinically by evaluating the lateral contour of the foot upon weight-bearing. If the high oblique midtarsal joint axis is present, the forefoot will abduct excessively, producing a characteristic angulation at the calcaneocuboid joint (Fig. 3.177).

The high oblique midtarsal joint axis may be responsible for injury, as it allows for a medial displacement of the talus relative to the calcaneus (Fig. 3.178). This unfortunately supplies body weight with a longer lever arm for pronating the subtalar joint, which usually maintains the rearfoot in a pronated position throughout the entire stance phase. Also, the nearly pure transverse plane motion of the forefoot may produce injury during propulsion, as it may disallow the normal locking of the calcaneocuboid joint necessary for stability: because abduction of the forefoot allows the cuboid to shift laterally, it is possible that the cuboid may escape the anatomical overhang of the calcaneus, thereby preventing the calcaneocuboid joint from locking during late midstance (216). The foot then behaves as a flexible lever arm that will buckle with the forces of propulsion.

To make matters worse, because the navicular simultaneously abducts with the cuboid, the talar head may escape medially from the navicular acetabulum, often allowing for the complete collapse of the medial longitudinal arch. Signs and symptoms associated with this foot type include a marked lowering of the medial longitudinal arch upon weight-bearing (with acute angulation of the lateral column), marginal proliferation of the lateral calcaneocuboid joint, chronic tibialis posterior and tibialis anterior tendinitis, plantar fasciitis, spring ligament sprain, medial knee pain, diffuse hyperkeratotic lesion beneath the second and third metatarsal heads, and a hammering of the lateral digits secondary to a bowing of the flexor digitorum longus (refer back to Fig. 3.34).

Orthotic management in this situation is often difficult because, even with proper shoe gear, excessive transverse plane motion of the forefoot may continue, and the tissues beneath the medial longitudinal arch are often compressed into the orthotic shell. In fact, many practitioners feel that the high oblique midtarsal joint axis defies orthotic control and that treatment failure is a rule, rather than an exception.

This dismal treatment prognosis is not shared by Hice (222), who claims it is possible to effectively manage this deformity as long as the orthotic maintains the subtalar joint in a near neutral position during midstance. To accomplish

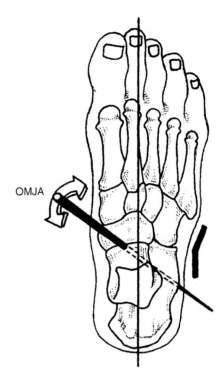

Figure 3.176. Normally, the oblique midtarsal joint axis (OMJA) allows for relatively equal amounts of transverse and sagittal plane motions.

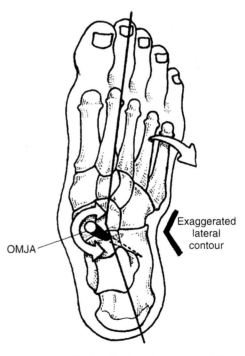

Figure 3.177. A vertically displaced oblique midtarsal joint axis (OMJA) allows for excessive abduction of the forefoot upon weight-bearing, as evidenced by the characteristic changes in the lateral contour of the calcaneocuboid joint.

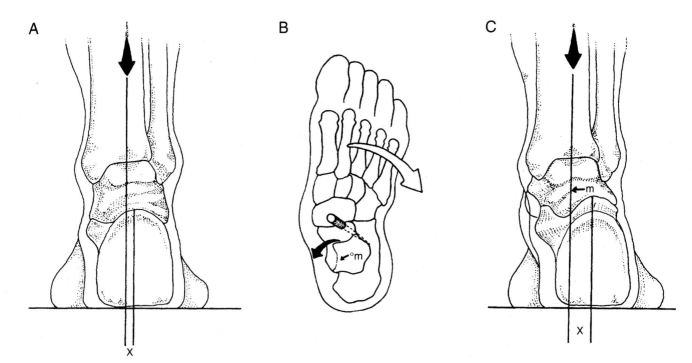

Figure 3.178. Normally, the talus is positioned almost directly over the calcaneus, thereby supplying body weight with a relatively small lever arm for pronating the subtalar joint (X in A). However, when a high oblique midtarsal joint axis is present (B), abduction of the forefoot occurs with simultaneous adduction of the rearfoot (arrows), which allows for a medial displacement of the talus relative to the calcaneus (arrow m in B and C). This in turn supplies body weight with a much more effective lever arm for pronating the subtalar joint (X in C).

this, a neutral position casting technique must be used, and the desired rearfoot and forefoot posts should be added together and placed beneath the distal medial aspect of the orthotic shell. (Remember that it is the orthotic shell that captures the rearfoot-to-forefoot relationship and that placement of the post merely determines how long the orthotic will remain functional.)

To give an example, imagine a patient with a high oblique midtarsal joint axis that requires a 3° forefoot varus post and a 4° rearfoot varus post. If the orthotic was posted in the usual manner with separate 3 and 4° posts placed beneath the forefoot and rearfoot, respectively, the subtalar joint would pronate an additional 4° as the patient's progression of forces passed anterior to the rock line of the orthotic (refer back to Fig. 3.92). This would allow the forefoot to abduct and the medial longitudinal arch to collapse just as the foot was approaching its propulsive period. The individual might complain that the distal orthotic seems to shift medially and/or the orthotic shell is digging into the soft tissues beneath the arch.

Hice (222) suggests that symptoms in this situation could have been avoided if a 7° forefoot varus post were added to the distal medial shell: this post angle would position the sagittal bisection of the rearfoot so that it is inverted 4° from perpendicular, which would allow for continued control of the subtalar joint until early propulsion. (This is essential for successful management of this deformity.) In almost all situations, the rearfoot of the orthotic shell should be posted flat for stability and, if necessary, a compressible post to sulcus may be added to allow for continued motion control throughout the propulsive period.

In situations in which there is no forefoot deformity and the individual presents with a combination rearfoot varus and high oblique midtarsal joint axis (which is a particularly difficult combination to treat), the desired rearfoot post should still be placed beneath the forefoot so it may continue to control motion during terminal stance phase. The use of the varus post placed beneath the distal medial shell is invaluable when treating this deformity, since it repositions the talus directly over the calcaneus, which effectively decreases the lever arm afforded body weight for pronating the subtalar joint.

In addition to foot orthoses, the use of firm, supportive shoe gear (with well-fitting heel counters), coupled with various proprioceptive and strengthening exercises, is usually necessary to treat a high oblique midtarsal joint axis successfully. The patient should be encouraged to "help the orthotic" by transferring the progression of forces along the lateral column and initiating a low gear push-off during propulsion. Also, because the chronically everted heel associated with this deformity often produces a functional forefoot varus deformity, manipulation of the tarsals should always be considered before prescribing a forefoot varus post.

DEVELOPMENTAL TRENDS IN LOWER EXTREMITY ALIGNMENT

At birth, rotational patterns of the lower extremity will differ significantly from those of the adult. During childhood and adolescence, the femur, tibia, and foot undergo very specific transformations in the transverse and frontal planes that will hopefully allow the adult to walk with a relatively straight gait pattern (i.e., the young adult should walk with an approximate 7° toe out gait pattern), with the tibia being nearly perpendicular to the ground at heel-strike. These developmental changes will be discussed separately, beginning with those occurring in the transverse plane.

Transverse Plane Alignment

In the infant, the femoral head is positioned in the acetabulum so that the femoral neck is angled approximately 60° posterior to the frontal plane (panel 1 in Fig. 3.179). Note that in panel 2, the femoral neck is internally rotated 35° to the transcondylar axis of the distal femur. This angle is referred to as the angle of femoral anteversion. (If the femoral neck were externally rotated relative to the distal femur, it would be referred to as femoral retroversion.) Because the 35° angle of femoral anteversion partially negates the 60° posterior positioning of the femoral head and neck in the acetabulum, the transcondylar axis of the knee joint is externally rotated 25° relative to the frontal plane (panel 3).

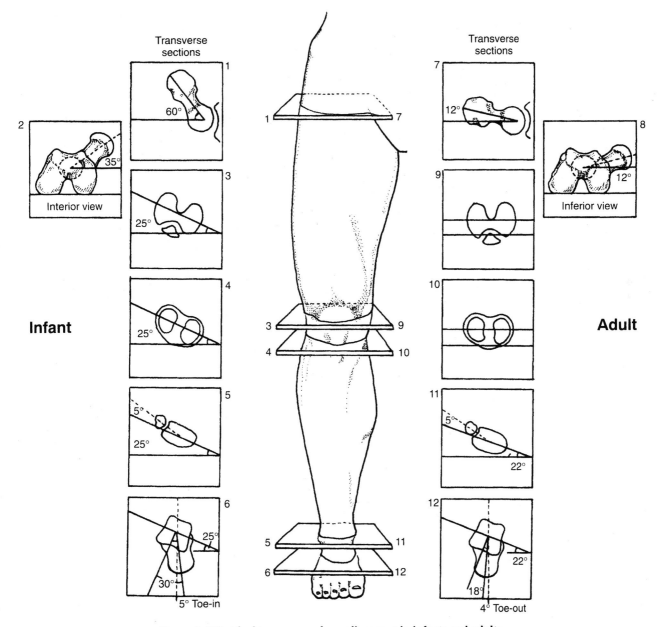

Figure 3.179. Ideal transverse plane alignment in infants and adults.

Panels 4 and 5 of Figure 3.179 demonstrate that the proximal and distal aspects of the tibia are well-aligned in the infant, i.e., there are 0° of tibial torsion. It is important to note that the degree of tibial torsion is difficult to evaluate without a CT scan or MRI and that on average, the degree of tibial torsion is approximately 5° less than the angle between the transmalleolar axis and the bisection of the proximal tibia. (Compare the dotted line in panel 5, which represents the transmalleolar axis, to the solid lines in panels 4 and 5, which represent actual tibial torsion.)

Panel 6 in Figure 3.179 illustrates the normal talar neck angle with respect to the superior articular surface of the body of the talus. This angle increases from 20° in the fetus to 30° in the infant (223). Since the entire foot follows the neck of the talus via the articulation with the navicular (223), the talar neck angle is an important, albeit often overlooked, component of transverse plane alignment.

By combining the various angles for each segment in the lower extremity, the average degree of toe-in should be approximately 5° (i.e., the talar neck in panel 6 deviates 5° medially from the sagittal plane). This is consistent with a study of 70 infants by Bleck (223) in which the mean normal internal rotation of the foot with reference to the line of progression was 4.4 ± 1.7°. Bleck noted that the internally rotated position of the foot in newborns is usually not noticed because most babies lie with their hips externally rotated. In fact, the prewalking child who is forced to stand will often turn his or her feet out by nearly 90° (224). This should not be considered abnormal, as it occurs only because the hips are maximally externally rotated. As the child begins to walk on its own, the normal toe in pattern becomes more apparent as all segments of the lower extremity rotate into their neutral positions during stance phase (223).

The ideal transverse plane alignment patterns in the adult are illustrated in panels 7–12. Note that in panels 7 and 8 the femoral neck is now positioned in the acetabulum approximately 12° posterior to the frontal plane, and the angle of femoral anteversion has reduced from 35° to 12° (8–15° is the norm). This allows the transcondylar axis of the distal femur to be positioned in the frontal plane (panel 9).

While complete derotation of the femoral neck generally occurs before the age of 8 (225), Bleck (223) claimed that the major reductions in femoral anteversion occur during the first 3 months of infancy, as extension and external rotation of the femur (which are necessary to reduce contracture of the hip flexors present at birth) produce an external rotational torque on the proximal end of the femur. Because this end of the femur is cartilaginous and is fixed to the rigid diaphysis, the external torque strain actually rotates the femoral neck relative to the shaft, producing a decrease in the angle of femoral anteversion. Apparently, this twist occurs in the subtrochanteric region where the plastic

cartilage of the proximal femur interfaces with the solid diaphysis (223).

Another important developmental change in alignment occurs in the tibia. By comparing the relative positions of the proximal and distal tibia in panels 10 and 11, you will note that the distal tibia becomes externally rotated 22° to the proximal tibia by adulthood. (The transmalleolar axis, which as mentioned is approximately 5° greater than the degree of tibial torsion, is positioned 27° to the frontal plane.) Jay (226) notes that the distal tibia rotates externally at a rate of 1–1.5°/year. This is clinically useful in determining the ideal degree of tibial torsion at a given age, in that a 10-year-old child should present with approximately 10° of external tibial torsion, with a transmalleolar axis of approximately 15°.

The final developmental change to be discussed occurs in the talar neck. From infancy to adulthood, the medial deviation of the talar neck should reduce from 30° to 18°, with the majority of these changes occurring by age 6 (223). Notice in panel 12 that after adding up the various transverse plane alignments, the adult should present with an approximate 4° toe out pattern when all segments are in neutral alignment. This angle of toe out is often deliberately increased, as most people externally rotate their hips in order to provide lateral stability during slower walking speeds.

While the developmental trends outlined in Figure 3.179 represent ideal ontogenic patterns, various genetic and/or developmental factors may either impair or exaggerate the rotational development at any or all segments of the lower extremity. While such torsional deformities may occasionally be inherited, they are more commonly developmental and typically result from faulty intrauterine positioning during the later months of pregnancy (224). Jay (226) noted that intrauterine constraints are more likely to detrimentally mold the fetal tissues when tight uterine muscles are present (as with a first-born child) or when a large fetus or multiple fetuses are present. Also, excessively tight abdominal muscles, a small pelvis, a prominent lumbar spine, uterine fibroids, or any fetal malposition (such as a breach or transverse lie position) all may impair normal rotation of the limb buds. The resultant torsional deformities are often maintained by various sitting and sleeping postures that act to perpetuate or even produce transverse plane malpositioning (Fig. 3.180).

In approximately 5–15% of the population, rotational patterns of infancy will persist beyond skeletal maturity (223). If the toe out gait pattern persists into adulthood (which usually is the result of femoral retroversion [228]), the individual is predisposed to injury because of the increase in pronatory forces placed upon the subtalar joint: normally, when the foot lands in a straight position, shear forces act to create a plantarflectory moment around the ankle axis. However, when the foot lands in a toe out gait

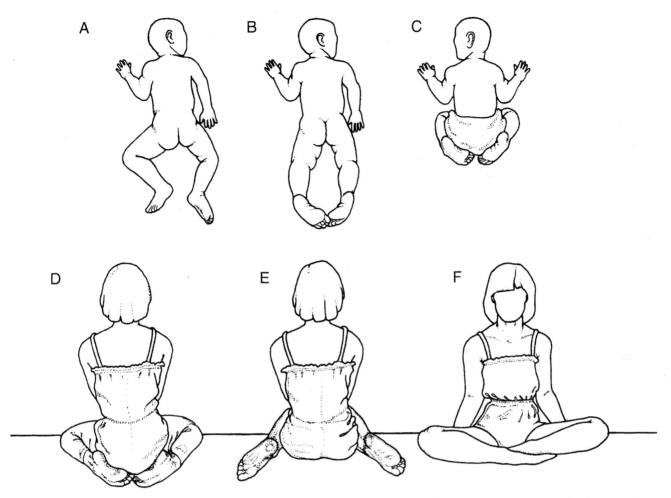

Figure 3.180. Sleeping and sitting postures that may perpetuate or produce various torsional deformities. (A) Prone frog leg: Abets external rotation deformity at hips, external tibial torsion, and valgus heels. **(B)** Prone, hips extended, feet adducted. Abets internal tibial torsion and varus heels. **(C)** Prone, hips flexed, feet adducted. Abets external rotation deformity at hips, internal tibial torsion, varus heels. **(D)** Sitting on adducted feet. Abets internal tibial torsion and varus heels. **(E)** Sitting with feet abducted (the "television position"). Abets excessive external tibial torsion and valgus heels. **(F)** Tailor's position. Abets external rotation deformity at hips and varus heels. With regard to these sitting and sleeping postures, Swanson et al. (227) stated that "the sleeping position which is initiated at birth and shortly thereafter may become a difficult habit to break and may carry over into the sitting and play postures and eventually into the walking postures of the child."

pattern, shear forces are applied more perpendicular to the subtalar axis and can therefore generate a strong pronatory force. It is for this reason that individuals with large ranges of external rotation at the hip are predisposed to medial tibial stress reactions (229).

A toe out gait pattern may also predispose to injury because it allows for a premature medial displacement of the normal progression of vertical forces (Fig. 3.181). This supplies body weight with an effective lever arm for maintaining the subtalar joint in a pronated position throughout midstance and propulsive periods. According to Davenport (230), excessive subtalar pronation associated with a toe out gait pattern may eventually result in loss of the medial longitudinal arch, adaptive shortening of the peroneals, im-

pingement of the talus upon the lateral aspect of the calcaneal sulcus (which often leads to a flattening and broadening of the lateral talar process), and a narrowing of the posterior talocalcaneal facet. Also, the first metatarsal head may also be damaged as the individual "rolls off" the medial forefoot; this forces the first ray into a dorsiflexed and inverted position and may predispose to tibial sesamoiditis, dorsal base exostosis, and dorsomedial bunion pain. It is for these reasons that MacConaill and Basmajian (228) claim that toe out gait patterns detrimentally affect mean levels of muscle activity much more than toe in patterns.

In the adult, a toe in gait pattern is relatively harmless, even though it forces the individual to maintain a low-gear push-off, which makes for a less efficient propulsion.

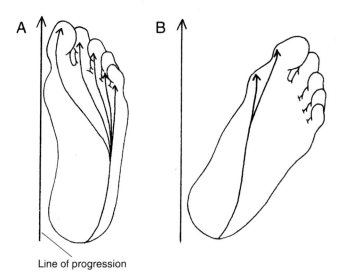

Line of progression

Figure 3.181. (A) Normal progression of forces; (B) progression of force with a toe out gait pattern.

The toe in gait pattern is more of a problem in children, as they learn to "correct" the deformity by abducting the forefoot upon the rearfoot. Although it gives the appearance of a straight toe gait pattern, this method of compensation is destructive, as it may permanently damage the architectural stability of the foot by obliterating the medial longitudinal arch. In fact, it is not uncommon for a child to outgrow the primary torsional component of the toe in, only to be left with a permanent flat foot deformity (231).

Because of the potential for deformity, Cailliet (94) claims that a toe in gait pattern should be encouraged and not discouraged or corrected, as it allows children to bear weight on the lateral border of the foot, which causes the foot to supinate, thereby allowing for the development of a functional medial longitudinal arch.

Treatment for the various torsional deformities is dependent on the location of the deformity and the age of the child. The segment or segments responsible for a toe in or out gait pattern can be identified with any of several different evaluation techniques. To begin with, a brief gait evaluation should be performed to determine the presence of femoral anteversion: If the knee joint points inwardly relative to the line of progression, then femoral anteversion is present. This will produce a toe in gait pattern unless compensatory external tibial torsion is present. It should be noted that it is not uncommon for multiple deformities to either negate or amplify one another, e.g., femoral anteversion with external tibial torsion produces a relatively straight gait pattern, while femoral anteversion with medial talar torsion and/or internal tibial torsion produces an extreme toe in gait pattern. The gait evaluation should be completed by recording the approximate deviation of each foot relative to the line of progression.

The position of the femoral neck may also be evaluated with the child positioned prone with the knee flexed 90°. By internally and externally rotating the femur and noting the position of the tibia when the greater trochanter is parallel to the examination table, the approximate degree of femoral ante or retroversion is easily determined (Fig. 3.182). This testing position is also useful for noting the degree of internal and external femoral rotation (Fig. 3.183).

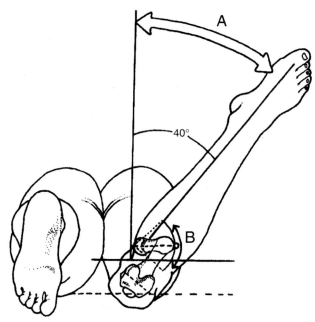

Figure 3.182. Craig's test. The examiner grasps the patient's ankle and rotates the femur **(A)** until the opposite hand palpates the greater trochanter as being parallel to the examining table (B). By noting the position of the tibia relative to vertical, it is possible to determine the degree of femoral ante or retroversion, i.e., in this case, the femoral neck is anteverted 40°. (Partially adapted from Magee DJ. Orthopedic Physical Assessment. Philadelphia: Saunders, 1987: 252.)

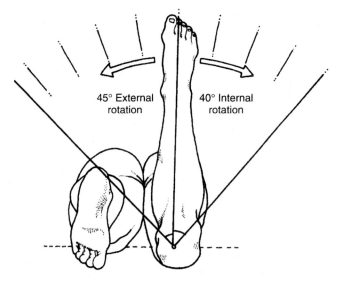

45° External rotation   40° Internal rotation

Figure 3.183. Determining relative degree of internal and external femoral rotation.

The diagnosis of excessive femoral anteversion can be made if the range of internal rotation exceeds 70° and the range of external rotation is less than 25° (224). While many investigators use the term "internal femoral torsion" to denote a pathological range of anteversion (i.e., internal femoral torsion exists when the degree of version or twist in a long bone exceeds by more than 2 SDs the norm for that age group), this text has deliberately avoided use of this term because of discrepancies in the literature regarding norm and inconsistencies in the term "torsion": internal or external tibial torsion does not denote pathology while internal or external femoral torsion does. Also, because variations in joint laxity may alter values for norm (224), subjective adjustments must be made if the overall range of motion is excessive (greater than 110°) or restricted (less than 75°).

If excessive femoral anteversion is present, the use of shoe modifications, twister cables, and night splints should be discouraged since they do not alter the natural history of gradual correction (233). In fact, twister cables only serve to promote the development of a pathological range of external tibial torsion (223) while the use of night splints may result in aseptic necrosis of the femoral head or hip dislocation if the respective external or internal force produced by the device is excessive (234, 238). Although excessive femoral anteversion was at one time blamed for the development of osteoarthrosis, bunion formation, flat feet, low back pain, and impaired athletic performance (235), these beliefs have long since been disproved (236).

Conservative treatment should consist of recommendations for changes in sitting and sleeping habits that neutralize or reverse the torsional deformity. Also, physical activities such as roller or ice skating and cross-country skiing are effective ways to teach a child to function with the hips in a more midline position. Classical ballet lessons, as long as they are initiated before the age of 11, may actually allow for a reduction in the degree of femoral anteversion (237). (Sammarco [237] cautioned that if an excessive turnout is forced on the adolescent after that age, the resultant increased range of motion is due to microscopic ruptures of the anterior hip capsule, not changes in the degree of femoral anteversion.)

Finally, although they do not alter the progression of femoral anteversion or retroversion, foot orthoses should be considered if excessive subtalar pronation is present. Because of an unacceptably high rate of complications, surgical intervention should be avoided (223).

Evaluation of tibial torsion requires that the child sit on the edge of an examining table with the knees flexed 90°. A goniometer is then used to measure the relationship between the transmalleolar axis of the ankle and the transcondylar axis of the knee (which, for all practical purposes, is represented by the edge of the table; see Fig. 3.184). The degree of tibial torsion is then determined by subtracting 5° from the formed angle. The resultant number

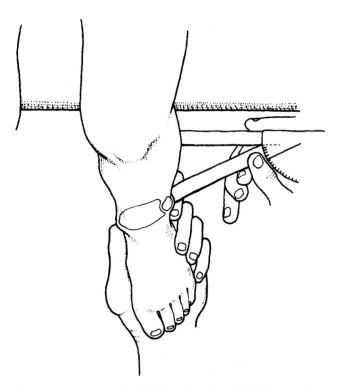

Figure 3.184. Measuring tibial torsion. (Modified from a photograph in Bleck EE. Developmental orthopaedics. III. Toddlers. Dev Med Child Neurol 1982; 24: 533–555.)

should be compared to the child's age. (Remember that the distal tibia externally rotates from a starting position of 0° at birth approximately 1–1.5°/year.)

If even slight tibial torsion is present, recommendations should be made for changes in sitting or sleeping habits (i.e., habitually sitting on adducted feet is a common cause for internal tibial torsion). If greater than 5° of tibial torsion is present between the ages of 6 and 12 months, correction may be possible with serial long leg casts (which extend from the toes to above the knees). Approximately once every 4 weeks, circumferential cuts are made at the proximal tibial junction, and the distal aspect of the cast is rotated 2 cm. This process is repeated several times until correction has been achieved.

Although the efficacy of night braces has not been thoroughly evaluated, most authorities recommend their use between the ages of 16 months and 3 years. The Langer Counter Rotation System (Fig. 3.185) is particularly well-tolerated by the child because it allows for reciprocal motion of the right and left lower extremities, enabling the child to crawl (238). When using night braces, care must be taken to maintain the subtalar joint in an inverted position, as failure to do so would allow the external rotational force created by the brace to abduct the forefoot, thereby creating flatfoot deformity.

While most authorities claim that internal tibial torsion is the most common cause of a toe in gait pattern (224,

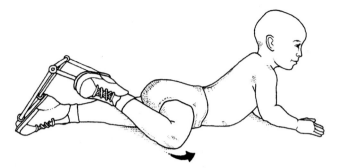

Figure 3.185. The Langer Pediatric Counter Rotation system. (Modified from a photograph in The Langer Group Newsletter. Deer Park, NY: Langer Biomechanics Group, May 1987; 14 (2): 15.)

226), Bleck (223) claims that when measured carefully, internal tibial torsion is a rare phenomenon and that medial talar torsion is the most common cause. It is possible to determine the degree of medial talar torsion by measuring the thigh-foot angle as the patient lies prone with the knees flexed 90° (Fig. 3.186). Because this angle represents the combined degree of both tibial and talar torsion, the approximate angle of medial talar torsion can be determined by noting the difference between the previously determined degree of tibial torsion and the thigh-foot angle.

For example, an adult with 22° of external tibial torsion and a thigh-foot angle of +4° will possess approximately 18° of medial talar torsion (as in panels 11 and 12 in Fig. 3.179). Ideally, since medial talar torsion reduces as external tibial torsion increases, the thigh-foot angle should gradually increase from approximately −10° in the 6 year old to +4° in the adult. (Unfortunately, details regarding the exact rate of derotation are scant and unreliable.)

If excessive medial talar torsion is present (i.e., greater than 30–40° in the infant and 15–20° in 3- to 6 year olds), recommendations should be made for changes in sitting and sleeping postures, and night braces should be considered. (These are particularly useful for 0- to 18-month-old infants.) Also, twister cables may be an effective form of treatment when used on 3- to 6-year-old children (223).

Interestingly, foot orthoses and/or shoe gear that inhibit midtarsal pronation about the oblique axis may impair the normal reduction in the degree of medial talar torsion. According to Bleck (223), abduction of the navicular during stance phase may be necessary to pull the neck of the talus laterally, thereby reducing the medial angulation of the talar neck. Because of this situation, foot orthoses that disallow the normal range of midtarsal pronation should be avoided, and only flexible, straight-lasted shoes should be allowed.

Of course, if destruction of the medial longitudinal arch occurs secondary to excessive subtalar or midtarsal joint pronation, then a partially controlling foot orthosis may be necessary to prevent permanent deformity. Because

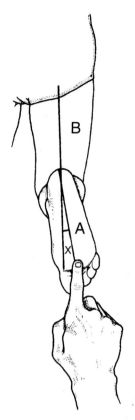

Figure 3.186. Measuring the thigh-foot angle. The subtalar joint is placed in its neutral position, and the forefoot is gently depressed with the index finger. The thigh-foot angle (**X**) is measured at the intersection of a line that parallels the medial mid and forefoot (**A**) and the continuation of a line that bisects the thigh (**B**). This angle is noted as positive if the forefoot is abducted with respect to the thigh bisection (as in this illustration), whereas a negative angle indicates that the forefoot is adducted. Care must be taken when marking the foot, as failure to maintain subtalar neutrality will result in gross error while the presence of a forefoot deformity, such as metatarsus adductus, will also result in inaccurate measurement. In the case of forefoot malalignment, accurate measurement may still be achieved by bisecting the rearfoot only.

the angle of medial talar torsion becomes fixed by age 6, functional foot orthoses after that age may be invaluable in maintaining a normal medial longitudinal arch until the foot reaches skeletal maturity during the early teens.

Although it has only briefly been mentioned, it is also possible that an in toe gait pattern is the result of a metatarsus adductus. In this condition, which is often mistakenly referred to as metatarsus varus, the metatarsals are angled medially, relative to the longitudinal bisection of the rearfoot. Because the medial angulation may occur at either the tarsometatarsal or midtarsal joint, some investigators distinguish between metatarsus adductus and forefoot adductus (Fig. 3.187). It is possible to categorize the extent of a metatarsus or forefoot adductus by noting where the longi-

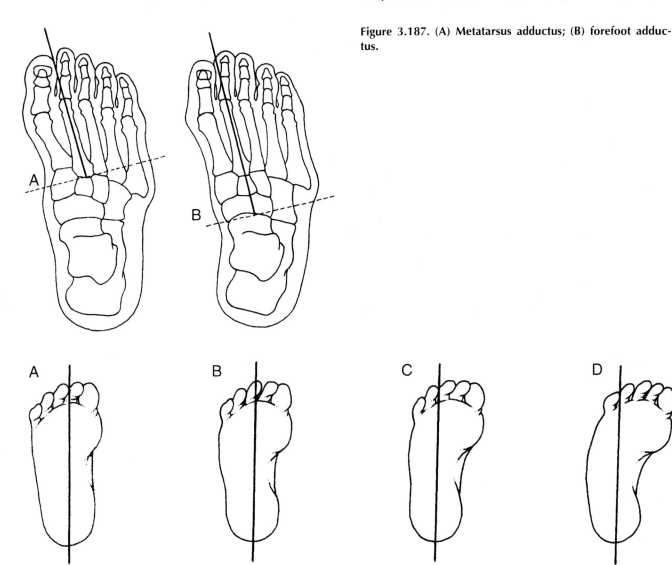

Figure 3.187. (A) Metatarsus adductus; (B) forefoot adductus.

Figure 3.188. In the normal foot, a line bisecting the heel should pass between the second and third digits (A). If a mild metatarsus or forefoot adductus is present, the line will pass through the third digit. In moderate and marked deformities (C and D), the heel bisector will pass between the third and fourth and fifth digits, respectively. (Modified from Bleck EE. Developmental orthopaedics. III. Toddlers. Dev Med Child Neurol 1982; 24: 533–555.)

tudinal bisection of the rearfoot intersects with the metatarsal heads (Fig. 3.188). Also, the flexibility of the foot should be evaluated by passively abducting the forefoot against the stabilized rearfoot. If the deformity is flexible, the forefoot may be abducted beyond midline; if semiflexible, it can be moved to midline only, and a rigid deformity cannot be moved to midline.

Unfortunately, there is no clear-cut criteria for determining which deformities continue through osseous maturity: often, a marked semiflexible deformity resolves during childhood while a mild flexible deformity may become permanent. As a general rule, it is suggested that mild deformities receive no treatment other than recommendations for changes in sitting and sleeping postures, wearing shoes on opposite feet and a gentle stretching procedure where the parent abducts the forefoot against the stabilized heel. These stretches should be maintained for 40 seconds and be repeated a minimum of 10 times daily.

Because it is difficult to correct a metatarsus adductus or forefoot adductus after infancy, it is suggested that moderate and marked deformities be treated with serial plaster casts (preferably before 8 months and ideally at the age of 4 months). This treatment involves wearing a plaster cast that maintains the heel in varus while the forefoot is molded into abduction. Two or three of these casts, changed every 1 or 2 weeks, are usually sufficient to achieve correction.

While many investigators feel that conservative treatment in the form of casts, braces, shoe gear, and/or stretches is no longer effective after the age of 2, Staheli (224) claims that a long leg cast may produce correction of the deformity if used before the age of 5. Operative correction is practically never appropriate because poor results are common and because an untreated metatarsus adductus has little potential for disability. A point of interest is that a metatarsus adductus deformity is often mistaken for a hallux adductus or "searching toe" in which hyperactivity of the abductor hallucis muscle produces a dynamic adduction of the hallux during gait.

Because of the potential for permanent impairment, it is important to differentiate a metatarsus adductus from a club foot deformity (talipes equinovarus). Unlike metatarsus adductus, a club foot is characterized by an inverted heel that does not evert to midline and a nonreducible ankle equinus. These combined deformities force the child to stand with full body weight centered beneath the fifth metatarsal head. This condition, which represents a defect in prenatal development, requires immediate plaster casting to reduce the forefoot varus and adductus and, after these have been corrected, the equinus. If the cast treatment is not successful during the first 4 months of life, surgical correction may be necessary. A complete description of this condition is well beyond the scope of this text. Suffice it to say that whether surgically treated or not, the clubbed foot is a common cause for uncompensated rearfoot varus deformities.

In addition to osseous causes for toe in or toe out gait patterns, it is also possible that, despite ideal osseous alignment, soft tissue contracture in the thigh or pelvis may produce an altered gait pattern. For example, contracture of the medial hamstring musculature will force the entire lower extremity into an internally rotated position during late swing phase (which is often maintained throughout the stance phase) while contracture of the biceps femoris muscle will have the exact opposite effect.

If it had been the iliopsoas musculature that was abnormally shortened, the lower extremity will often externally rotate during the propulsive period, as the spine is simultaneously forced into hyperextension. Also, children who sit in the tailor's position will often present with contracture in the hip external rotators that produces a toe out gait pattern. It is clear that comprehensive evaluation of torsional deformities should include examination for adaptive shortening of all the muscles in the lower extremity and pelvis.

In closing this section on transverse plane deformity, it should be emphasized that the role of foot orthoses is not to correct an osseous malformation, but rather, to prevent destruction of the medial longitudinal arch that might otherwise have occurred during growth years. A common treatment regimen is to use a polyethylene orthotic shell that is formed with long lateral and medial flanges and a deep heel seat (see Fig. 6.3). A minimum 5° rearfoot varus post is recommended to prevent abnormal pronation (231). Because

these orthotics will prevent excessive abduction of the forefoot, parents of children with toe in gait patterns should be informed that the orthotics might actually increase the appearance of the toe in deformity and that the purpose of the orthotic is to maintain the integrity of the medial longitudinal arch while normal ontogeny hopefully allows the torsional deformity to resolve itself. Because they prevent normal derotation of the forefoot about the longitudinal midtarsal joint axis, forefoot varus posts should be avoided in children less than 6 years old (239).

Although some orthotic laboratories recommend that gait plates be used to treat torsional deformities (Fig. 3.189), these devices should be avoided with toe out deformities and are of questionable value with toe in deformities since the resultant propulsive period pronation, although visually appealing to the parents, will not facilitate correction of the deformity.

Comprehensive conservative care should always include recommendations for changes in sitting and sleeping postures, along with recommendations for home stretches and exercises. Even if ineffective, these exercises give the parents a sense of control and may ease anxiety over the eventual development of the deformity. Sleeping in a side-lying position with a pillow placed beneath the head to maintain spinal alignment should be encouraged, since it prevents aspiration with regurgitation while also maintaining the limbs in a neutral position (240). This position, with sides alternated after each feeding, is particularly important during the first 3 months of life when movements are minimal and deformity is more likely to be maintained. Swanson et al. (227) claim that children who sleep in a side-lying position most often present with their legs parallel and little internal or external rotation.

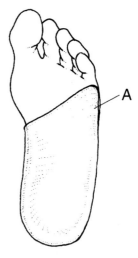

Figure 3.189. The gait plate for toe in deformities. By extending a rigid orthotic shell distally beneath the fourth and fifth metatarsal heads **(A)**, the child is unable to effectively push-off without abducting the forefoot in order to roll off of the medial forefoot.

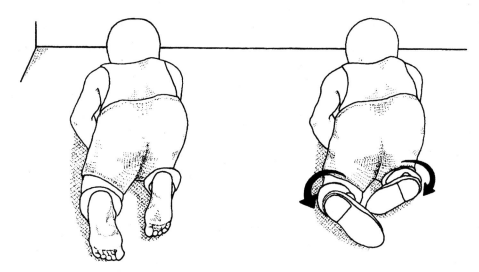

Figure 3.190. Stiff-soled shoes may force the crawling child to internally or externally rotate the legs. (Modified from photographs in Schuster RO. The effects of modern foot gear. J Am Podiatry Assoc 1978: 68 (4): 235.)

Final recommendations should be made for shoe gear: the lasts should not maintain the deformity (i.e., the child with metatarsus adductus should not be wearing a curve-lasted shoe), and the soles should be flexible. As noted by Schuster (241), it is not unusual for a child's shoe to require more bending force than the child actually weighs. In his evaluation of sole stiffness, this investigator demonstrated that various shoes require anywhere from 4–70 lbs of pressure to bend at the ball. A stiff-soled shoe forces the crawling child to progress with an in or out toe pattern (Fig. 3.190) and may delay onset of walking for weeks (241). A stiff- soled shoe may also increase torsional deformity in the walking child, as it inhibits dorsiflexion of the toes at the metatarsophalangeal joints. This effectively increases the length of the foot, and the child often develops a toe in or toe out gait pattern in order to roll off the medial or lateral aspect of the shoe (thereby shortening the functional length of the foot).

Frontal Plane Alignment

In addition to the specific changes occurring in the transverse plane, it is also essential that certain developmental changes occur in the frontal plane that allow the tibia to be nearly perpendicular to the ground at heel strike. The ideal frontal plane developmental trends are described in Figure 3.191.

As noted in the section describing the rearfoot varus deformity, defects in frontal plane alignment may occur if premature walking is initiated when the physiological varum is at its peak. Because most cases of tibial or genu varum reduce spontaneously, treatment before the age of 18 months is seldom necessary (13). If after 18 months the physiological varum has not improved (i.e., the medial femoral condyles are more than 4 cm apart when the medial malleoli are placed together, and radiographs show a medial beaking of the proximal tibial metaphysis), then a Danish night splint should be considered (Fig. 3.192).

Although it is less common, it is also possible that abnormal development of the lower extremity will result in a genu valgum. While the most common cause for this deformity is renal osteodystrophy (13), it may also be the result of infection, tumor, trauma, or various paralytic conditions. According to Kling (13), treatment for children less than 7 years of age may be safely ignored unless the condition is asymmetrical, excessive (i.e., the tibiofemoral angle is greater than 15°), or if the child presents with a short stature.

Children with a genu valgum secondary to trauma may be treated with a knock-knee brace that should be worn for approximately 1 year. Bleck (223) claimed that 1% of genu valgum deformities persist beyond the age of 10. If at this age the malleoli are more than 3 inches apart when the knees are positioned together, then stapling of the medial distal epiphysis should be considered. As with torsional deformities, foot orthoses for individuals with genu valgum are recommended to prevent deformity of the foot during growth years. Gould et al. (243) noted a significant correlation between the presence of valgus knees and hyperpronated feet. They stated that all of the subjects in their study who presented without valgus knees had normal arches. The medial longitudinal arch is predisposed to collapse in the presence of a genu valgum because those individuals walk with a wide base of gait that allows body weight to fall medially to the talus, thereby creating a strong pronatory force at the subtalar joint. The same biomechanical scenario also exists with rearfoot valgus deformities (Fig. 3.193), in extremely obese individuals and in women during the 3rd trimester of pregnancy who walk with a wide base of gait.

Orthotic management in all of these situations is to get under the pronatory force from above by using an extrinsic rearfoot post with a high medial heel cup and a medial outflare on the post. (These additions are described in the laboratory preparation section.) Gould (245) noted that the rearfoot varus post should slowly reduce the genu val-

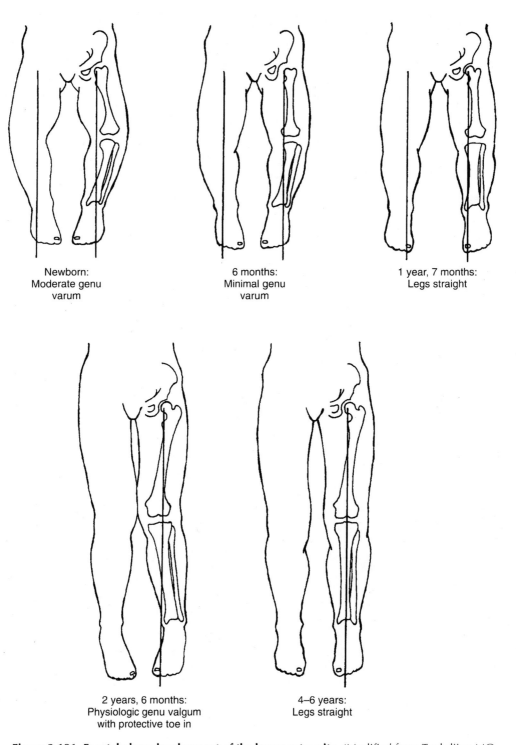

Newborn:
Moderate genu
varum

6 months:
Minimal genu
varum

1 year, 7 months:
Legs straight

2 years, 6 months:
Physiologic genu valgum
with protective toe in

4–6 years:
Legs straight

Figure 3.191. Frontal plane development of the lower extremity. (Modified from Tachdjian MO. Pediatric Orthopedics. Philadelphia: Saunders, 1972: 1463.)

gum deformity, possibly because it externally rotates the tibia, thereby allowing for improved functional alignment at the knee. Langer (246) suggested that effective treatment may require changes in shoe gear such as adding a medial outflare to the heel of the shoe and, if necessary, reinforcing the medial aspect of the heel counter with stiffening

material. It should be emphasized that some individuals present with a base of gait that is so wide that it is physically impossible to create an orthotic that can support medial to the application of body weight. This being the case, a rearfoot post on an orthotic may actually act to increase pressure on the medial plantar heel, which is already sup-

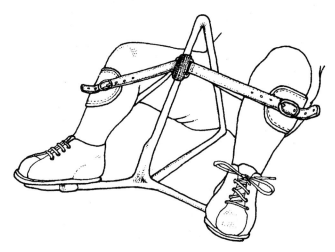

Figure 3.192. The Danish night splint may be used to correct an excessive physiological varum. Unfortunately, this splint (which may be worn until age 3) is ineffective at treating the adolescent form of Blount's disease, which typically produces tibial varum in obese black males between the ages of 5 and 14. Surgical correction with valgus osteotomy may be the only way to maintain normal mechanical alignment in these cases. (Adapted from Blount W. Tibia vara: osteochondrosis deformans tibiae. In: Adams JP (ed). Current Practice in Orthopedic Surgery. St. Louis: C.V. Mosby, 1966: 141–156.)

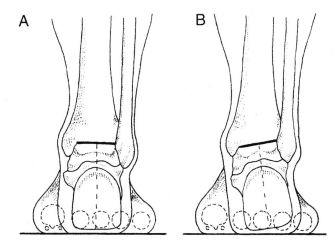

Figure 3.193. Normally, the ankle joint will form in such a way that its articular surface is perpendicular to the tibial shaft (A). It is, however, possible for the ankle joint to be inverted or everted relative to the tibial shaft (244). An everted ankle joint results in the formation of a subtalar valgus deformity **(B).** (Note that this is a relatively rare phenomenon.)

porting too much weight. This may result in iatrogenic injury to the medial calcaneal condyle and/or tissues beneath the calcaneal incline angle. These injuries may be avoided by taking weight-bearing foot impressions with the patient standing in a normal base of gait while maintaining talonavicular congruency. Orthotics made from these impressions

should not be posted and should serve primarily as supports necessary to prevent destruction of the medial longitudinal arch.

Development of the Medial Longitudinal Arch

The last prerequisite for normal function is that ontogeny allow for the development of a functional medial longitudinal arch. Not only is deflection of the medial arch necessary for adequate shock absorption but the restraining ligaments that stabilize the arch are invaluable during locomotion since they store and return elastic energy during the early and latter periods of stance phase, respectively. Gould et al. (243) studied development of the medial longitudinal arch in 125 beginning walkers and noted that the development of a neutral arch required a well-developed sustentaculum tali (Fig. 3.194), a healthy tibialis posterior tendon and muscle, an adequate deltoid ligament, a non-constricted achilles tendon and a properly placed inferior calcaneonavicular ligament. These investigators noted that the development of the arch, which was proven to be accelerated with the use of arch supports, is not complete until age 8. They also noted that hyperpronation (most often secondary to genu valgum) was the norm for 5 year olds. This discredits previous anecdotal reports, claiming that younger children possess a healthy medial longitudinal arch that is obliterated by a fat pad.

As with frontal and transverse plane malpositions of the lower extremity, various congenital and/or developmental factors may impair development of the medial longitudinal arch, thereby resulting in the formation of a flatfoot deformity. The four most common types of flatfoot defor-

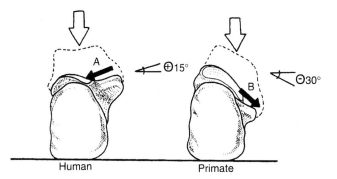

Figure 3.194. As viewed in the frontal plane, the sustentaculum tali should be angled in such a way that it supports the talus, displacing it laterally with superimposed body weight (A). Inman (247) stated that the sustentaculum tali in a neutral foot will show a positive angle between 5 and 15°. Notice how the sustentaculum tali in the primate is angled inferiorly, thereby allowing for a plantar medial migration of the talus **(B).** Gould et al. (243) noted that a hyperpronated foot will present with a 0° or negative angle of the sustentaculum tali. They also noted that the sustentaculum tali should be fully ossified by age 7.

mity are described in the following section. Note that the first two types of flatfoot deformity are mentioned only for purposes of exclusion since they are relatively rare and are treated with aggressive casting techniques and/or surgery during the first few months of life.

Convex pes valgus.   Also known as a vertical talus or rocker bottom foot, this uncommon condition can be identified in the newborn by the dorsiflexed and abducted forefoot that is rigid and does not reduce. It represents a primary dislocation of the talonavicular joint in which the talus is locked in a plantarflexed position, with the navicular articulating with the dorsal aspect of the talus. (A crease actually forms along the dorsal talonavicular space.) This causes the sole of the foot to appear convex as the talar head bulges plantarly. Although the etiology for this condition remains uncertain, it is believed to be the result of neuromuscular disease or defects in tarsal evolution that are aggravated by intrauterine molding (248). It is unfortunate that conservative treatment for this deformity with casting and manipulation is seldom effective, and operative correction is almost always necessary.

Talipes calcaneovalgus.   This condition is often referred to as congenital flatfoot and is similar to the vertical talus in that the forefoot is dorsiflexed and everted. (The foot actually appears to be folded laterally upon itself.) Because this deformity is always flexible, it responds well to a conservative treatment program of taping, manipulation, and casting as long as treatment is initiated before 18 months of age (249). As with the vertical talus, the etiology remains uncertain but is mostly likely the result of intrauterine positioning or neuromuscular disease.

Peroneal spastic flatfoot.   Also known as rigid flatfoot, the peroneal spastic flatfoot is associated with spasm of the lateral compartment musculature, which maintains the heel in a fixed position of valgus. (The heel is resistant to both active and passive inversion.) In approximately 70–80% of these cases, the etiology can be related to various tarsal coalitions that may be osseous (synostosis), cartilaginous (synchondrosis), fibrous (syndesmosis), or a combination thereof. The most common coalitions occur between the talus and the calcaneus with calcaneonavicular coalitions being the second most common. Because of difficulties in identifying the various coalitions with x-rays, CT or MRI may be essential. The remaining 20–30% of cases with peroneal spastic flatfoot may be related to any of several factors, including trauma (fracture or sprain/strain), tuberculosis of the tarsals, rheumatoid arthritis, nonspecific tarsal synovitis, tenosynovitis of the peroneals or tibialis posterior, osteoarthrosis, neoplasm, or subtalar arthrodesis (250). For whatever reason, the diminished subtalar joint motion somehow creates a cycle of pain, peroneal spasm, and calcaneovalgus, which becomes progressively more rigid with time. Although the peroneal spastic flatfoot is often present from birth, it rarely produces symptoms before adolescence, when excessive activity or a sudden

sprain disrupts the adhesions, sometimes producing incapacitating pain.

Conservative treatment for the peroneal spastic flatfoot should include manipulation, immobilization (short or long leg cast may be used), and/or foot orthotics. Subotnick (251) recommended that foot orthotics be made by casting the foot in its most comfortable position and then using the appropriately sized forefoot and/or rearfoot posts to maintain this position during ambulation. Although there is much conflicting information in the literature regarding the efficacy of conservative care, such treatments should always be considered since they are safe and very often effective (particularly in cases of acute trauma and inflammatory arthritis [250]). In many cases, however, conservative treatment affords only temporary relief, as it does not correct what is most often the underlying cause of the peroneal spastic flatfoot: tarsal coalitions. If symptoms persist despite comprehensive conservative care, surgical excision of the coalition may be necessary. Surgical intervention is more likely to produce a favorable result if the coalition is narrow and the patient is young, i.e., less than 20 years old.

Hypermobile flatfoot.   As previously mentioned, the hypermobile flatfoot may be secondary to anatomical variation in the shape of the sustentaculum tali or to generalized ligamentous laxity. It can be readily identified by the extreme lowering of the medial longitudinal arch upon weight-bearing, the increased range of forefoot inversion, medial displacement of the talus relative to the calcaneus, and the dramatically reduced range of ankle dorsiflexion. The severity of the deformity can be determined by measuring the talometatarsal angle on lateral weight-bearing x-rays: If the talometatarsal angle is between 1 and 15°, a mild deformity is present; a 16–30 ° angle represents moderate deformity; and an angle greater than 30° is considered a severe deformity (Fig. 3.195).

Orthotic treatment should only be considered after the age of 3 since ages 1–3 represent a holding period during which no specific treatment is needed, other than firm, supportive shoe gear with a small arch support (252). Children with moderate or severe deformities are candidates for foot orthoses, particularly if there is a family history of flatfoot. Successful orthotic treatment necessitates that an off-weight-bearing plaster cast be taken in which all segments are maintained in their neutral position (252). A polypropylene shell is then molded over the positive model (note that the medial longitudinal arch is not lowered), and the child is instructed to wear the orthotics constantly, preferably in high-top shoes with long stiff heel counters. Lateral weight-bearing x-rays should be taken with the orthotic in the shoe to ensure that proper correction has been achieved. If the talometatarsal angle has not been reduced, the orthotic must be refabricated. Bordelon (252) has demonstrated that when worn constantly, the orthotics produce a rate of correction in the talometatarsal angle of approximately 5°/year.

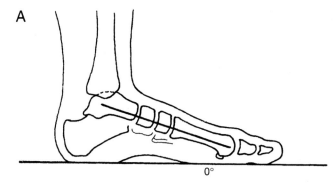

A

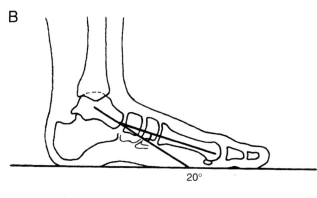

B

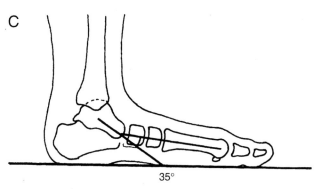

C

Figure 3.195. Measurement of the lateral talometatarsal angle. **(A)** Normal; **(B)** moderate deformity; **(C)** severe deformity. (Adapted from Bordelon RL. Hypermobile flatfoot in children. Clin Orthop Related Res 1983; 181: 7–14.)

Because the improvement in the talometatarsal angle persists even after the orthotic has been discontinued, it can be assumed that these are permanent osseous changes, as is consistent with the laws of Heuter-Volkmann, Davis, and Wolff. If the deformity remains unchanged despite constant use of the orthotic for several years, and the severity of the achilles tendon contracture remains unchanged, surgery should be considered. Arthrodesis (particularly of the subtalar joint) should be avoided whenever possible, as the procedure of choice is an achilles tendon lengthening with osteotomy of the calcaneus to align the heel (252). After operative correction, the patient should continue to wear the

foot orthoses until approximately 13 years of age in females and 15 years in males.

References

1. McPoil TG, Knecht HG, Schuit D. A survey of foot types in normal females between the ages of 18 and 30 years. J Orthop Sports Phys Ther 1988; 9: 406–409.
2. Hlavac H. Compensated forefoot varus. J Am Podiatr Assoc 1970; 60: 229–233.
3. Root MC, Orion WP, Weed JH. Normal and Abnormal Function of the Foot. Los Angeles: Clinical Biomechanics, 1977.
4. Salenius P, Vankka E. The development of the tibiofemoral angle in children. J Bone Joint Surg 1975; 57A: 259–261.
5. Yochum TR, Rowe LJ. Essentials of skeletal radiology. Baltimore: Williams & Wilkins, 1987: 1014.
6. Cockshott WP: Dactylitis and growth disorders. Br J Radiol 1964; 36:19.
7. Watson RJ, Burko H, Megas H, et al. Hand-foot syndrome in sickle cell disease in young children. Pediatrics 1963; 31: 975.
8. Bateson EM. The relationship between Blount's disease and bow legs. Br J Radiol 1968; 41: 107–114.
9. Bathfeld CA, Beighton PH. Blount's disease: a review of etiological factors in 110 patients. Clin Orthop 1978; 135: 29–33.
10. Kessel L. Annotations on the etiology and treatment of tibia vara. J Bone Joint Surg 1970; 52B: 93–99.
11. Cook SD, Lavernia CJ, Burke SW. A biomechanical analysis of the etiology of tibia vara. J Pediatr Orthop 1983; 3: 449–454.
12. Golding JSR, MacNeil-Smith JDG. Observations on the etiology of tibia vara. J Bone Joint Surg 1963; 45B: 320–325.
13. Kling TF. Angular deformities of the lower limbs in children. Orthop Clin North Am 1987; 4: 513–527.
14. Scranton PE, et al. Support phase kinematics of the foot. In Bateman JE, Trott AW (eds). The Foot and Ankle. New York: Thieme-Stratton, 1980.
15. Viitasolo JT, Kvist M. Some biomechanical aspects of the foot and ankle in athletes with and without shin splints. Am J Sports Med 1983; 11: 125–130.
16. Clarke TE, Frederick EC, Hamill CL. The effects of shoe design parameters on rearfoot control in running. Med Sci Sports Exercise 1983; 15: 376–381.
17. James SL, Bates BT, Osternig LR. Injuries to runners. Am J Sports Med 1978; 6:40–50.
18. Brown LP, Yavorsky P. Locomotor biomechanics and pathomechanics: a review. J Orthop Sports Phys Ther 1987; 1:7.
19. Messier SP, Pittala KA. Etiologic factors associated with selected running injuries. Med Sci Sports Exercise 1988; 5: 501–505.
20. Cavanagh PR, et al. An evaluation of the effect of orthotics on force distribution and rearfoot movement during running. Paper presented at the American Orthopaedics Society Sports Medicine Meeting, Lake Placid, NY, 1978.
21. Inman VT, Mann RA. DuVries Surgery of the Foot. St. Louis: CV Mosby, 1970.
22. Matheson GO, Clement DB, McKenzie DC. Stress fractures

in athletes. A study of 320 cases. Am J Sports Med 1987; 15: 46–58.

23. Riegger C. Mechanical properties of bone. In: Gould JA, Davies GJ (eds). Orthopaedic and Sports Physical Therapy. St. Louis, Mosby, 1985; 3–49.

24. Lutter LD. Foot related knee problems in the long distance runner. Foot Ankle 1980; 1: 112–116.

25. McKenzie DC, Clement DB, Taunton JE. Running shoes, orthotics and injuries. Sports Med 1985; 2: 334–347.

26. Noble CA. Iliotibial band friction syndrome in runners. Am J Sports Med 1980; 8:232–234.

27. D'Amico JC, Rubin M. The influence of foot orthoses on the quadriceps angle. J Am Podiatr Med Assoc 1986; 76: 337–339.

28. Kegerreis S, Malone T, Johnson F. The diagonal medial plica: an underestimated clinical entity. J Orthop Sports Phys Ther 1988; 9: 305–309.

29. Huberti HH, Hayes WC. Patellofemoral contact pressures. J Bone Joint Surg 1984; 66A: 715–724.

30. Manter JT. Movements of the subtalar and transverse tarsal joints. Anat Rec 1941; 80: 397–409.

31. Carrier PA, Janigan JD, Smith SD, Weil LS. Morton's neuralgia: a possible contributing etiology. J Am Podiatry Assoc 1975; 65: 315–321.

32. Langer S, Wernick J. A Practical Manual for a Basic Approach to Biomechanics. New York: Langer Acrylic Laboratory, 1972.

33. Dahle KH, Mueller M, Delitto A, Diamond JE. Visual assessment of foot type and relationship of foot type to lower extremity injury. J Orthop Sports Phys Ther 1991; 2: 71.

34. Hlavac HF. The Foot Book. Mountain View, CA: World Publications, 1977: 187.

35. Taunton JE, Clement DB, McNicol K. Plantar fasciitis in runners, a study of 40 cases. Med Sci Sports Exercise 1980; 2: 137.

36. Neale D, Hooper G, Clowes C, Whiting MF. Adult foot disorders. In: Neale D (ed). Common Foot Disorders Diagnosis and Management: A General Clinical Guide. Edinburgh: Churchill Livingstone, 1981: 56–57.

37. Gehlsen GM, Seger A. Selected measures of angular displacement, strength and flexibility in subjects with and without shin splints. Res Q Exerc Sport 1980; 51: 478–485.

38. Mann RA. Biomechanics of running. In: Pack RP (ed). Symposium of the Foot and Leg in Running Sports. St. Louis: Mosby, 1982: 28.

39. Bates BT, Osternig LR, Mason B. Foot orthotic devices to modify selected aspects of lower extremity mechanics. Am J Sports Med 1979; 6: 338–342.

40. Smith LS, Clarke TE, Hamill CT, Santopietro F. The effects of soft and semirigid orthotics upon rearfoot movement in running. J Am Podiatr Med Assoc 1986; 76: 227–233.

41. Smart GW, Taunton JE, Clement DB. Achilles tendon disorders in runners—a review. Med Sci Sports Exercise 1980; 4: 231–243.

42. Schoenhaus HD, Jay RM. Cavus deformities, conservative management. J Am Podiatry Assoc 1980; 5: 235–238.

43. D'Ambrosia RD. Orthotic devices in running injuries. Clin Sports Med 1985; 4: 611–618.

44. Eggold JF. Orthotics in the prevention of runner's overuse injuries. Phys Sports Med 1981; 9: 124–128.

45. Novick A, Kelley DL. Position and movement changes of the foot with orthotic intervention during the loading response of gait. J Orthop Sports Phys Ther 1990; 7: 301–312.

46. Donatelli R, Hulbert C, Conaway D, St. Pierre R. Biomechanical foot orthotics: a retrospective study. J Orthop Sports Phys Ther 1988; 6: 205–212.

47. Straus WL. Growth of the human foot and its evolutionary significance. Contrib Embryol 1927; 101: 95.

48. McPoil T, Cameron JA, Adrian MJ. Anatomical characteristics of the talus in relation to forefoot deformities. J Am Podiatr Med Assoc 1987; 7: 77–81.

49. Tax HR. Podopediatrics. Baltimore: Williams & Wilkins, 1980: 59.

50. Coplan JA. Rotational motion of the knee: a comparison of normal and pronating subjects. J Orthop Sports Phys Ther 1989; 10: 366–369.

51. Tiberio D. The effect of excessive subtalar pronation on patellofemoral mechanics: a theoretical model. J Orthop Sports Phys Ther 1987; 9: 160–165.

52. Glancy J. Orthotic control of ground reactive forces during running (a preliminary report). Orthot Prosthet 1984; 3: 12–40.

53. Cavagna GA, Dusman B, Margaria R. Positive work done by a previously stretched muscle. J Appl Physiol 1968; 24(1): 21.

54. Cavagna GA, Saibene FP, Margaria R. Effect of negative work on the amount of positive work performed by an isolated muscle. J Appl Physiol 1965; 20(1): 157–160.

55. Murphy PC, Baxter DE. Nerve entrapment of the foot and ankle in runners. Clin Sports Med 1985; 4: 753–763.

56. Przylucki H, Jones CL. Entrapment neuropathy of the muscle branch of the lateral plantar nerve: a cause of heel pain. J Am Podiatry Assoc 1981; 71: 119–124.

57. Newell SG, Miller SJ. Conservative treatment of plantar fasciitis. Phys Sportsmed 1977; 5: 68–73.

58. Smith S. Fatigue perturbation of the calcaneus. Foot and Leg Function. Deer Park, NY: Langer Biomechanics Group, 1989; 4: 2.

59. Williams PL, Smibert JG, Cox R, Mitchell R, Klenerman L. Imaging study of the painful heel syndrome. Foot Ankle 1987; 7: 345–349.

60. Hughes LY. Biomechanical analysis of the foot and ankle for predisposition to developing stress fractures. J Orthop Sports Phys Ther 1985; 3: 96–101.

61. Ross FD. The relationship of abnormal foot pronation to hallux abductovalgus—a pilot study. Prosthet Orthot Int 1986; 10: 72–78.

62. Jordan HH, Brodsky AE. Keller operation for hallux valgus and hallux rigidus. AMA Arch Surg 1951; 62: 586–596.

63. Rogers WA, Joplin RJ. Hallux valgus, weakfoot and the Keller operation: an end result study. Surg Clin North Am 1947; 27: 1295–1302.

64. O'Connor PL, Baxter DE. Developmental disorders: adult foot. In: Gould JS (ed). The Foot Book. Baltimore: Williams & Wilkins, 1988: 207.

65. Mann RA. Surgery of the Foot. Ed 5. St. Louis: Mosby, 1986.

66. Subotnick SI. Biomechanics of the subtalar and midtarsal joints. J Am Podiatry Assoc 1975; 65: 756–764.

67. Haber L, Winthrop L, Weiner SS. Biomechanical findings in

a random survey of fifth toe abnormalities. J Am Podiatry Assoc 1975; 3: 206–213.

68. Mann R, Inman VT. Phasic activity of intrinsic muscles of the foot. J Bone Joint Surg 1964; 46A(3): 469–481.

69. Glancy J. Orthotic control of ground reactive forces during running (a preliminary report). Orthot Prosthet 1984; 3:12–40.

70. Curchod G. Sciatic pain and the feet. Ann Swiss Chirop Assoc 1971; 5: 207–213.

71. Nakeno KK. Sciatic nerve entrapment: the piriformis syndrome. J Musculoskeletal Med 1987; Feb: 33–37.

72. Burns MJ. Non-weightbearing cast impressions for the construction of orthotic devices. J Am Podiatr Assoc 1977; 67: 790–795.

73. Bojsen-Moller F. Calcaneocuboid joint and stability of the longitudinal arch of the foot at high and low gear push off. J Anat 1979; 129: 165–176.

74. Sgarlato TE. A Compendium of Podiatric Biomechanics. San Francisco: California College of Podiatric Medicine, 1971.

75. Lutter LD. Cavus foot in runners. Foot Ankle 1981; 1: 225–228.

76. Dwyer FC. The present status of the problem of pes cavus. Clin Orthop Related Res 1975; 106: 254–275.

77. Lariviere JY, Miladi L, Dubousset JF, Seringe R. Medial pes cavus in children: a study of failures following Dwyer's procedure. Rev Chir Orthoped 1985; 71: 563–573.

78. Bruckner J. Variations in the human subtalar joint. J Orthop Sports Phys Ther 1987; 8: 489–494.

79. Schoenhaus HD, Jay RM. Cavus deformities, conservative management. J Am Podiatry Assoc 1980; 70: 235–238.

80. Builder MA, Marr SJ. Case history of a patient with low back pain and cavus feet. J Am Podiatry Assoc 1980; 6: 299–301.

81. Cangialosi CP, Schall SJ. The biomechanical aspects of anterior tarsal tunnel syndrome. J Am Podiatry Assoc 1980; 70: 291–292.

82. Radin EL. Tarsal tunnel syndrome. Clin Orthop Related Res 1983: 167–170.

83. Wapner KL, Sharkey PF. The use of night splints for treatment of a recalcitrant plantar fasciitis. Foot Ankle 1991; 12(3): 135.

84. Carrier PA, Janigan JD, Smith SD, Weil LS. Morton's neuralgia: a possible contributing etiology. J Am Podiatry Assoc 1975; 65: 315–321.

85. Brantingham JW, Snyder R, Michaud T. Morton's neuroma. J Manipulative Physiol Ther 1991; 5: 317–322.

86. Carroll RL. Vertebrate Paleontology and Evolution. New York: Freeman: 469.

87. Morton TG. A peculiar and painful affliction of the fourth metatarsophalangeal articulation. Am J Med Sci 1876; 71: 37–45.

88. Bossley CJ, Cairney PC. The intermetatarsophalangeal bursa—its significance in Morton's metatarsalgia. J Bone Joint Surg 1980; 62B: 184–187.

89. Goldman F. Intermetatarsal neuromas: light and electron microscopic observation. J Am Podiatr Med 1980; 70: 265–276.

90. Cowan D, Jones B, Robinson J, Polly D. Medial longitudinal arch height and risk of training associated injury. Med Sci Sports Exercise 1989; 2: 60.

91. Sarrafian SK, Topouzian LK. Anatomy and physiology of the extensor apparatus of the toes. J Bone Joint Surg 1969; 51A(4): 669–679.

92. Bordelon RL. Surgical and Conservative Foot Care. Thorofare, NJ: Slack: 55.

93. Bojsen–Moller F, Flagstad KE. Plantar aponeurosis and internal architecture of the ball of the foot. J Anat 1976; 121(3): 599–611.

94. Cailliet R. Foot and Ankle Pain. Philadelphia: Davis, 1968.

95. Betts LO. Morton's metatarsalgia: neuritis of the fourth digital nerve. Med J Aust 1940; 1: 514–515.

96. Rathbun JB, MacNab I. The microvascular pattern of the rotator cuff. J Bone Joint Surg 1970; 52B: 540–553.

97. Ljungqvist R. Subcutaneous partial rupture of the Achilles tendon. Acta Orthop Scand Suppl 1968: 118.

98. Lambert KL. The weight-bearing function of the fibula. J Bone Joint Surg 1971; 53A(3): 507–513.

99. Langer S. Problem of the month. In: Foot and Leg Function. Deer Park, NY: Langer Biomechanics Group, 1988; 1: 14.

100. Subotnick S. Podiatric Sports Medicine. Mt. Kisco, NY: Futura Publishing, 1975.

101. Roncarati A, McMullen W. Correlates of low back pain in a general population sample: a multi-disciplinary study. J Manipulative Physiol Ther 1988; 3:158–164.

102. Denslow, Korr I. Third International Seminar, The International Federation of Orthopaedic Manipulative Therapists. Vail, CO: 1977.

103. Wosk J, Voloshin AS. Low back pain: conservative treatment with artificial shock absorbers. Arch Phys Med Rehabil 1985; 66: 145–148.

104. D'Ambrosia R, Drez D. Prevention and Treatment of Running Injuries. Thorofare, NJ: Slack, 1989.

105. Lutter LD. Orthopedic management of runners in the foot and ankle. In: Bateman JE, Trott AW (eds). The Foot and Ankle. New York: Thieme–Stratton, 1980.

106. Bojsen-Moller F. Anatomy of the forefoot, normal and pathologic. Clin Orthop Related Res 1979; 142: 10.

107. Cavanagh PR, Rodgers MM, Iiboshi A. Pressure distribution under symptom-free feet during barefoot standing. Foot Ankle 1987; 7:262–276.

108. Langer S. Forefoot valgus, plantarflexed first ray. Clarification please. In: Langer Biomechanics Newsletter. Deer Park, NY: Langer Biomechanics Group, 1977: 4; 2–6.

109. Schuster R. Foot types and the influence of environment on the foot of the long distance runner. Ann NY Acad Sci 1977: 301, 881–887.

110. Valmassy R. Orthoses. In: Subotnick S (ed). Sports Medicine of the Lower Extremity. New York: Churchill Livingstone, 1989: 432.

111. Wood Jones F. Structure and function as seen in the foot. London: Bailliere, Tindall, & Cox, 1944.

112. Betts RP, Franks CI, Duckworth T. Analysis of pressure and loads under the foot. Part II. Quantitation of the dynamic distribution. Clin Phys Physiol Meas 1980; 1:113–124.

113. Grieve DW, Rashdi T. Pressures under normal feet in standing and walking as measured by foil pedobarography. Ann Rheum Dis 1983; 43: 816–818.

114. Gross TS, Bunch RP. A mechanical model of metatarsal stress fracture during distance running. Am J Sports Med 1989; 5: 669–674.

115. Teitz CC. Sports medicine concerns in dance and gymnastics. Pediatr Clin North Am 1982; 29: 1399–1421.

116. Gould JS (ed). The Foot Book. Baltimore: Williams & Wilkins, 1988: 220.

117. Glover MG. Plantar warts. Foot Ankle 1990; 3: 172–178.

118. Holmes GB, Timmerman L. A quantitative assessment of the effect of metatarsal pads on plantar pressures. Foot Ankle 1990; 3: 141–145.

119. Morton DJ. The Human Foot. New York: Columbia University Press, 1935.

120. Harris RI, Beath T. The short first metatarsal, its incidence and clinical significance. J Bone Joint Surg 1949; 31A: 553–565.

121. Rodgers MM, Cavanagh PR. Pressure distribution in Morton's foot structure. Med Sci Sports Exercise 1989; 21(1): 23.

122. Mosley HG. Static disorders of the ankle and foot. Clin Symp 1957; 9: 85.

123. Travell JG, Simons DG. Myofascial Pain and Dysfunction: the Trigger Point Manual. Baltimore: Williams & Wilkins, 1983: 112.

124. Dananberg HG. Letter to the editor. The kinetic wedge. J Am Podiatr Med Assoc 1988, 78(2).

125. Subotnick SI. The biomechanics of running: implications for the prevention of foot injuries. Sports Med 1985; 2: 144–153.

126. Rothbart BA, Estabrook L. Excessive pronation: a major biomechanical determinant in the development of chondromalacia and pelvic lists. J Manipulative Physiol Ther 1988; 5: 373–379.

127. Ford LT, Goodman FG. X-ray studies of the lumbosacral spine. South Med J 1966; 59: 1123–1128.

128. Porterfield JA. The sacroiliac joint. In: Gould JA, Davies GJ (eds). Orthopaedic and Sports Physical Therapy. St. Louis: Mosby, 1985: 555.

129. Schuit D, Adrian M, Pidcoe P. Effects of heel lifts on ground reactive force patterns in subjects with structural leg-length discrepancies. Phys Ther 1989; 69: 41–48.

130. Press SJ. A report of clinical applications of computers in analysis of gait spinal imbalances. Chiropract Sports Med 1987; 1:30.

131. Sanner WH, Page JC, Tolboe HR, et al. A study of ankle joint height changes with subtalar joint motion. J Am Podiatry Assoc 1981; 3: 158–161.

132. Hiss JM. Functional Foot Disorders. Los Angeles: The Oxford Press, 1949.

133. Novick A, Kelly DL. Position and movement changes of the foot with orthotic intervention during the loading response of gait. J Orthop Sports Phys Ther 1990; 11(7): 301–312.

134. Cyriax J. The Textbook of Orthopedic Medicine. Vol I, Ed 5. London: Bailliäre, Tindall, & Cassell, 1969.

135. Taillard W. Lumbar spine and leg length inequality. Acta Orthop Belg 1969; 35: 601.

136. Subotnick S. Case history of unilateral short leg with athletic overuse injury. J Am Podiatr Med Assoc 1980; 5: 255–256.

137. Redler I. Clinical significance of minor inequalities in leg length. New Orleans Med Surg J 1952; 104: 308–312.

138. Subotnick S. Skiing injuries In: Subotnick S (ed). Sports Medicine of the Lower Extremity. New York: Churchill Livingstone, 1989: 611.

139. Hickey DE, Hukins DW. Relation between the structure of the annulus fibrosis and the junction and failure of the intervertebral disc. Spine 1980; 5: 106–115.

140. Schultz AB, Warwick DN, Berkson, MH, Nachemson AL. Mechanical properties of human lumbar spine motion segments. Part 1. Responses in flexion, extension, lateral bending and torsion. J Biomech Eng 1979; 101: 46–52.

141. Inman VT, Ralston HJ, Todd F. Human walking. Baltimore: Williams & Wilkins, 1981.

142. Lillich JS, Baxter DE. Common forefoot problems in runners. Foot Ankle 1986; 7: 145–151.

143. Hughes LY. Biomechanical analysis of the foot and ankle for predisposition to developing stress fractures. J Orthop Sports Phys Ther 1985; 3: 96–101.

144. Close JR. Some applications of the functional anatomy of the ankle joint. J Bone Joint Surg 1956; 38A(4): 761–781.

145. O'Donoghue DH. Impingement exostoses of the talus and tibia. J Bone Joint Surg 1957; 39A(4): 835–852.

146. Adelaar, RS, Dannelly EA, Meunier PA, Stelling FH, Calvard DF. A long-term study of triple arthrodesis in children (Proceedings of the American Academy of Orthopedic Surgeons). J Bone Joint Surg 1976; 58A: 724.

147. Outland T, Murphy ID. The pathomechanics of the peroneal spastic flatfoot. Clin Orthop 1963; 27: 64–73.

148. Engsberg JR, Allinger TL. A function of the talocalcaneal joint during running support. Foot Ankle 1990; 2: 93–96.

149. Sandoz R. Some physical mechanisms and effects of spinal adjustments. Ann Swiss Chirop Assoc 1976; 6: 91.

150. Mennell J. Joint Pain. Boston: Little Brown, 1964.

151. Rahlmann JF. Mechanisms of intervertebral joint fixation: a literature review. J Manipulative Physiol Ther 1987; 4: 177–187.

152. MacConail MA, Basmajian JV. Muscles and Movements: a Basis for Human Kinesiology. Baltimore: Williams & Wilkins, 1969.

153. Schafer RC, Faye LJ. Motion Palpation and Chiropractic Technique--Principles of Dynamic Chiropractic. Huntington Beach, CA: The Motion Palpation Institute, 1990.

154. Hammer WI. Functional Soft Tissue Examination and Treatment by Manual Methods. Gaithersburg, MD: Aspen Publishers, 1991.

155. Kaltenborn FM. Mobilization of the Extremity Joints. Oslo: Olaf Norlis Bokhandel, 1980.

156. Greenman PE. Principles of Manual Medicine. Baltimore: Williams and Wilkins, 1989.

157. Maitland GD. Peripheral Manipulation. London: Butterworths, 1977.

158. Condon SA, Hutton RS. Soleus muscle electromyographic activity and ankle dorsiflexion range of motion during four stretching procedures. Phys Ther 1987; 67: 24–30.

159. Moore MA, Hutton RS. Electromyographic investigation of muscle stretching techniques. Med Sci Sports Exercise 1980; 5: 322–329.

160. Prentice WE. A comparison of static stretching and p.n.f. stretching for improving hip joint flexibility. Athletic Training 1983; 1: 56–59.

161. Sady SP, Wortman M, Blanke D. Flexibility training: ballistic, static or proprioceptive neuromuscular facilitation. Arch Phys Med Rehabil 1982; 6: 261–263.

162. Tanigawa MC. Comparison of hold-relax procedure and pas-

sive mobilization on increasing muscle length. Phys Ther 1972; 7: 725–735.

163. Safran MR, Garrett WE, Seaber AV, Glisson RR, Ribbeck BM. The role of warm-up on muscular injury prevention. Am J Sports Med 1988; 16: 123–129.

164. Suzuki S, Hutton RS. Postcontractile motoneuron discharge produced by muscle afferent activation. Med Sci Sports Exercise 1976; 4: 258–264.

165. Eldred E, Hutton RS, Smith JL. Nature of persisting changes in afferent discharge from muscle following its contraction. Prog Brain Res 1976; 44: 157–171.

166. Moore JC. The golgi tendon organ: a review and update. Am J Occup Ther 1984; 4: 227–236.

167. Astrand PO, Rodahl K. The Textbook of Work Physiology. Ed 2. New York: McGraw-Hill, 1970.

168. Holt ND (referenced in Altar MJ). Science of Stretching. Champaign, IL: Human Kinetics Books, 1988: 89.

169. Stanish WD, Hubley-Kozey CL. Neurophysiology of stretching. In: D'Ambrosia RD, Drez D (eds). Prevention and Treatment of Running Injuries. Thorofare, NJ: Slack, 1989.

170. Godges JJ, MacRae H, Longdon C, Tinberg C, MacCrae P. The effects of two stretching procedures on hip range motion and gait economy. J Orthop Sports Phys Ther 1989; 9: 350–357.

171. Sapega AA, Quedenfeld TC, Moyer RA, Butler RA. Biophysical factors in range-of-motion exercise. Phys Sports Med 1981; 12: 57–65.

172. Kendall FP, Kendall McCreary E. Muscles, Testing and Function. Ed 3. Baltimore: Williams & Wilkins, 1983.

173. Bruckner J. Variations in the human subtalar joint. J Orthop Sports Phys Ther 1987; 8: 489–494.

174. Harris RI. Rigid valgus foot due to talocalcaneal bridge. J Bone Joint Surg 1955; 37A(l): 169–183.

175. Wagner FW. Personal communication. In: Bordelon RL. Surgical and Conservative Foot Care. Thorofare, NJ: Slack, 1988: 111.

176. Schoitz EH, Cyriax J. Manipulation: Past and Present. London: William Heinemann Medical Books, 1978.

177. Palmer DD. The Science, Art and Philosophy of Chiropractic. Portland, OR: Portland Publishing, 1910: 56.

178. Woo SL-Y, Matthews JV, Akeson WH, Amiel D, Convery FR. Connective tissue response to immobility: correlative study of biomechanical and biochemical measurements of normal and immobilized rabbit knees. Arthritis Rheum 1975; 18: 257–264.

179. Maitland GD. Vertebral Manipulation. London: Butterworths, 1986: 96, 107.

180. Good AB. Spinal joint blocking. J Manipulative Physiol Ther 1985; 8: 1–8.

181. Paris SV. Spinal manipulative therapy. Clin Orthop 1983; 179: 55–61.

182. Maitland GD. The hypothesis of adding compression when examining and treating synovial joints. J Orthop Sports Phys Ther 1980; 2(1): 7–14.

183. Newell SG, Woodle A. Cuboid syndrome. Phys Sports Med 1981; 9: 71–76.

184. Goodwin GM, McCloskey DL, Matthews PBC. The persistence of appreciable kinesthesia after paralyzing joint afferents but preserving muscle afferents. Brain Res 1972; 37: 326.

185. Netter F. The Nervous System. Part One. Anatomy and Physiology. West Caldwell, NJ: The CIBA Collection of Medical Illustrations, 1983: 1985.

186. Gowitzke BA, Milner M. Scientific Bases of Human Movement. Ed 3. Baltimore: Williams & Wilkins, 1988.

187. Hufschmidt HJ. Demonstration of autogenic inhibition and its significance in human voluntary movement. In: Granit R. (ed). Muscle Afferents and Motor Control. New York: John Wiley & Sons, 1966.

188. O'Connell AL, Gardner EB. Understanding the Scientific Bases of Human Movement. Baltimore: Williams & Wilkins, 1972.

189. Robbins SE, Gouw GJ, Hanna AM. Running-related injury prevention through innate impact-moderating behavior. Med Sci Sports Exercise 1989; 21(2): 130–139.

190. Bremner JM, Lawrence JS, Maill WE. Degenerative arthritis in a Jamaican rural population. Ann Rheum Dis 1968; 27: 326–332.

191. Lentell GL, Katzman LL, Walters MR. The relationship between muscle function and ankle stability. JOSPT 1990; 11(12): 605–611.

192. Anderson O, Grillner S. On the feedback control of the cat's hindlimb during locomotion. In Taylor A, Prochazka A (eds). Muscle Receptors and Movement. New York: Oxford University Press, 1982: 427–432.

193. Rowinski MJ. Afferent neurobiology of the joint. In: Gould JA, Davies GJ. (eds). Orthopaedic and Sports Physical Therapy. St. Louis: Mosby, 1985: 50–63.

194. Freeman M, Dean M, Hanham I. The etiology and prevention of functional instability of the foot. J Bone Joint Surg 1965; 47B: 678–685.

195. Billek Sawhney B, Whitney SL, Sawhney R. Assessment of static balance. In: Orthopaedic Section Poster Presentations at the 1991 Combined Sections Meeting. J Orthop Sports Phys Ther 1991; 13(5): 252.

196. Cyriax J. Textbook of Orthopaedic Medicine. Vol 2, Ed 11. London: Bailliäre-Tindall, 1984.

197. Carrick FR. Lecture notes from NYCC diplomate in neurology program. Nov. 1987.

198. Korr IM. Neurobiologic Mechanisms in Manipulative Therapy. New York: Plenum, 1978: 247.

199. Voss DE, Ionta MK, Myers BJ. Proprioceptive Neuromuscular Facilitation. Ed 3. Philadelphia: Harper & Row, 1985.

200. Liebenson C. Active muscular relaxation techniques. Part Two. Clinical application. JMPT 1990; 13(1): 5.

201. Cavanagh PR, Lafortune MA. Ground reaction forces in distance running. J Biomech 1980; 13: 397–406.

202. Cavanagh PR. The biomechanics of lower extremity action in distance running. Foot Ankle 1987; 197–216.

203. Harris RI, Beath T. Hypermobile flatfoot with short tendo achilles. J Bone Joint Surg 1948; 30A(1): 116–138.

204. Robbins SE, Hanna AM. Running-related injury prevention through barefoot adaptations. Med Sci Sports Exercise 1987; 19(2): 148–156.

205. Perry J. Anatomy and biomechanics of the hindfoot. Clin Orthop Related Res 1983; 177: 9–15.

206. Janda V. Muscles, central nervous motor regulation and back problems. In: Korr IM (ed). The Neurobiologic Mechanisms in Manipulative Therapy. New York: Plenum, 1978: 27–41.

207. LeBlanc A, Gogia P, Schneider V, Krebs J, Schonfeld E,

Evans H. Calf muscle area and strength changes after five weeks of horizontal bed rest. Am J Sports Med 1988; 16: 624–629.

208. Gould N. Evaluation of hyperpronation and pes planus in adults. Clin Orthop Related Res 1983; 18: 37–45.

209. Cibulka M, Rose SJ, Delitta A, Sinacore D. A comparison of two treatments for hamstring strains. Phys Ther 1984; 64: 750.

210. Muckle DS. Associated factors in recurrent groin and hamstring injuries. Br J Sports Med 1982; 16: 37–39.

211. Lee DG. Tennis elbow: a manual therapist's perspective. J Orthop Sports Phys Ther 1986; 8: 134–142.

212. Alter J. Stretch and Strengthen. Boston: Houghton-Mifflin, 1986.

213. Aubrey BJ, Bernardone JJ, Connolly TJ. The prospective evaluation of invasive and non-invasive treatment protocols for plantar fasciitis. Rehabil Res Dev Prog Rep 1989; 50.

214. Seto JL, Brewster CE, Lombardo ST, Tibone JE. Rehabilitation of the knee after anterior cruciate ligament reconstruction. J Orthop Sports Phys Ther 1989; 11(1): 8–18.

215. Houk J, Henneman E. Response of golgi tendon organs to active contraction of the soleus muscle of the cat. J Neurophysiol 1967; 30: 466.

216. Vogler H. Biomechanics of talipes equinovalgus. J Am Podiatr Med Assoc 1987; 77(1): 21–28.

217. Bordelon RL. Hypermobile flatfoot in children. Clin Orthop Related Res 1983; 181: 7–14.

218. Olsen TR, Seidel M. The evolutionary basis of some clinical disorders of the human foot. A comparative survey of the living primates. Foot Ankle 1983; 3: 322–341.

219. Hutton WC, Dhanedran M. The mechanics of normal and hallux valgus feet—a quantitative study. Clin Orthop 1981; 157: 7–13.

220. Lee Dellon A. Deep peroneal nerve entrapment on the dorsum of the foot. Foot Ankle 1990; 11(2): 73–78.

221. Hicks JH. The mechanics of the foot. I. The joints. J Anat 1953; 87: 345.

222. Hice GA. Orthotic treatment of feet having a high oblique midtarsal joint axis. J Am Podiatry Assoc. 1984; 74(11): 577–582.

223. Bleck EE. Developmental orthopaedics. III. Toddlers. Dev Med Child Neurol 1982; 24: 533–555.

224. Staheli LT. Rotational problems of the lower extremity. Orthop Clin North Am 1987; 18(4): 503–512.

225. Fabry G, MacEwen GD, Shands AR. Torsion of the femur, a follow-up study in normal and abnormal conditions. J Bone Joint Surg 1973; 55A: 1726–1738.

226. Jay RM. In-toe secondary to medial tibial torsion. Foot and Leg Function. Deer Park, NY: Langer Biomechanics Group, 1989; 1(4): 8–14.

227. Swanson AB, Greene PW, Allis HD. Rotational deformities of the lower extremity in children and their clinical significance. Clin Orthop 1963; 27: 157–175.

228. MacConaill MA, Basmajian CJ. Muscles and Movements. Huntington, NY: Krieger, 1969.

229. Lilletuedt J, Kreighbaum E, Phillips RL. Analysis of selected alignment of the lower extremity as related to the shin splint syndrome. J Am Podiatr Med Assoc 1976; 69(3): 211–217.

230. Davenport J. The pathomechanics of the flatfoot deformity. Foot and Leg Function. Deer Park, NY: Langer Biomechanics Group, 1988: 1(1): 7.

231. Schoenhaus H. Torsional abnormalities in pediatrics. Foot and Leg Function. Deer Park, NY: Langer Biomechanics Group 1988; 1(1): 11.

232. Magee DJ. Orthopedic Physical Assessment. Philadelphia: Saunders, 1987: 252.

233. Fabry G, McEwen GD, Shands AR. Torsion of the femur: a follow-up study in normal and abnormal conditions. J Bone Joint Surg 1973; 55A: 1726.

234. Tax HR. Dangers posed to the hips of infants by counter splints used to treat internal rotation of the legs. J Am Podiatr Assoc 1975; 65(1): 54–56.

235. Alvik I. Increased anteversion of the femoral neck as the sole sign of dysplasia coxae. Acta Os 1960; 29: 301.

236. Staheli LT, Lippert F, Denotter P. Femoral anteversion and physical performance in adolescence and adult life. Clin Orthop 1977; 129: 213.

237. Sammarco GJ. The dancers hip. Clin Sports Med 1983; 2(3): 485–498.

238. Valmassy RL, Lipe L, Falconer R. Pediatric treatment modalities of the lower extremity. J Am Podiatr Med Assoc 1988; 78(2): 69–80.

239. Spencer A. Practical Podiatric Orthopedic Procedures. Cleveland, OH: Ohio College of Podiatric Medicine, 1978: 124.

240. Schoenhaus HD, Poss KD. The clinical and practical aspects in treating torsional problems in children. J Am Podiatr Assoc 1977; 67(9): 62.

241. Schuster RO. The effects of modern foot gear. J Am Podiatr Assoc 1978; 68(4): 235.

242. Tachdjian MO. Pediatric Orthopedics. Philadelphia: Saunders, 1972: 1463.

243. Gould N, Moreland M. Alvarez R, Trevino S, Fenwick J. Development of the child's arch. Foot Ankle 1989; 9(5): 241.

244. Isman RE, Inman VT. Anthropometric studies of the human foot and ankle. Bull Prosthet Res, Spring 1969.

245. Gould N. Positional anomalies and early patterns of gait. In: Gould JS: The Foot Book. Baltimore: Williams & Wilkins, 1988: 128.

246. Langer S. Genu valgum, obesity, pregnancy and losing control of pronation. The Langer Biomechanics Newsletter. Langer Biomechanics Group, Deer Park: New York, May 1987; 14: 24.

247. Inman VT. The Joints of the Ankle. Baltimore: Williams & Wilkins, 1975.

248. Adelaar RS, Williams RM, Gould JS. Congenital convex pes valgus: results of an early comprehensive release and a review of congenital vertical talus at Richmond Crippled Children's Hospital and the University of Alabama in Birmingham. Foot Ankle 1980; 1: 62.

249. McGillicuddy DM, Jones ET, Hensinger RN. The early treatment of talipes equinovarus with adhesive taping. Orthopedics 1980; 3: 33.

250. Gould N. Flatfoot: spastic. In: Gould JS. The Foot Book. Baltimore: Williams & Wilkins, 1988: 185.

251. Subotnick S. Foot injuries. In: Subotnick S (ed). Sports Medicine of the Lower Extremity. New York: Churchill Livingstone, 1989: 268.

252. Bordelon RL. Hypermobile flatfoot in children. Comprehension, evaluation and treatment. Clin Orthop Related Res 1983; 181: 7.

Chapter Four

Biomechanical Examination

Successful management of any biomechanical abnormality requires a thorough evaluation of the entire kinetic chain in which the various angular relationships, ranges of motion, and dynamic interactions are carefully measured and recorded. Since improper measuring techniques lead to faulty treatment, practitioners should be sufficiently skilled so that the examination yields accurate and reproducible results. This chapter will review the components of a biomechanical examination, as divided into supine, prone, standing, and dynamic evaluations.

SUPINE EXAMINATION

This examination should begin by motion palpating the various lower extremity articulations. The presence of joint dysfunction should be noted, and any fixations should be gently mobilized. In addition to relaxing the patient, this helps to reduce any functional deformities that might adversely affect measurements. The relative lengths of the metatarsals are then determined by plantarflexing the digits and noting the locations of the dorsal metatarsal heads. A standard goniometer or tractograph is then used to measure the range of hallux dorsiflexion (Fig. 4.1). Of interest, a definite correlation exists between a decreased range of hallux dorsiflexion and plantar fascia pain (2).

After the range of hallux dorsiflexion has been noted, the position of the first metatarsal head and range of first ray motion may then be evaluated (refer back to Fig. 3.68). At this time, it is also possible to evaluate the range of forefoot inversion available about the longitudinal midtarsal joint axis (Fig. 4.2).

The range of ankle dorsiflexion is measured by resting one arm of a goniometer parallel to the fibula while the opposite arm parallels the plantar lateral foot (Fig. 4.3). This measurement should be taken with the knee extended and flexed to differentiate between gastrocnemius and soleus contracture. If significant muscle tension is noted during this evaluation, the measurements should be repeated after several hold/relax stretches have been performed. This gives a more accurate reading of the degree of ankle dorsiflexion available during locomotion.

While a limited range of ankle dorsiflexion may be responsible for injury secondary to midtarsal compensation, Blake (4) noted that an exaggerated range of ankle dorsiflexion (i.e., greater than 15° with knee straight and 20° with knee flexed) may also be responsible for injury secondary to inadequate muscular stabilization. He emphasizes that in this situation, treatment should consist of strengthening, and not stretching, exercises. For similar reasons, an exaggerated range of ankle plantarflexion may also be responsible for injury secondary to inadequate muscular stabilization afforded by an overly flexible tibialis anterior (5). Messier and Pittala (5) noted that a range of ankle plantarflexion exceeding 60° is a good determinant for predicting plantar fascia pain.

Structural leg length discrepancies should be evaluated by using Alli's test (see Fig. 3.107) and anterior superior iliac spine (ASIS) to medial malleolus measurements. If necessary, various manual techniques should be used prior to recording these measurements in order to rule out functional leg length discrepancy. A series of treatments and/or home stretches may be necessary before it is possible to accurately differentiate a structural from a functional leg length discrepancy.

The degree of tibial torsion may be evaluated by positioning the femoral condyles in the frontal plane and measuring the transmalleolar position (Fig. 4.4).

The range of internal and external femoral rotation should then be recorded. If the range of external femoral rotation is limited when the lower extremity is straight, the measurement should be repeated with the hip flexed, as contracture in the anterior hip capsule will produce a lessened range of external rotation that dramatically increases as the hip is flexed. (Flexion reduces tension on the Y ligament of Bigelow.) Also, if knee injury is present, the range of tibiofemoral rotation should be evaluated with the knee flexed in various positions. Remember that excess subtalar pronation produces a laxity of the knee-restraining ligaments that results in an increased range of rotation, particularly when the knee is flexed between 0 and 30° (6).

The range of knee flexion and extension should then be recorded: genu recurvatum is often associated with ankle equinus, while flexion contracture at the knee often results in achilles tendinitis and/or plantar fascia pain secondary to the increased dorsiflectory requirements placed upon the ankle. Tightness in the hamstring musculature can be evaluated by performing straight leg raises with varying degrees of internal and external hip rotation. A tight medial hamstring will result in a lessened straight leg raise when the hip is externally rotated, while a tight biceps femoris muscle will restrict the height of a straight leg raise when the hip is internally rotated. Such contracture may be responsible for an in or out toe gait pattern, as previously mentioned.

Figure 4.1. Measuring hallux dorsiflexion with a goniometer. Note that unless the first metatarsophalangeal joint has been injured, the range of hallux plantarflexion need not be measured, as this is a vestigial function that serves no purpose in locomotion (1).

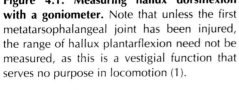

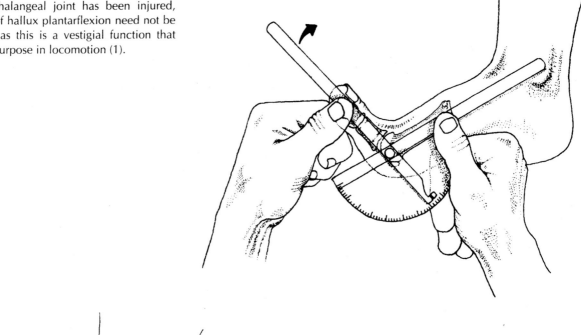

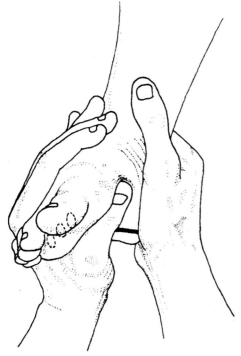

Figure 4.2.   Measuring forefoot inversion about longitudinal midtarsal joint axis. With the foot placed in its neutral position, the examiner stabilizes the heel with one hand while inverting the forefoot with the other. The relationship between the central three metatarsal heads and the plantar heel is then noted. Unfortunately, methods for quantifying first ray and midtarsal motions are relatively inexact and need to be improved (3). Of note, Klave et al. (23) recently demonstrated that if the first ray dorsiflexes more than 9.3 mm above the second metatarsal, the individual is likely to develop bunion pain (the average range present in their asymptomatic population was 5.3 mm).

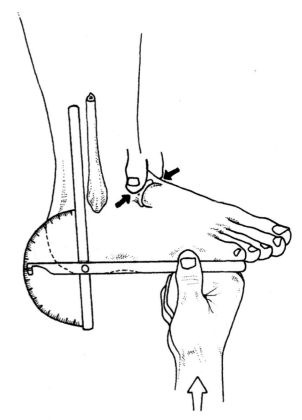

Figure 4.3.   Measuring ankle dorsiflexion. While talonavicular congruency is maintained to prevent midtarsal compensation, the forefoot is forced into a maximally dorsiflexed position, and the measured number of degrees is recorded.

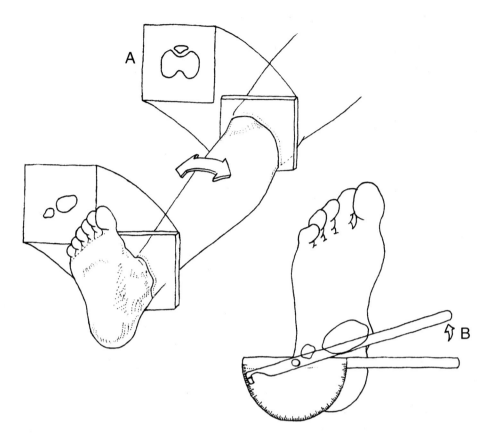

A

Figure 4.4. Measuring tibial torsion.
The leg is rotated until the posterior femoral condyles rest parallel to the examining table **(A).** To ensure that the condyles are positioned properly, the examiner should slightly flex the patient's knee. When the femoral condyles are parallel to the table, the knee will move straight up. A goniometer may then be used to measure the transmalleolar position **(B).**

B

The final portion of the supine exam should include a manual evaluation of muscle strength.

PRONE EXAMINATION

The patient is placed in a prone position and the lower extremity is rotated to bring the posterior surface of the calcaneus into the frontal plane. (This may require placing a folded towel beneath the contralateral pelvis.) The calcaneus is then bisected by pinching the plantar aspects of the medial and lateral condyles and drawing a line that is perpendicular to the line connecting these points (Fig. 4.5). The plantar skin contour should not be used as a reference for bisecting the heel, as a chronically pronated foot will deform the plantar heel so that the skin appears inverted relative to the plantar condyles. (The opposite is true with a chronically supinated rearfoot.)

Also, although it has become standard practice to bisect the calcaneus using the medial and lateral surfaces for reference, this practice should only be considered when the size of the fat pad or thickness of the skin negates bisecting the calcaneus via palpation of the plantar condyles. Because the outline of the posterior calcaneus most often forms a trapezoid, marking the calcaneus by bisecting the medial and lateral surfaces would produce a line that deviates from the perpendicular bisection of the plantar condyles (Fig. 4.6). Since it is the location of the condyles that determines stance phase motion of the subtalar joint, the condyles

should always be the reference points. If the medial and lateral surfaces of the calcaneus must be used, bony deformities (such as Haglund's deformity or an abnormally shaped calcaneus) should be ignored.

It cannot be overstressed that adequate marking of the calcaneal bisection is essential for proper evaluation and treatment, as an incorrect bisection would produce error in both the rearfoot and forefoot measurements, e.g., the rearfoot bisection in Figure 4.6 that uses the medial and lateral contours of the calcaneus for references (dashed line) gives the impression of a combined subtalar varum/forefoot valgus deformity while the true bisection (solid line) clearly demonstrates a neutral forefoot and rearfoot.

Once the calcaneus has been marked, the distal one-third of the leg may be bisected. The alignment between the posterior calcaneus and the distal leg may now be measured (Fig. 4.7). Although Root et al. (7) originally maintained that the neutral position of the subtalar joint should be determined by noting the overall range of motion available to the subtalar joint and then placing the calcaneal bisection in a position that is one-third of the way from its fully pronated position, this technique has been all but abandoned because variation in subtalar range of motion makes for much inconsistency.

Also, while most authorities recommend measuring the range of subtalar eversion with the patient in a prone position, more recent investigation demonstrates that off-weight-bearing measurements of subtalar eversion are not

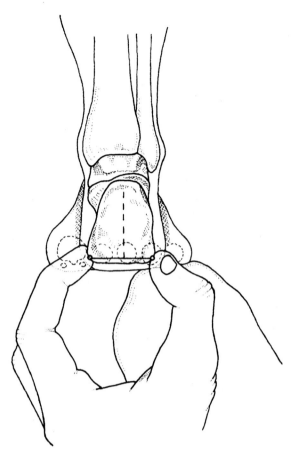

Figure 4.5.   Bisecting the calcaneus. With the foot maintained in its neutral position, the examiner visually bisects the medial and lateral calcaneal condyles **(solid line)** and then draws a line perpendicular to this one on the patient's heel **(dotted line).** To free the marking hand, while maintaining the lateral column in its locked position, the seated examiner uses a knee to apply pressure beneath the fourth and fifth metatarsal heads. The transition from hand pressure to knee pressure should be smooth, with no change in forefoot or rearfoot relationships.

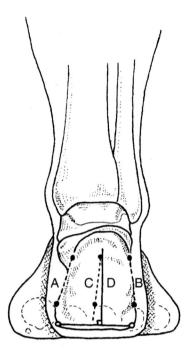

Figure 4.6.   Using the medial and lateral surfaces of the calcaneus for references (A and B) usually results in a heel bisection that is inverted (C) relative to the true bisection (D).

valid (8). Because of this, these measurements, which are useful when evaluating uncompensated foot types, should be performed during static stance. (Lattanza et al. [9] noted a 37% increase in subtalar eversion when its range is measured in a weight-bearing position.)

After subtalar alignment has been recorded, the forefoot/rearfoot relationship can be measured (Fig. 4.8). Even though this measurement requires eyeing the various relationships between the measuring arms and the plantar forefoot and rearfoot, even inexperienced practitioners are able to achieve a high degree of consistency in these measurements. In fact, Kaye and Sorto (10) demonstrated that four out of five examiners were able to correctly identify forefoot relationships within 1°.

An important point of concern regarding forefoot measurements is the frequency with which practitioners find forefoot varus deformities. Although present in less than 9% of the population (11), many experienced practitioners report forefoot varus deformities in excess of 80% of the patient population. Burns (12) offers a possible explanation for this by stating: "It seems most clinicians looking at pronated feet think that forefoot varus is the most probable cause, and with this preconditioning set in one's mind, it is much easier to find a forefoot varus."

An incorrect measurement of a forefoot varus deformity may be the result of various errors in examination. The most common mistakes can usually be traced to either inadequate loading of the fourth and fifth metatarsal heads while placing the foot in its neutral position or to an incorrect marking of the posterior calcaneus, e.g., using a line that is parallel to the lateral surface of the calcaneus when bisecting the heel will result in a false forefoot varus measurement, as this line will be everted relative to the true bisection. Also, determining the neutral position of the subtalar joint with the method described by Root et al. (7) is likely to produce a false forefoot varus measurement, as it is not uncommon for the inversion/eversion ratio of subtalar motion to be 4:1, instead of the ideal 2:1. This results in the forefoot/rearfoot relationship being measured while the subtalar joint is being held in a supinated position. Because of a decreased parallelism of the midtarsal axes, this results in a false forefoot varus measurement (Fig. 4.9).

Other factors that may result in an incorrect forefoot varus measurement include the presence of a dorsiflexed first ray and/or a functional forefoot varus deformity. If

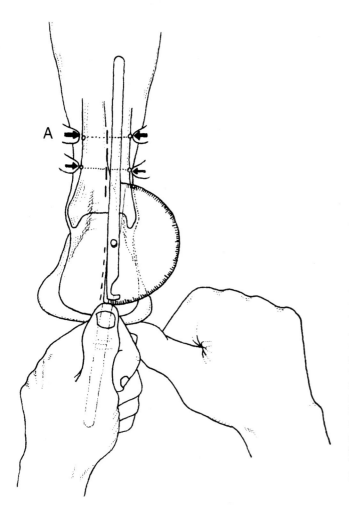

Figure 4.7. Measuring neutral subtalar alignment. To begin with, the lower leg is bisected. This requires first palpating, then bisecting a 3-inch section of the tibia and fibula just proximal to the malleoli (A). The malleoli should not be used, and asymmetrical muscle mass and the achilles tendon should be ignored. The longitudinal axis of the foot is then positioned perpendicular to the floor and the degree of subtalar varum is then measured while maintaining foot neutrality. It should be stressed that the importance of this angle is often overrated as it is relatively small compared to the degree of tibiofibular varum.

Another important consideration is that several studies (24, 25) have demonstrated poor interrater reliability for this measurement. Inconsistencies with this measurement can almost always be related to difficulties associated with bisecting the lower leg; i.e. failure to position the foot perpendicular to the floor and/or difficulties with visually bisecting the lower leg on obese people often allows for non-reproducible bisection lines. These problems, however, may be minimized with practice (e.g., it is sometimes necessary when evaluating obese individuals to bisect the lower leg with a line that is parallel to a particularly straight section of the distal tibia) as experienced examiners are capable of achieving high levels of intra (26) and interrater reliability (27). Of note, it has been recently demonstrated that a simple qualitative measurement of neutral subtalar alignment (i.e., noting if the subtalar joint is in varus or valgus) has demonstrated an acceptable interrater reliability with varus deformities being correlated with a previous history of medial tibial stress syndrome (28). Furthermore, Powers at al. (29) demonstrated that individuals possessing a subtalar varus deformity (as measured off-weight-bearing) were more likely to present with retropatellar pain than a control population. These researchers were also able to obtain acceptable levels of intrarater reliability when taking this measurement.

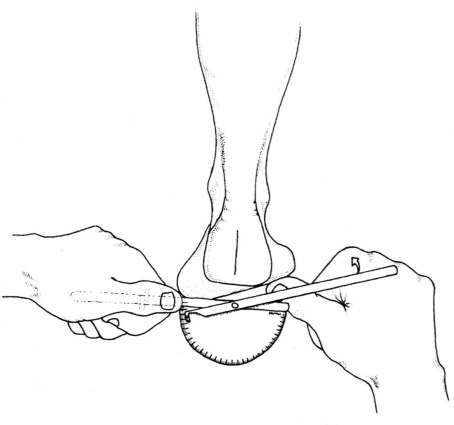

Figure 4.8. Measuring forefoot alignment. With the foot maintained in its neutral position, one arm of a goniometer is placed parallel to the plantar forefoot while the other arm is resting perpendicular to the calcaneal bisection.

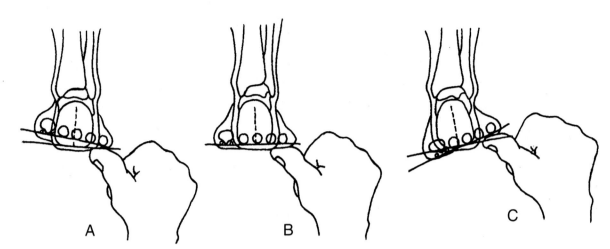

Figure 4.9. Because the range of midtarsal joint motion is dependent on the position of the subtalar joint, measuring the forefoot/rearfoot relationship with the subtalar joint supinated will result in a false forefoot varus measurement (A) while evaluating the forefoot/rearfoot relationship with the subtalar joint pronated will result in a false forefoot valgus measurement (C).

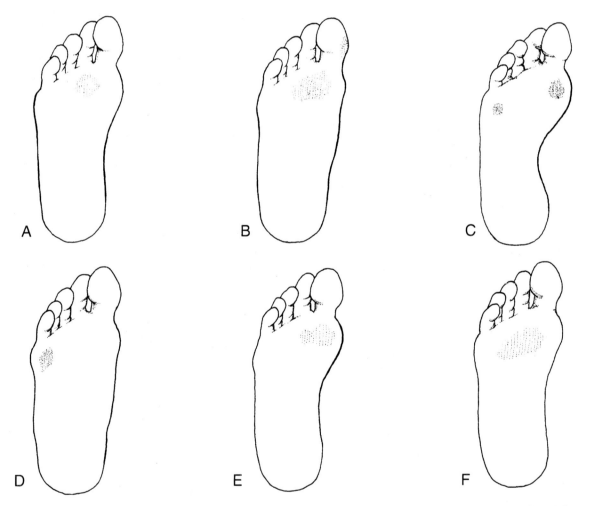

Figure 4.10.   Plantar callus patterns. These patterns show compensated rearfoot varus (A), compensated forefoot varus (B), rigid plantarflexed first ray (C), uncompensated rearfoot/forefoot varus (D), flexible plantarflexed first ray (E), and compensated equinus deformity (F).

there is any doubt as to the position of the first metatarsal head, the practitioner should use only the central three metatarsal heads for reference. Also, a suspected functional forefoot varus should be vigorously mobilized prior to measuring the forefoot/rearfoot relationship.

With the forefoot maintained in its neutral position, alignment of the metatarsals should then be recorded, and the range of first ray dorsiflexion and plantarflexion should be noted. Hip range of motion is readily evaluated by flexing the knees 90° and observing tibial positions as the hip is maximally internally and externally rotated. The legs are then straightened, and the range of hip extension and knee flexion is checked. Note than when evaluating hip extension, one hand should be placed over the sacrum to ensure that motion is coming only from the hip and not through compensatory sacroiliac or spinal extension. A suspected leg length discrepancy should be evaluated and, if indicated, specific muscles should be checked for contracture and/or weakness.

The final portion of the prone exam should include careful examination of plantar callus patterns, as these patterns provide invaluable information regarding the degree of shear and compressive forces present during stance phase (Fig. 4.10).

STANDING EXAMINATION

The patient is asked to stand, and the integrity of the medial longitudinal arch is noted on and off weight-bearing. This information is useful in identifying various foot types. For example, an individual with a forefoot varus deformity will classically present with a loss of the medial longitudinal arch both on and off weight-bearing while the rigid plantarflexed first ray deformity will typically result in a medial longitudinal arch that is elevated both on and off weight-bearing. Although interrater reliability for evaluating arch height is low (13), this information should still be recorded, as it helps corroborate other examination findings and tests the integrity of the subtalar and midtarsal restraining ligaments.

One method to quantify changes in arch height more accurately is to measure the navicular differential as the foot moves from its neutral position to a position of relaxed static stance. (The navicular differential refers to the change in height of the navicular tuberosity relative to the floor.) This method allows for quantifiable changes in arch height to be recorded.

The practitioner should then stand behind the patient and note the amount of shank rotation as the patient actively inverts and everts the rearfoot. As mentioned previously, a high subtalar joint axis will allow much tibial rotation with relatively insignificant amounts of obligatory calcaneal inversion/eversion, while a low subtalar joint axis will have the opposite effect. The range of subtalar joint inversion

and eversion may now be measured by placing the subtalar joint in its neutral position and noting the location of the calcaneal bisection relative to the ground. The patient is then asked to evert the heel maximally and the change in angulation is noted. The procedure is reversed to measure the range of inversion and is repeated bilaterally. This position also allows for measurement of the weight-bearing neutral rearfoot position, the neutral subtalar position and the subtalar joint angle present during relaxed calcaneal stance and single leg stance (see Fig. 4.ll).

The standing evaluation continues with observation of the lateral contour of the foot during relaxed stance: a vertically positioned oblique midtarsal joint axis will result in an acute angulation at the calcaneocuboid joint (refer back to Fig. 3.177) while a foot with an inadequate sustentaculum tali or single articulated subtalar joint will present with a straight lateral column, despite the medial displacement of the talus relative to the calcaneus.

The possible effects of a leg length discrepancy should be noted by checking for lateral deviation of the spine, as well as the levels of the iliac crests, greater trochanters, tibial plateaus, and medial malleoli. A functional leg length discrepancy secondary to asymmetrical pronation will result in an excessive lowering of one medial malleolus relative to the other. The standing evaluation can be completed by performing an equinus compensation test (Fig. 4.12), a modified Romberg's test, and by noting displacement of the fat pad upon weight-bearing (Fig. 4.13).

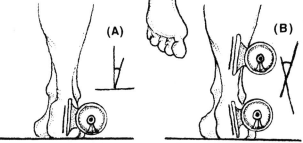

Figure 4.ll. By placing the patient in the proper angle and base of gait while the talonavicular joint is maintained in its close-packed position, the neutral position of the rearfoot (A) can be measured by noting the angle formed between the calcaneal bisection and the ground. This is an important angle as it represents the combined degree of the lower leg and neutral subtalar measurements; e.g., a four degree lower leg varum plus a two degree subtalar joint varum should produce a six degree rearfoot varus deformity. This angle helps determine the size of the rearfoot post (see page 2ll) as it often represents the position of the calcaneus at heel strike (although the actual position of the rearfoot at heel strike varies depending upon factors such as speed, base of gait, strength, and the use of orthotics; e.g., orthotics increase the degree of rearfoot inversion present at heel strike while strengthening exercises [30] and a wider base of gait [31] may decrease rearfoot inversion at heel strike). After noting the neutral rearfoot position, the weight-bearing neutral subtalar joint angle can be measured by noting the angle formed between the calcaneal and lower leg bisections. This angle, which should match the off-weight-bearing measurement, is then remeasured as the patient first moves to a relaxed double limb calcaneal stance position and finally to a single leg stance position. As noted by McPoil and Cornwall (32), the angle formed by the rearfoot and lower leg during single leg stance (B) serves as an indicator of the degree of maximum eversion possible during walking (although typically the subtalar joint will pronate to an end range somewhere between the resting calcaneal stance and single leg stance angle). Depending upon the source, hyperpronation exists when the difference between the neutral subtalar angle and the single leg stance angle exceeds I4 degrees. (Keep in mind that some authors question the significance of frontal plane rearfoot measurements as transverse plane shank rotation appears to be a more accurate indicator of subtalar pronation [33].)

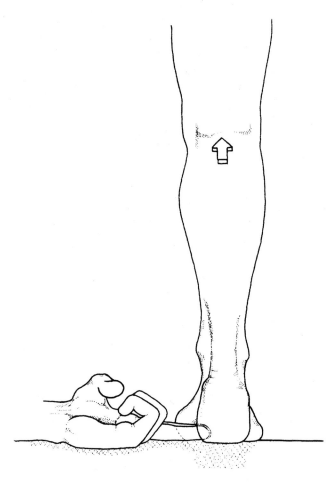

Figure 4.12.   Equinus compensation test. As with measuring subtalar eversion off-weight-bearing, measuring ankle dorsiflexion in an off-weight-bearing position may not accurately reflect the available range of motion during ambulation. To confirm the effect of a limited range of ankle dorsiflexion as measured off-weight-bearing, the patient is asked to stand with knees extended and the subtalar joint in its neutral position. The examiner then places fingers beneath the midtarsal joint and asks the patient to flex the knees: a true equinus that is secondary to a bony restriction or soleus contracture will produce compensatory midtarsal motion as the proximal tibia moves forward with knee flexion. Conversely, contracture in the gastrocnemius muscle will produce compensatory midtarsal motion as the straightened lower extremity is moved forward.

DYNAMIC EXAMINATION

The gait evaluation basically serves as a double-check system to confirm your neutral position measurements, i.e., a patient with a 10° forefoot varus deformity should remain pronated throughout propulsion with the rearfoot everted during heel lift, etc. In order to perform this evaluation, a clear, level walkway is needed that is at least 20 feet long. Keep in mind that the gait evaluation is the most difficult part of the exam, as many movements take place in frac-

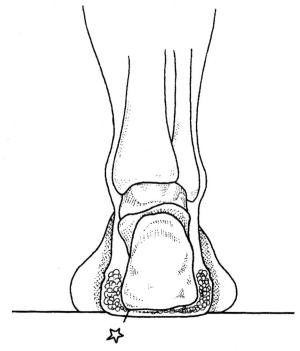

Figure 4.13.   Normally, the infracalcaneal fat pad will deform medially and laterally upon weight-bearing, allowing for an approximate 25% reduction in height. It is clinically interesting that individuals presenting with heel pain will often allow for as much as a 50% reduction in the height of the fat pad upon weight-bearing. This may result in injury to the infracalcaneal bursa and/or medial calcaneal condyle **(star)** as the plantar calcaneus is forced to dissipate ground-reactive forces over a smaller surface area. The ability of the fat pad to dampen ground-reactive forces lessens with age (14) and repeated trauma (15). Also, Jorgensen and Bojsen-Moller (15) note that the fat pad, which absorbs shock 2.1 times better than sorbothane, possesses an open plexus of veins that allows compression of the pad to enhance the countergravitational return of blood.

tions of a second, with multiple structural interactions occurring simultaneously. To compound the problem, many patients will consciously or unconsciously modify their gait pattern when they know someone is watching them.

With these factors taken into consideration, it is easy to see why gait observations are frequently wrought with inaccuracy, as even the most experienced practitioners have to avoid seeing what they want to see. In fact, some individuals claim the eye is an inadequate tool for gait evaluation (16). To simplify these problems, and to ensure that the visual examination yields clinically significant results, it is suggested that one concentrate on singling out isolated events during the gait cycle as they occur in one specific plane of motion.

For example, after having the patient walk up and down the walkway until he or she is relaxed, one should note the precise frontal plane position of the calcaneus at the time of heel strike, full forefoot load, heel lift, and toe off. Typical comments recorded during this evaluation might read: "Heel-strike occurs with the rearfoot excessively inverted, with rapid subtalar pronation occurring during early contact. The calcaneus remains moderately everted throughout mid and early propulsion (the rearfoot is everted approximately 5° at heel lift) with a low gear push-off returning the calcaneus to a slightly inverted position by midpropulsion. The final push-off occurs through the transverse axis, with the swing phase motions nonremarkable."

Observation of frontal plane movements of the calcaneus has become the most commonly used method for quantifying subtalar motion during gait, as the calcaneus is the least mobile segment, the easiest to record, and its movement accurately reflects subtalar motions (16, 22). Although it is difficult to quantify without video equipment, the range of frontal plane rearfoot motion should always be recorded as accurately as possible. Because it is impossible to use exact degrees while performing the visual exam, describing motions as mild (0–5°), moderate (5–10°), and marked (greater than 10°) will suffice.

In all situations, the information obtained during the gait evaluation should be consistent with your examination findings. In the rare case that your measurements do not match the observed gait pattern, it is suggested that one repeat any questionable portions of the exam that might be responsible for the discrepancy. (Problems associated with muscular strength, decreased proprioception, and/or soft tissue contracture are notorious for producing unanticipated gait patterns.)

In addition to noting frontal plane motions of the rearfoot, the examiner should also record the various structural interactions as they occur during each successive portion of the gait cycle. During the contact period, the approximate position of the knee at heel strike should be noted (any abnormalities, such as an hyperextended knee or an excessively flexed hip, should be recorded), and the range of knee flexion during contact period should be estimated and compared bilaterally. (An individual often compensates for a structural leg length discrepancy by hyperflexing the long-leg knee during the contact period.) Any toe in or toe out gait pattern should be recorded and compared to the anticipated angle of gait as estimated by the off-weight-bearing measurements (i.e., combined talar, tibial, and femoral rotations). An in or out toe gait pattern that occurs when osseous deformities are not present suggests the presence of soft tissue imbalance.

Because of difficulties with observation, it is suggested that transverse plane motions of the thigh and shank be observed as the patient walks towards the examiner: excessive subtalar pronation should produce a corresponding increase in internal tibial rotation, while femoral anteversion often results in an extreme medial displacement of the patella during contact and midstance periods. The frontal plane position of the forefoot at heel strike and full forefoot

load should also be noted, and muscular control of contact period ground-reactive forces should be observed: Is there a particularly smooth and steady rate of ankle plantarflexion/subtalar pronation, or does heel strike occur as a hard and jarring action secondary to inadequate muscular stabilization?

The structural interactions occurring during the midstance period are the most difficult to evaluate. As the contact period ends, in addition to noting the frontal plane position of the calcaneus at full forefoot load, the examiner should be observing the contralateral swing phase leg externally rotating the stance phase leg: the external rotatory moment created by the swing leg should begin to supinate the subtalar joint by late midstance. Remember that during midstance, the subtalar joint is maintained in a pronated position as muscles and ligaments of the foot and leg are storing energy that will be returned during propulsion.

The frontal plane position of the calcaneus during heel lift should be noted, and the amount of hip and knee extension, as well as the degree of ankle dorsiflexion present during terminal midstance, should be recorded. Remember that ideally, the hip will be extended 10°, the knee should be straight and the ankle dorsiflexed 10° at heel lift. Any deviation from this pattern, such as a premature heel lift and/or midtarsal compensation for an ankle equinus, should be noted. It should be emphasized that many individuals differ from the ideal in that they move into the propulsive period with the subtalar joint markedly pronated. As long as he/she is able to supinate the subtalar joint during early propulsion (i.e., heel lift releases the calcaneus from ground-reactive forces, thereby allowing the subtalar joint to rapidly supinate with the initiation of a low gear push-off), this pattern of gait should not be considered pathological, as it may represent a variation of norm (17).

The final observations made during the midstance period should include evaluation of pelvic motions. Ideally, the contralateral innominate should drop 4–6° as the torso moves over the stance phase leg (18). Pelvic motions are an excellent indicator of structural leg length discrepancies, as the center of mass on the long-leg side appears to pole-vault over the midstance period lower extremity. Furthermore, osteoarthrosis of the stance phase hip often produces a gluteus medius gait pattern in which the entire torso tilts laterally over the midstance period femur (Fig. 4.14). Also, although uncommon, it is possible that extreme weakness of the hip extensors will allow the entire torso to hyperextend over the pelvis during early stance phase (Fig. 4.15).

As the foot moves into its propulsive period, there should be a visible transition into a low-gear push-off (it is often possible to see the plantar fascia tense) with the calcaneus continuing to invert as the ankle simultaneously plantarflexes. At this time, the contralateral pelvis should continue to rotate forward, and the medial longitudinal arch should increase in height. The presence of an abductory twist at heel lift should be noted and related to possible tor-

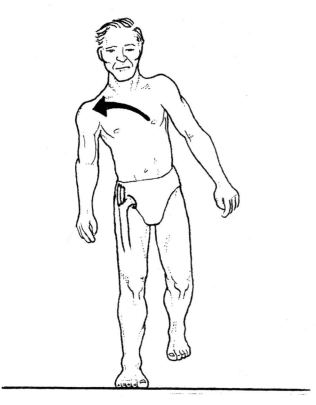

Figure 4.14. The gluteus medius gait pattern. (Modified from Hoppenfeld S. Physical Examination of the Spine and Extremities. New York: Appleton-Century-Crofts, 1976: 139.)

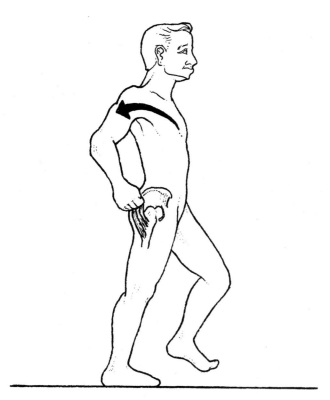

Figure 4.15. The gluteus maximus gait pattern. (Modified from Hoppenfeld S. Physical Examination of the Spine and Extremities. New York: Appleton-Century-Crofts, 1976: 139.)

sion injuries, i.e., stress fracture of the distal tibia, overuse synovitis of the ankle or knee, etc.

As the foot moves into the latter portion of its propulsive period, the shift into a high-gear push-off should be noted as the rearfoot slightly everts from its inverted position. Finally, by observing the patient as he or she walks towards the examiner, one can evaluate the position of the first ray during terminal propulsion. If the subtalar joint remains pronated throughout propulsion with the first ray maintained in a dorsiflexed and inverted position (which strains the medial band of the plantar fascia as seen from a side view), it is suggested that the range of hallux dorsiflexion be measured during static stance, with the subtalar joint maintained in the approximate position of function present during terminal stance phase. This helps identify a functional hallux limitus that might otherwise have been overlooked.

Evaluation of the swing phase leg should include noting the approximate ranges of hip and knee flexion, as well as the range of ankle dorsiflexion necessary to produce ground clearance during midswing. It should be remembered that tibialis anterior is an ankle dorsiflexor during early swing phase and a forefoot invertor during late swing phase (20).

The swing phase should ideally end with the foot positioned so that the rearfoot is slightly inverted and the forefoot is fully inverted prior to heel strike. Also, the swing leg innominate should shift from its lowered position during midswing to a neutral position at heel strike. It should be noted that final portion of swing phase is another excellent time to evaluate the effect of structural leg length discrepancy: the swing phase leg often appears to drop an excessive amount prior to heel strike on the side of the short leg.

The gait evaluation may now be concluded by noting the distance between each foot during an average stride, i.e., by noting the base of gait. Tibiofibular varum can then be measured by placing the patient in the average base and angle of gait and measuring the relationship between the bisection of the distal leg and the ground (Fig. 4.16). If a functional tibiofibular varum is present (e.g., contracture in the adductor musculature resulting in a cross-over gait pattern), appropriate measures should be taken to reduce the soft tissue imbalance.

In addition to the visual information obtained at the time of the examination, many practitioners opt for the more reliable information obtained with various video/cinematography equipment. For purposes of measuring contact period eversion of the rearfoot, standard home video cameras are effective (these recorders shoot approximately 30 frames/sec) as the subtalar joint moves through its full range of motion during the first 50% of the contact period, then has a dwell at its end-point that allows for accurate measurement (16). Also, this equipment allows for slow motion analysis of the complex structural interactions. The information obtained via video evaluation may also be invaluable, as it allows for pre- and posttreatment compar-

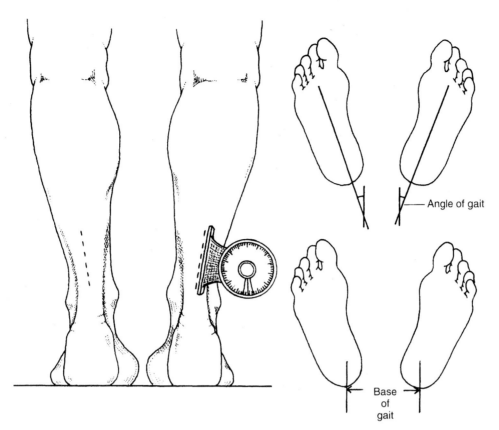

Figure 4.16. Measuring tibiofibular varum. Prior to recording this measurement, the patient must be positioned with feet in the proper angle and base of gait. Although once considered essential, it is not necessary to maintain subtalar neutrality when taking this measurement, as best results are achieved with the foot in a resting calcaneal stance position (21).

isons, a feature that is particularly useful when dealing with soft tissue contractures.

In addition to video equipment, many practitioners have come to rely on more sophisticated methods of gait evaluation such as the EDG (electrodynogram). This device, which was developed by Langer Laboratories, consists of 7 plantar foot sensors that accurately measure shoe/foot interfaces at each site. Although unable to measure absolute force, the EDG supplies reproducible information regarding the duration of time that each sensor is exposed to pressure, as well as subtle changes related to relative increases or decreases in pressure (22). This information is clinically useful, as it allows for numerical quantification that may be compared to an established norm. The significance of this information cannot be understated, as the EDG allows for objective pre- and posttreatment evaluation. Furthermore, because the equipment is portable and carried by the patient (flat wires connect the sensors to a ram pack anchored to the patient's belt), biomechanical data relative to foot/shoe or foot/orthoses can be obtained in virtually any environment.

References

1. Hiss JM. Functional Foot Disorders. Los Angeles: The Oxford Press, 1949.
2. Creighton DS, Olson VL. Evaluation of range of motion of the first metatarsophalangeal joint in runners with plantar fasciitis. J Orthop Sports Phys Ther 1987; 8(7): 357.
3. Rodgers MM, Cavanagh PR. Pressure distribution in Morton's foot structure. Med Sci Sports Exerc 1989; 21(1): 23.
4. Blake RL. Common Sports Injuries and Their Treatment. Foot and Leg Function. Deer Park, NY: Langer Biomechanics Group, 1989; 9(3): 7.
5. Messier SP, Pittala KA. Etiologic factors associated with selected running injuries. Med Sci Sports Exerc 1988; 5: 501–505.
6. Coplan JA. Rotational motion of the knee: a comparison of normal and pronating subjects. J Orthop Sports Phys Ther 1989; 10: 366–369.
7. Root MC, Orion WP, Weef JH. Biomechanical Examination of the Foot. Vol. I. Los Angeles: Clinical Biomechanics, 1971.
8. Smith-Oricchio K, Harris BA. Interrater reliability of subtalar neutral, calcaneal inversion and eversion. J Orthop Sports Phys Ther 1990; 12(1): 10.
9. Lattanza L, Gray G, Kanther R. Closed versus open kinematic chain measurements of subtalar joint eversion: implications for clinical practice. J Orthop Sports Phys Ther 1988; 9(9): 310.
10. Kaye JM, Sorto LA. The K square. A new biomechanical measuring device for the foot and ankle. J Am Podiatr Assoc 1979; 69(1): 58.
11. McPoil TG, Knecht HG, Schuit D. A survey of foot types in

normal females between the ages of 18 and 30 years. J Orthop Sports Phys Ther 1988; 9: 406–409.

12. Burns MJ. Non-weightbearing cast impressions for the construction of orthotic devices. J Am Podiatr Assoc 1977; 67(11): 790.

13. Jones B, Cowan D, Robinson J, Polly D, Berrey H. Clinician assessment of medial longitudinal arch from photographs. Med Sci Sports Exerc 1989; 21(2): 60.

14. Perry J. Anatomy and biomechanics of the hindfoot. Clin Orthop Related Res 1983; 177: 9.

15. Jorgensen Uffe, Bojsen-Moller F. Shock absorbency of factors in the shoe/heel interaction—with special focus on the role of the heel pad. Foot Ankle 1989; 9(11): 294.

16. Cavanagh PR. The shoe-ground interface in running. In: Mack RP (ed). Symposium of the Foot and Leg in Running Sports. St. Louis: CV Mosby, 1982: 30–44.

17. Campbell KR, Grabiner MD, Hawthorne DL, Alexander IJ. Three-dimensional kinematic analysis of tibial-calcaneal motions during the support phase of gait. Med Sci Sports Exerc 1989; 21(2): S88.

18. Schaefer RC. Clinical Biomechanics. Musculoskeletal Actions and Reactions. Ed. 2. Baltimore: Williams & Wilkins:113.

19. Hoppenfeld S. Physical Examination of the Spine and Extremities. New York: Appleton-Century-Crofts, 1976:139.

20. Basmajian JV, DeLuca CJ. Muscles Alive: Their Functions Revealed by Electromyography. Ed. 5. Baltimore: Williams & Wilkins, 1985.

21. McPoil TG, Schuit D, Krecht HG. A comparison of three positions used to evaluate tibial varum. J Am Podiatr Med Assoc. 1988; 78(1): 22.

22. Stuck RM, Moore JW, Patwardhan AG. Forces under the hallux rigidus foot with surgical and orthotic intervention. J Am Podiatr Med Assoc 1988; 78(9): 465.

23. Klave K, Hansen ST, Masquelet AC. Clinical, quantitative assessment of first tarsometatarsal mobility in the sagittal plane and its relation to hallux valgus deformity. Foot Ankle Int. 1994; I: 9-13.

24. Elveru RA, Rothstein JM, Lamb RJ. Goniometric reliability in a clinical setting: Subtalar and ankle joint measurements. Phys Ther 1988; 68: 672-677.

25. Picciano AM, Rowlands MS, Worrell T. Reliability of open and closed kinetic chain subtalar joint neutral positions and navicular drop test. J Orthop Sports Phys Ther 1993; 18 (4): 553-558.

26. Astrom M, Arvidson T. Alignment and joint motion in the normal foot. J Orthop Sports Phys Ther 1995; 22(5): 216-222.

27. Diamond JE, Mueller MJ, Delitto A, Sinacore DR. Reliability of a diabetic foot evaluation. Phys Ther 1989; 69(10): 797-802.

28. Sommer HM, Vallentyne SW. Effect of foot posture on the incidence of medial tibial stress syndrome. Med Sci Sports Exercise 1995; 27(6): 800-804.

29. Powers CM, Maffucci R, Hampton S. Rearfoot posture in subjects with patellofemoral pain. J Orthop Sports Phys Ther 1995; 22(4): 155-159

30. Feltner ME, Macrae HS, Macrae PG et al. Strength training effects on rearfoot motion during running. Med Sci Sports Exercise 1994; 26(8): 1021-1027.

31. Williams KR, Ziff, JL. Changes in distance running mechanics due to systematic variations in running style. Int J Sports Biomech 1991; 7: 76-90.

32. McPoil, TG, Cornwall, MW. Relationship between three static angles of the rearfoot and the pattern of rearfoot motion during walking. J Orthop Sports Phys Ther 1996; 6: 370-375.

33. Nawoezenski DA, Cook TM, Saltzman CL. The effect of foot orthotics on three-dimensional kinemetics of the leg and rearfoot during running. J Orthop Sports Phys Ther 1995; 6: 317-327.

Chapter Five

Casting Techniques

After the examination has been completed and it has been determined that use of foot orthoses is indicated, the practitioner must now decide which casting technique best suits the patient's biomechanical needs. Because the most common cause for orthotic failure is incorrect positioning of the foot during the casting process (1), it is essential that the negative impression be accurate. Surprisingly, there is a fair amount of controversy regarding which technique most accurately allows for ideal function: Some authorities claim weight-bearing casts are necessary to capture plastic deformation of the soft tissues while others advocate that non-weight-bearing plaster casts are superior, as they allow for maximal control of motion.

In order to clear up some of the confusion, the following sections will review the principles and procedures associated with each of the various techniques and relate this information to the clinical objectives involved in making an orthotic. The advantages and disadvantages associated with each technique will be summarized at the end of each section. The final decision as to which technique should be used is based upon treatment goals, examination findings, and the treating doctor's experience and/or preference.

The primary casting methods are outlined as follows:

1. Full-weight-bearing polystyrene foam step-in.
2. Neutral position, semi-weight-bearing polystyrene foam step-in.
3. Neutral position, off-weight-bearing plaster casts.
4. Hang technique plaster casts.
5. In-shoe vacuum techniques.

FULL-WEIGHT-BEARING POLYSTYRENE FOAM STEP-IN

Method

The patient is instructed to stand in a tray of polystyrene foam with full-weight equally distributed between both feet.

Rationale

Laboratories advocating this technique advocate that it is superior to all others, as it captures the degree of soft tissue deformation associated with static stance. This information is then used to choose a specific height for the medial longitudinal arch.

Discussion

The concept of noting plastic deformity in a cast is valid, as it provides information regarding the integrity of the bony and ligamentous restraining mechanisms. However, the need to verify this information with a weight-bearing cast is of questionable value since it may more accurately be measured by noting the navicular differential as the foot shifts from its neutral position to its resting stance position. Furthermore, full-weight-bearing casting techniques also capture a picture of the foot in its fully compensated position: since resistance from the polystyrene foam causes the plantar forefoot and rearfoot to shift to the same transverse plane (which obliterates flexible forefoot deformities), it forces the midtarsal joint to collapse and enables a hypermobile first ray to dorsiflex and invert. An orthotic fabricated from such an impression maintains all of the positional pathologies associated with this aberrant compensation.

Note that some laboratories claim they prefer a compensated picture so the medial arch can be built up from that position. However, without the foot in front of them, the orthotic laboratory has no idea where neutral position is and, therefore, must guess as to the ideal arch height necessary for correction. Such nonspecific buildup of the medial longitudinal arch risks undercorrection (with continued symptomatology) or worse, overcorrection, which may be extremely destructive, as an oversized arch support randomly inverts the entire foot. This may lead to a variety of injuries, as inversion of the forefoot often prevents plantarflexion of the first ray during propulsion (which may eventually lead to destruction of the first metatarsophalangeal joint) while inversion of the rearfoot may prevent deflection of the midtarsals and limit the range of subtalar pronation necessary for shock absorption.

As noted by Robbins et al. (2, 3), excessive buttressing of the medial longitudinal arch may produce proprioceptive deficits (potentially producing a neurotrophic arthropathy) and, by stimulating cutaneous receptors under the medial longitudinal arch, may eventually lead to injury of the metatarsal heads secondary to impaired muscular stabilization. Furthermore, Glancy (4) stated that because an exaggerated medial arch support will block the storage and eventual return of elastic energy during the contact period, the long and short digital flexors may be chronically strained as they attempt to compensate for the weakened calf musculature by firing vigorously during midstance and propulsion (i.e., tibialis posterior is especially weakened by the complete blockage of rearfoot eversion). An excessively high arch support may also damage the tissues directly beneath the medial longitudinal arch, as it may contuse the abductor hallucis muscle and create a bowstring effect that increases tensile strain placed on the plantar fascia (5). An excessively high arch support may also produce a neuropraxia of the medial and lateral plantar nerves that can take 4–6 weeks to heal, even after the arch support has been removed (6).

For the above-mentioned reasons Root et al. (7) cautioned against nonspecific buildup of the medial longitudinal arch. They claimed that although such inserts will initially reduce symptoms associated with ligamentous sprain (they reduce tension on the stretched calcaneonavicular ligament), they should always be avoided, as they may eventually lead to permanent osseous deformity of the first metatarsophalangeal joint.

Keep in mind that the main goal of orthotic therapy is to allow for noncompensated function about all joints of the foot and ankle during all phases of stance. To accomplish this, the laboratory must receive a model of the foot in its neutral position. This position serves as a reference point for ideal function that enables the orthotic to control motion precisely about all axes during the contact, midstance, and propulsive periods of gait: the rearfoot post and calcaneal incline angle of the orthotic shell will control subtalar motion during contact period; the rearfoot post and medial arch support will control subtalar and midtarsal motion during midstance (the arch is lowered to allow for deflection of the midtarsals necessary for shock absorption and proprioception); and forefoot posting (if needed) controls midtarsal and subtalar movements during the propulsive period (and indirectly, during swing phase).

By properly posting the rearfoot and forefoot segments during the various periods of stance phase, a well-made orthotic enables the medial longitudinal arch to support itself, without unnecessary buttressing via extrinsic supports (8). Laboratories that insist on full-weight-bearing casts typically base their evaluation on static function, with support of the medial arch the primary goal of treatment. This approach is outdated and inappropriate, as it allows for effective control of abnormal foot function only during midstance: the arch support is nonfunctional during the contact and propulsive periods of gait, as the arch does not firmly contact the foot during these periods.

The inability of arch supports to effectively control biomechanical abnormalities was demonstrated in a particularly interesting study that compared the effectiveness of arch supports and functional orthotics (i.e., semirigid plastic orthotic shells with dense rubber posts) (9). The authors of this study demonstrated that after failure with arch supports, 81.2% of the 35 patients had successful resolution of symptoms when treated with the functional orthoses. This clearly

demonstrated that an effective orthotic must do much more than merely support the medial arch.

NEUTRAL POSITION SEMI-WEIGHT-BEARING POLYSTYRENE FOAM STEP-IN

Method

With the patient standing next to the examining table, the feet are positioned at their proper angle and base of gait, as determined during the gait evaluation. The patient is then asked to sit, and the practitioner places a tray of polystyrene foam under each foot. While maintaining talonavicular congruency, a firm downward force is applied, first on top of the knee, then on top of the metatarsal heads and toes (Fig. 5.1). The finished impression must be at least 2 inches deep so that the laboratory can fill it with enough plaster to obtain an adequate positive model of the patient's foot. This technique may also be performed by wrapping the patient's foot in plaster as it rests on a soft foam bed.

Rationale

Maintaining the subtalar joint in its neutral position gives the laboratory a reference point for ideal position.

Discussion

This technique affords a fast, simple, and effective method for capturing a picture of the foot with ideal subtalar joint positioning. Because a semi-weight-bearing impression is used, there is adequate displacement of the plantar soft tissues, which negates the need for filling-out or "fudging" around borders of the cast, as is necessary with all off-weight-bearing techniques. Schuster (10) claimed that any modification of the positive model to allow soft tissue expansion upon weight-bearing is guesswork and should be avoided. Schuster (10) also claims that semi-weight-bearing techniques allow for a more tolerable orthotic.

The only drawback to this technique is that it distorts flexible forefoot deformities (particularly the flexible forefoot valgus and plantarflexed first ray), as resistance from the polystyrene foam causes the plantar forefoot to shift from its neutral position. While Schuster (10) maintained that semi-weight-bearing impressions are able to capture forefoot/rearfoot relationships accurately, this has been recently disproved by McPoil et al. (11), as they demonstrated that only neutral position off-weight-bearing techniques were able to duplicate forefoot/rearfoot relationships accurately. Because of this, semi-weight-bearing techniques are used primarily in the treatment of rearfoot varus deformities and/or rigid deformities. (A rigid forefoot varus or valgus will not shift from its fixed position upon meeting resistance from the polystyrene foam.)

The semi-weight-bearing techniques are particularly

individuals and the laboratory does not allow for adequate soft tissue expansion, the edges of the orthotic shell will often dig into the patient's plantar soft tissues.) Schuster (10) claimed that the average foot will lengthen 5%, widen 11% at the ball and 13% at the heel, and the navicular will drop 8–10 mm upon weight-bearing.

NEUTRAL POSITION OFF-WEIGHT-BEARING PLASTER CASTS

Method

As the name implies, this technique involves taking a plaster cast with the patient's foot maintained in a neutral position. This process requires four strips of extra-fast-setting plaster splints (each strip is folded in half), a tray of warm water, and a towel to clean up the mess. First, the patient's lower extremity is rotated so that the foot rests in a vertical position. (This may require placing a towel beneath the patient's hip.) Although this procedure may be done with the patient prone or supine, for simplicity, only the supine techniques are illustrated. (Both prone and supine casting techniques produce comparable results [11].)

With the foot in a vertical position, the subtalar joint is placed in its neutral position, and a firm dorsiflectory force is placed on the fourth and fifth metatarsal heads (Fig. 5.2). The patient is instructed to keep the foot as close to this position as possible while the plaster is being applied; this prevents buckling of the plaster when the foot is later repositioned and loaded. A plaster splint is prepared for application by folding a dry splint into the palm of the hand while pinching the free end between the thumb and index

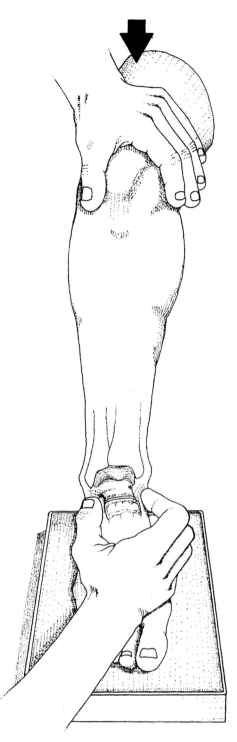

Figure 5.1.   The neutral position semi-weight-bearing impression technique.

useful for treating equinus conditions (it is often difficult to determine how much to lower the medial longitudinal arch when using off-weight-bearing techniques) and for individuals whose foot structure changes markedly upon weight-bearing. (If off-weight-bearing techniques are used on these

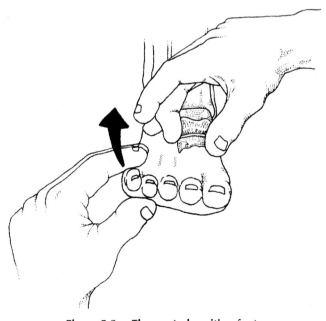

Figure 5.2.   The neutral position foot.

Figure 5.3.   Off-weight-bearing plaster casting techniques.

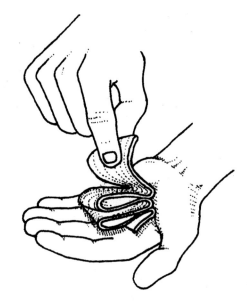

Figure   5.4.   Off-weight-bearing plaster casting techniques.

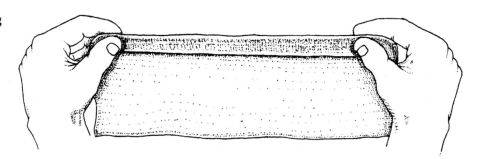

finger (Fig. 5.3). The plaster strip is then submerged into a tray of warm water (for approximately 3 seconds), gently squeezed, and removed from the water. The plaster of Paris is then mixed thoroughly through the cloth by repeatedly squeezing the wet plaster strip in the palm of the hand. It is important that the free end be firmly held throughout this process, as doing so allows unfolding of the wet plaster strip.

Once the plaster has mixed with the cloth, the plaster strip is opened, and the upper border of the strip is folded approximately 1/4 inch, thereby creating a lip along the entire upper edge (Fig. 5.4). The plaster is then applied to the foot by wrapping it around the heel and "tacking" it down to the top of the first and fifth metatarsal heads (Fig. 5.5). The hanging plaster is then smoothed against the medial arch (Fig. 5.6), then overlapped by the lateral strip. The small v-shaped flat that forms at the base of the heel is then smoothed against the cast (Fig. 5.7). The second piece of plaster is applied by draping it over the forefoot (the plaster on the dorsal foot is tacked against the previous strip) and folding it as illustrated in Figures 5.8 and 5.9. The patient is then asked to relax, and the forefoot is loaded by pressing up on the fourth and fifth metatarsal heads while maintaining talonavicular congruency with the opposite hand (Fig. 5.10).

Because of the dangers associated with capturing a supinated impression, it is suggested that a slight abductory

force be used while loading the metatarsal heads and that talonavicular congruency be maintained in a position in which the head of the talus is slightly more palpable on its medial side. The foot is held in this position while the plaster hardens (for approximately 2 minutes).

An alternate method of loading the forefoot is with the suspension technique (12, 13). This popular technique requires that the practitioner firmly grasp the proximal phalanges of the fourth and fifth digits between the thumb and index finger (Fig. 5.11A). The forefoot is then loaded by gently plantarflexing the fourth and fifth digits until they parallel the long axis of the foot (this allows the respective metatarsal heads to dorsiflex slightly, black arrow in Fig. 5.11B) while simultaneously applying an upward and slightly lateral force in order to lock the calcaneocuboid joint. Throughout this process, the toes are tractioned in long axis extension (the relaxed foot is actually suspended from the table), which allows for proper elongation of the plantar soft tissues.

The finished cast is removed by pinching the skin on the dorsum of the foot (white arrows in Fig. 5.12) and pulling down on the heel. The practitioner then carefully pushes the cast forward, gently shaking it until the cast glides off the forefoot (Fig. 5.13).

The accuracy of the negative impression may now be

Figure 5.5. Off-weight-bearing plaster casting techniques.

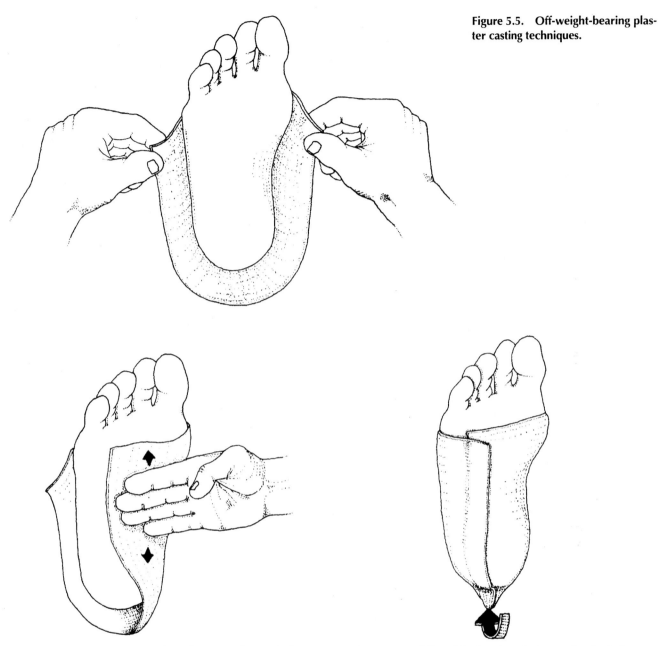

Figure 5.6. Off-weight-bearing plaster casting techniques.

Figure 5.7. Off-weight-bearing plaster casting techniques.

evaluated by placing the impression on a level surface and noting the frontal plane position of the heel: if a forefoot varus is present, the bisection of the rearfoot should be everted; if a neutral forefoot is present, the rearfoot should stand vertical; if a forefoot valgus or plantarflexed first ray is present, the bisection should be inverted (Fig. 5.14).

The most important criterion to consider when evaluating the negative model is that the plaster impression should match in every detail the shape of the neutral position foot (Fig. 5.15). Deviation from the anticipated foot shape most commonly results from insufficient loading of the lateral column (which gives the false impression of a plantarflexed lateral column or forefoot varus), taking the impression with the subtalar joint supinated or pronated

(which will result in a false forefoot varus or valgus, respectively), and/or faulty use of the suspension technique (inappropriate dorsiflexion of the toes will result in a plantarflexed lateral column while excessive pressure from the thenar eminence may produce a false forefoot adductus secondary to inadvertent supination of the forefoot about the oblique midtarsal joint axis). If for any reason the neutral foot and negative impression do not match, the cast should be retaken.

Rationale

This technique captures a picture of the foot in its most stable position: the subtalar joint is in neutral and the

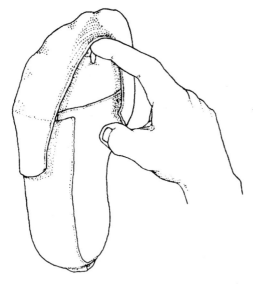

Figure 5.8.   Off-weight-bearing plaster casting techniques.

Figure 5.10.   Off-weight-bearing plaster casting techniques.

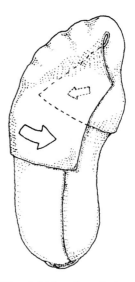

Figure 5.9.   Off-weight-bearing plaster casting techniques.

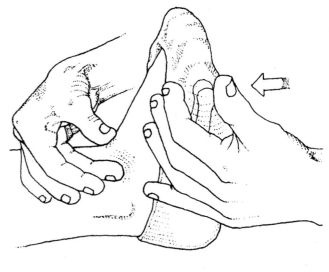

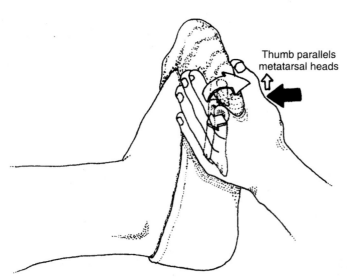

Thumb parallels
metatarsal heads

A

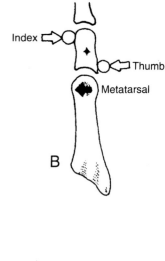

Index

Thumb

Metatarsal

B

Figure 5.11.   The suspension technique. Note that when one uses this method, the thumb should always parallel the lesser metatarsal heads and should not encroach upon the second or third digits (13).

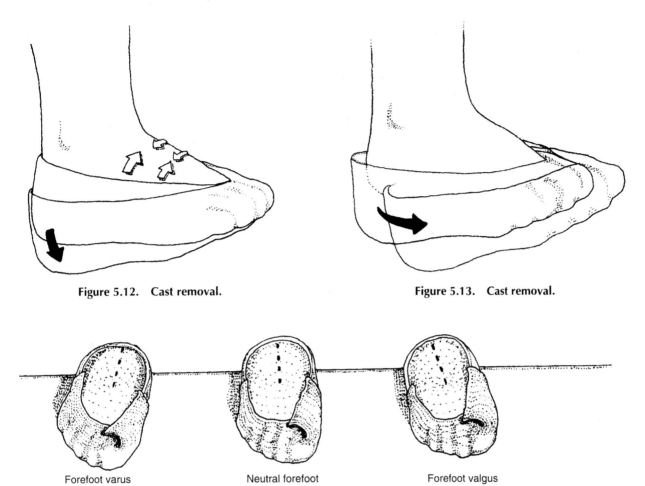

Figure 5.12.   Cast removal.

Figure 5.13.   Cast removal.

Forefoot varus   Neutral forefoot   Forefoot valgus

Figure 5.14.   **Evaluating forefoot/rearfoot relationships.**

calcaneocuboid joint is in its close-packed position, thereby stabilizing the forefoot against the rearfoot. This gives the laboratory a reference point for ideal positioning of all articulations.

Discussion

This is the most accurate technique for capturing forefoot/rearfoot relationships (11). An orthotic made from this impression allows for precise control of motion during all periods of stance. The only problem with this technique is that it requires practice before accurate reproduction of the neutral foot is possible (particularly with the suspension technique) and necessitates that plaster be added to the positive model to allow for soft tissue expansion upon weightbearing.

HANG TECHNIQUE PLASTER CAST

Method

This technique requires taking a plaster cast while the patient lies supine with the foot and leg resting in a com-

fortable position. There is no loading of the forefoot or positioning of the subtalar joint during the casting procedure.

Rationale

It has been suggested that a negative impression made using this technique closely duplicates the contours of a neutrally positioned foot.

Discussion

Although the hang technique was popular in the 1940s, it has for the most part been abandoned. The reason for this is that the increased tension commonly found in the muscles responsible for decelerating subtalar and midtarsal pronation have a tendency to maintain the resting foot in a position where the forefoot is inverted about the longitudinal midtarsal joint axis while the rearfoot is supinated about the subtalar joint axis.

Unless substantial modifications are made on the positive impression (which would seriously compromise the accuracy of the positive model), an orthotic molded to this

Figure 5.15.   Criteria for evaluating negative casts (14). 1) The frontal plane position of the heel should be within 2° of the measured forefoot/rearfoot relationship. 2) The transverse plane relationship between the forefoot and rearfoot should exactly match the patient's foot, i.e., an individual with a rectus foot should present with a straight lateral column (**A**), while an individual with a metatarsus adductus should demonstrate a medial angulation of the forefoot (**B**). 3) If the suspension technique is used, the thumbprint, which should always parallel the sulcus (**C**), should not contact the third digit, and the thenar eminence should not be imprinted on the lateral aspect of the cast. Also, the fourth and fifth digits should be neither dorsiflexed nor plantarflexed (**D**). 4) The contour of the lateral arch (**E**) should duplicate the contour of the patient's neutral position foot. 5) Examination of the interior of the cast should reveal well-defined skin lines, and the plantar impressions of the first and fifth metatarsal heads should be clear.

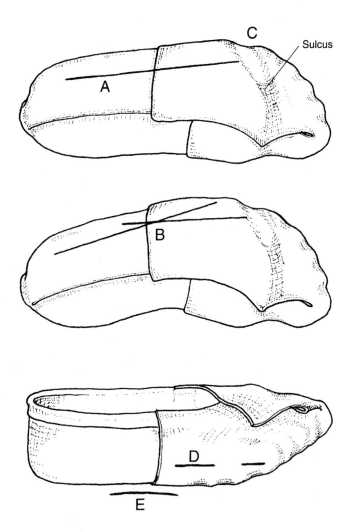

Figure 5.16.   In-shoe vacuum cast technique. When performing this casting technique, Valmassy (13) recommends using a loose-fitting running shoe.

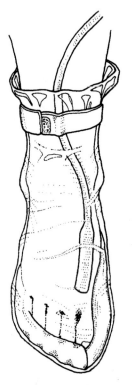
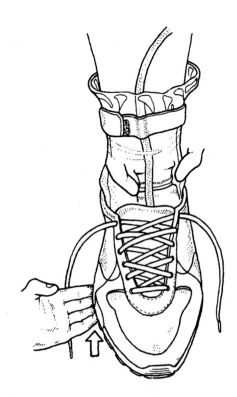

impression would maintain the entire foot in a supinated position. As mentioned previously, this may result in a variety of injuries. Also, because this technique makes no attempt to load the lateral forefoot, it captures all functional foot deformities (the most common being the functional forefoot varus) that are typically not treated with posting techniques.

Because the problems associated with this technique may be avoided simply by maintaining the foot in its neutral position for the 2 minutes it takes the plaster to harden, it is suggested that the hang technique be completely abandoned.

IN-SHOE VACUUM TECHNIQUES

Method

The foot is wrapped in plaster and placed in a plastic bag. The cast is then vacuum-molded to the patient's foot while he/she is wearing a specific shoe (Fig. 5.16). A variation of this technique involves vacuum-molding a heat-malleable orthotic shell (usually Plastazote) directly to the patient's foot as he/she sits on an examining chair. The subtalar joint is typically maintained in its neutral position, and the forefoot may or may not be loaded.

Rationale

To precisely control motion, the orthotic must conform both to the patient's foot and to his/her shoe gear.

Discussion

The concept that an orthotic must conform to the patient's shoe gear is particularly valid when considering shoes with extreme heels and curved shanks. If an orthotic made from a neutral position impression is worn in such a shoe, the shell would be forced to bend or rock at the high point of the shank, thereby irritating tissues beneath the midtarsal joint. Although use of the vacuum technique would avoid this problem as it captures a picture of the foot as it rests in the shoe, this technique has serious drawbacks, as it most often captures a picture of the foot with the forefoot adducted and the midtarsal joint supinated (13).

This risks iatrogenic injury from overcorrection unless substantial modifications are made on the positive. Also, while Brown and Smith (15) claim that it is possible to capture forefoot/rearfoot relationships accurately with this technique, it seems unlikely since the sole of the shoe acts to maintain the plantar forefoot and rearfoot on the same transverse plane.

CAD-CAM TECHNIQUES

Method

CAD-CAM is an acronym for Computer Aided Design - Computer Aided Manufacturing. In the past, this technology was utilized primarily by the automobile industry as the CAD could only be run on very large and expensive computers. Fortunately, advances in microcomputer technology have allowed for more widespread use of CAD-CAM techniques. In fact, automated orthoses are now being manufactured by more than 15 labs.

Basically, the process involves using magnetic resonance (MR), white light or laser to scan an image of the patient's foot (or cast) into a computer. According to Black (16), the MR method involves passing a magnetic field across a cast and recording the image. The image is then compared to over 10,000 previously recorded casts to select the most appropriate orthotic shape. This information is then sent to a milling machine for production of the final orthotic (which is typically made from a fairly rigid plastic).

The white light technique involves taking a number of photographic images that are analyzed and modified by a computer software program that interprets its shape and ultimately mills a device.

By far, the most sophisticated method of CAD-CAM technology is the laser scanner. Developed by John Bergmann, DPM, the process involves passing a laser light source over a patient's foot or cast (the patient's foot is usually maintained in its neutral position using the suspension technique). As the laser passes over the foot, a video camera records the image. Because the camera and laser are positioned at specific angles, it is possible to calculate the x, y, and z coordinates at any given point along the entire surface (usually, data samplings are recorded at 2 mm intervals). The computer then analyzes this information and creates a graphic display of the foot on a computer screen.

The next step involves manipulating the graphic image to allow for soft tissue expansion with weight-bearing and/or for the addition of virtually any modification including balances, forefoot platforms, pocket accommodations, deep heel cups, etc.

Once the image has been modified to the desired shape, it is sent over a computer network to a milling area. The milling machine resembles a drill press that exactly duplicates the final computer image out of an intermediate material (usually wax). This intermediate serves as a positive model upon which any shell material may be molded, e.g., leather, Plastazote, graphite, etc. If a plastic orthotic is desired, first the top is milled to the desired shape, then the material is inverted to mill the bottom. As with designing the superior surface, it is possible to mill the plantar surface into any shape, thereby incorporating intrinsic/extrinsic forefoot and/or rearfoot posts, medial grind-offs, etc.

In addition to MR, white light and laser scanning, another popular CAD-CAM technique is contact digitizing. This method involves having the patient step on a tray containing 576 four millimeter wide pistons that are maintained in an elevated position by a stream of controlled air pressure. As the patient's foot displaces the pistons, a computer analyzes the information and produces a 3D image that can be modified. The final image is then sent to a milling machine and converted into an orthotic. Presently, orthotics manufactured with the contact digitizing technique are limited to a compressed EVA material.

Rationale

CAD-CAM technology was developed to provide practitioners with a fast and accurate method of duplicating a patient's foot and precisely modifying it to control motion and/or redistribute pressure.

Discussion

When performing a scan, the patient's foot may be maintained in a neutral off-weight-bearing position (as with the laser optical scan) or a semi-weight-bearing or full-weight-bearing position (as with contact digitizing techniques). Because some critics point out that the off-weight-bearing impressions require substantial modification of the positive model (this is true whether a laser scan or plaster cast is taken), Bergmann Orthotic Laboratory provides a glass plate to compress the patient's foot during the scan (thereby duplicating a semi-weight-bearing impression).

In regards to orthotic production, a major criticism of some CAD-CAM labs relates to the limited selection of shell materials; i.e., MR techniques are typically limited to the rigid plastics while labs utilizing contact digitizers provide only compressed EVA. (Although labs providing contact digitizers correctly point out that it is not the material that makes an orthotic functional, it is the post angles.) Because laser scanning incorporates an intermediate model, the practitioner may choose from the same materials available with manual production techniques, e.g., leather, graphite, etc.

Another criticism of CAD-CAM devices relates to the accuracy of the milling machines. Some of the early CAM systems required constant recalibration or the completed orthotic would be different than the one displayed on the computer screen (this could result in iatrogenic injury as an incorrectly sloped arch would contuse the corresponding soft tissues). This, however, is no longer a problem as advances in microcomputer-milling interactions allow for exact duplication of the desired images. (This is why remake rates for CAD-CAM and manually produced orthotics are the same.) The primary advantages of the CAD-CAM systems relate to speed of use (a foot can be scanned in seconds) and accuracy (the laser optical system captures the forefoot/rearfoot relationship within 1/100th of a degree). The primary disadvantage relates to cost: the laser optical systems sell for approximately 8,000 dollars, while a contact digitizer can be leased for about 160 dollars per month. Of note, in the not too distant future, in-office milling machines will be available (this will allow for same day turnover).

References

1. Brown D, Smith C. Vacuum casting for foot orthoses. J Am Podiatr Assoc 1976; 66(8): 582.
2. Robbins SE, Hanna AM. Running-related injury prevention through barefoot adaptations. Med Sci Sports Exerc 1987; 19(2): 148–156.
3. Robbins SE, Gouw GJ, Hanna AM. Running-related injury prevention through innate impact-moderating behavior. Med Sci Sports Exerc 1989; 21(2): 130–139.
4. Glancy J. Orthotic control of ground reaction forces during propulsion: a preliminary report. Orthot Prosthet 1984; 38: 12.
5. Campbell JW, Inman VT. Treatment of plantar fasciitis and calcaneal spurs with the UC-BL shoe insert. Clin Orthop Related Res 1974; 103: 57.
6. Waller JF. Hindfoot and midfoot problems of the runner. In: Mack RP (ed). Symposium of the Foot and Leg in Running Sports. St. Louis: CV Mosby, 1982: 71.
7. Root MC, Orion WP, Weed JH. Norman and Abnormal Function of the Foot. Los Angeles: Clinical Biomechanics, 1977.
8. D'Amica JC. Prescribing foot orthoses: the decision making process. Foot and leg function. Deer Park, NY: Langer Biomechanics Group 1988; 1(1): 3.
9. Vitek M, Kerkoc P. Treatment of positional anomalies of the foot with a functional supportive inlay. Orthopade (Berlin) 1989; 127(1): 15–21.
10. Schuster RO. Neutral plantar impression cast-method and rationale. J Am Podiatr Assoc 1976; 66(6): 422.
11. McPoil TG, Schuit D, Krecht HG. Comparison of three methods used to obtain a neutral plaster foot impression. Phys Ther 1989; 69: 448.
12. Burns MJ. Non-weightbearing cast impressions for the construction of orthotic devices. J Am Podiatr Assoc 1977; 67(11): 790.
13. Valmassy RL. Advantages and disadvantages of various casting techniques. J Am Podiatr Assoc . 1979; 69(12): 707.
14. Ross AS, Jones L. Non-weightbearing negative cast evaluation. J Am Podiatr Assoc 1982; 72(12): 634.
15. Brown D, Smith C. Vacuum casting for foot orthoses. J Am Podiatr Assoc 1978; 66(8): 582.
16. Black E. Automated lab technology. Biomechanics 1995; 4: 77-78.

Chapter Six

Laboratory Preparation and Orthotic Fabrication

Although the practitioner need not be familiar with all stages of orthotic fabrication, a cursory understanding of the various materials, posting techniques, and orthotic additions is necessary for the clinician to prescribe the most appropriate orthotic. To familiarize the reader with this information, this chapter will review each step in the process of manufacturing an orthotic.

MODIFICATION OF POSITIVE MODEL

To begin with, a positive model must be obtained from the negative impression. This is accomplished by positioning the negative impression so that the bisection of the rearfoot is vertical (which, when forefoot deformity is present, requires placing a wedge under the medial or lateral metatarsal heads) and, then pouring a mixture of plaster and water into the negative impression.

After the plaster has hardened (which requires approximately 5 to 10 minutes), the negative slipper is torn off and the plantar surface of the positive model is smoothed by wet-rubbing it with a wire mesh or wet sandpaper. The positive cast is then placed upright and gently rubbed in a circular motion against the table. This determines the weight-bearing contact points of the first metatarsal head and the plantar heel (Fig. 6.1A and B). The weight-bearing point beneath the first metatarsal head serves as a reference for determining the outline of the orthotic shell, as a mark is placed 1 cm proximal to this point, thereby indicating the medial distal border of the shell (Fig. 6.1C). A horizontal line is then extended from this point across the plantar surface of the positive cast until it bisects with the fifth metatarsal shaft (Fig. 6.1D). A mark is then made 1/2 cm proximal to this intersection to indicate the distal lateral border of the orthotic shell (Fig. 6.1E).

The lateral edge of the orthotic is determined by extending a line laterally from the weight-bearing point of the heel (B) to a point approximately 14 mm from the supporting surface (Fig. 6.1F). A line connecting this point to the previously determined mark located proximal to the fifth metatarsal head (E) serves as a reference line for the lateral aspect of the orthotic shell.

INTRINSIC FOREFOOT POSTING

If forefoot posting is desired, it is now possible to make modifications that allow for what is referred to as an intrinsic forefoot post. Although it has not yet been discussed, a forefoot deformity may be treated either by adding wedges to the exterior surface of the shell (referred to as extrinsic forefoot posting) or by making modifications to the shape of the positive impression so that the shell itself is able to control the forefoot deformity (referred to as intrinsic forefoot posting).

In order to intrinsically post a forefoot, two small nails are driven into the positive model just proximal to the first and fifth metatarsophalangeal joints. If a forefoot varus deformity is present, the nail beneath the fifth metatarsophalangeal joint is driven to a point where it is flush with the cast while the medial nail is driven only deep enough so that when resting upright, the bisection of the heel rests in a vertical position (Fig. 6.2A). If a forefoot valgus deformity is present, the medial nail would be driven flush while the lateral nail captures the forefoot deformity.

A metatarsal platform is then made by adding plaster to the plantar forefoot (covering the nails and extending over the heads of all the metatarsals; Fig. 6.2B). The positive impression is then placed upright onto a sheet of wax paper, and the medial and lateral sides of the metatarsal platform are packed tight (Fig 6.2C). When the plaster is semi-dry, the excess is removed, leaving a 2-cm platform that maintains the exact height necessary for full correction of the forefoot deformity (Fig. 6.2D). To allow for adequate soft tissue displacement on weight-bearing, additional plaster is placed along the entire lateral aspect of the positive model (referred to as the lateral expansion). Also, additional plaster is added beneath the medial longitudinal arch in order to allow adequate deflection of the midtarsal joints during the contact period. Although the lab typically adds 1/4 inch of plaster to the arch area (referred to as an MLA fill-in), the practitioner may request either an 1/8 or 1/2 inch fill-in to allow for a greater or lesser amount of midtarsal motion during early stance phase.

Finally, the metatarsal platform is smoothly blended into the arch contour (Fig. 6.2E), and a small region of plaster beneath the lateral column is filed away to ensure a constant pronatory force on the fifth ray during gait (Fig. 6.2F). An orthotic shell that is molded to this model will have a bend at its distal medial edge that allows the shell to support the forefoot varus deformity intrinsically, without the use of added wedges (Fig. 6.2G). Note that if a forefoot valgus deformity were present, the bend would have been in the distal lateral portion of the orthotic shell.

A point of clinical concern relates to how far back the metatarsal platform should be blended into the arch. In most

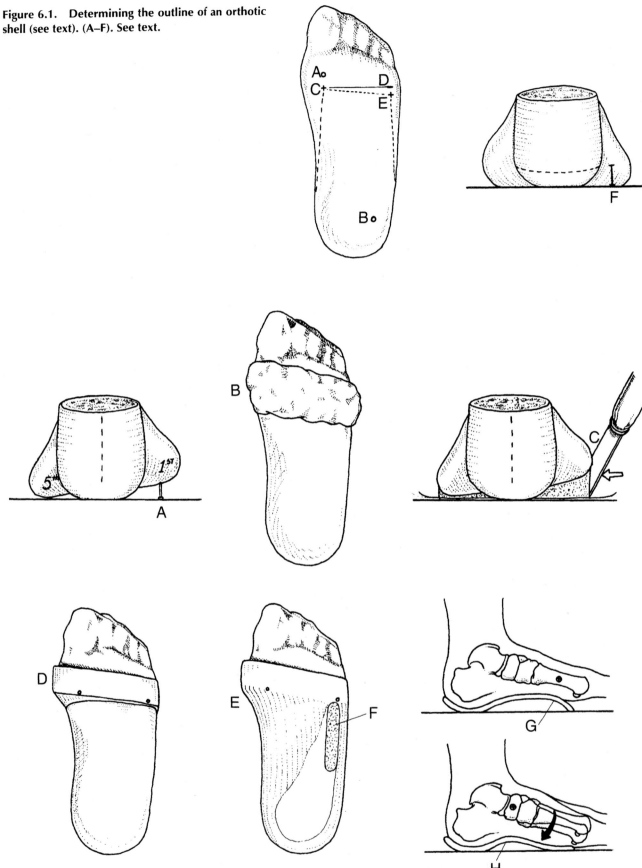

Figure 6.1. Determining the outline of an orthotic shell (see text). (A–F). See text.

Figure 6.2. (A–H) Method for intrinsically posting the forefoot.

situations, the platform is blended so that it merges with the center of the metatarsal shafts (black dot in Fig. 6.2G). This being the case, the intrinsic post will remain functional until the early propulsive period when the progression of forces pass distal to this point. Some orthotic laboratories, however, recommend that the metatarsal platform be blended as far back as the navicular (Fig. 6.2H). This creates problems, as the formed orthotic shell will be unable to control the forefoot deformity beyond early midstance, as the first ray will actively plantarflex in order to make ground contact. Because of this, it is suggested that intrinsic posts be blended no more proximally than the center of the metatarsal shafts.

SHELL SELECTION

With the intrinsic posting completed and the final modifications made to the positive model, the practitioner must now decide which material is to be used for the orthotic shell. The more commonly used materials include the acrylic rohadur (a rigid, glass-like material), the semirigid graphite laminates and thermoplastics (polyethylene and polypropylene), and the very soft and compressible polyethylene foams (e.g., various densities of Plastazote). These materials have the ability to decrease shear forces, redistribute body weight, and/or alter motion about the various axes of the foot and ankle. The decision as to which material should be used is based upon examination findings (foot motions, patient weight, etc.) and treatment goals.

As a general rule, the softer materials are used when control of motion is not a concern and the primary goal of treatment is to decrease shear force and/or redistribute body weight away from painful plantar lesions (as with diabetic individuals). Orthotics made for this purpose are referred to as accommodative devices since no attempt is made to alter motion. These orthotics are typically made from negative impressions taken with the foot in its compensated position, as with full-weight-bearing techniques.

Conversely, the semirigid and rigid materials are used when controlling abnormal movement is the primary concern. Such orthotics, which are categorized as functional orthotics, are designed to allow for near neutral position function of the subtalar joint, which necessitates that only neutral position casting techniques be used.

An important factor to consider when choosing materials is that it is not so much the choice of shell material that determines whether an orthotic is functional or accommodative, as it is the shape of the impression to which the shell is molded (i.e., Is the positive impression made from a neutral position cast or full-weight-bearing impression?) and the amount of forefoot and/or rearfoot posting used. This was demonstrated by McPoil et al. (1), as they noted no difference in center of pressure recordings when the same subjects wore flexible, semirigid and then rigid or-

thoses. This is not to say that there is no difference between these orthotic materials. Smith et al. (2) compared the velocity and range of rearfoot motion between subjects using identically posted soft and semirigid orthotic shells. They noted that while both types of orthotics decreased velocity of pronation by 15%, the semirigid shell more effectively decreased the range of calcaneal eversion. The clinical significance of this information is that either material may be used when the goal of treatment is merely to slow down the velocity of rearfoot motion (as with a medial tibial stress reaction associated with a rearfoot varus deformity). However, when controlling the range of pronation is a concern (as with a hallux abductovalgus deformity secondary to a collapse of the medial longitudinal arch during midstance and propulsion), then use of the more rigid materials is indicated.

A word of caution regarding the use of the more rigid shells is that because these materials are so controlling, they must be molded to a positive impression that exactly duplicates the patient's neutral position foot. If an error was made during the casting process, it is more likely to produce iatrogenic injury when using the less forgiving rigid shells. Because of this, the novice should initially stick to softer shells until he or she feels comfortable with casting techniques. Also, experience has demonstrated that the faster an individual pronates (as occurs with proprioceptive deficits or muscle weakness), the less likely he or she will be able to tolerate a rigid shell.

After the material has been selected for the shell, it is formed directly over the prepared positive model. If a leather shell is to be used, it is first saturated with water and molded to the positive model, then allowed to air dry for 24–48 hours. The more popular thermoplastics and graphite laminates are molded by first placing the chosen material in a convection oven (which makes it pliable for pressing) and immediately molding the heated shell over the positive model in an orthotic press. Once the shell has cooled, it is removed from the press and trimmed to the desired shape (Fig. 6.3A-N). Note that the thermoplastic shells are available in 1/8, 5/32, and 3/16 inch thicknesses (the lab chooses a shell thickness based upon the patient's weight).

EXTRINSIC FOREFOOT AND TIP
POSTING TECHNIQUES

With the outline of the shell properly contoured, a forefoot deformity that was not treated with intrinsic posting techniques may now be addressed with either extrinsic posting or tip posting techniques. The tip post is the easiest method of treating a forefoot deformity, as it merely requires pressing a fingertip down in the center of the heel seat so that either the distal medial or lateral edge of the shell lifts off the table. (The medial edge will lift up with a forefoot varus deformity while the lateral edge will lift up with a forefoot valgus deformity.) With the shell stabilized in this position, a heat gun is used to warm the elevated

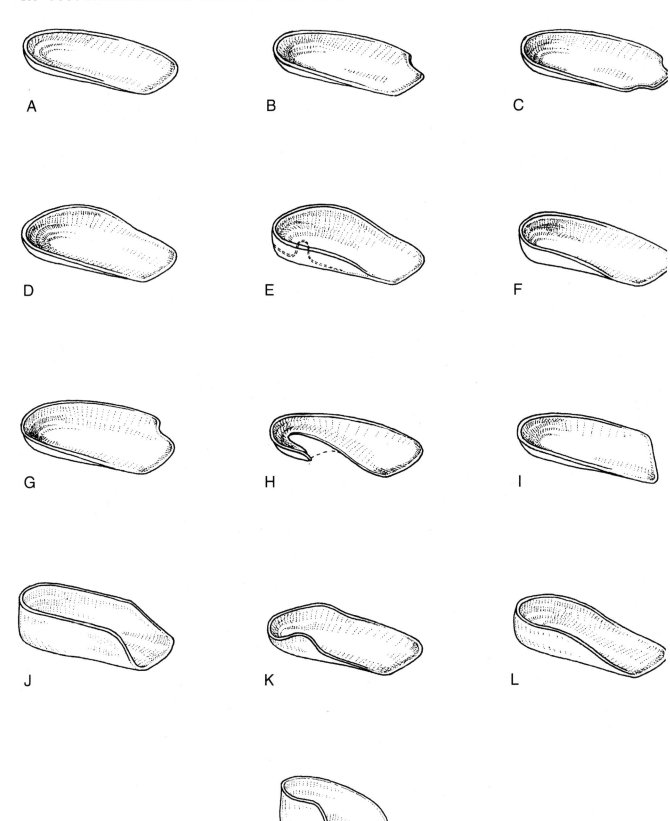

A

B

C

D

E

F

G

H

I

J

K

L

M

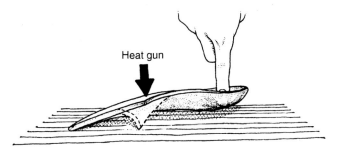

Figure 6.4.   Tip posting a forefoot varus deformity.

edge, allowing it to become so pliable that it drops to the supporting surface (Fig. 6.4). The shell proximal to the bent edge now serves as a point of contact that supports the forefoot deformity. A well-made tip post accomplishes the same thing as an intrinsic forefoot post, only there is no need to alter the positive model with a metatarsal platform.

The final method of posting the forefoot is the extrinsic post. As illustrated in Figure 6.5, this technique requires first scuffing the distal plantar edge of the orthotic shell (tape is used to protect the proximal shell [A]) and then gluing the posting material to the shell (B). A firm crepe is

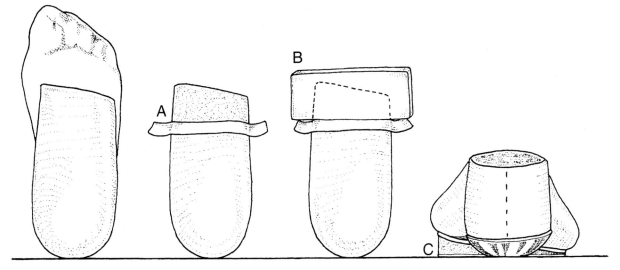

Figure 6.5.   Method for extrinsically posting the forefoot.

Figure 6.3.   Possible variations in shell shape. (A) The standard shell, cut to the specifications outlined in Figure 6.1. **(B)** The first ray cut-out is used to treat a plantarflexed first ray deformity. When treating large plantarflexed first ray deformities, it is suggested that a 2–5 bar post be used (which may be extended to the sulcus) in conjunction with a sub 1 balance for lesion. **(C)** A first and fifth ray cut-out is used to treat plantarflexed first and fifth rays. **(D)** The high medial flange is incorporated to buttress the longitudinal arch and may be used to treat excessive pronation associated with a genu valgum, an out-toe gait pattern, and/or a high oblique midtarsal joint axis. **(E)** High medial and lateral flanges more effectively stabilize the subtalar and midtarsal joints and may be used when more effective control of motion is desired. The *dotted line* illustrates the shape of a lateral clip that is typically used in children with toe-in deformities to prevent them from sliding off of the orthotic. **(F)** The deep heel seat. This modification is used to prevent displacement of the infracalcaneal fat pad. This pad, which consists of columnar arrangements of sealed fat, serves to distribute ground-reactive forces over the entire plantar heel, thereby protecting the more prominent portions of the calcaneus from trauma. As noted by Jorgensen and Bojsen-Moller (4), confinement of the pad increased its shock-absorbing capabilities by as much as 49%. **(G)** The bunion flange may be used to protect a sensitive hallux abductovalgus deformity. **(H)** The slim orthotic shell is used to allow for a better fit in dress shoes. It may be requested that the area of the shell corresponding to the lateral column be removed *(dotted line)* or that this area plus the center of the heel seat be removed. (Note that although removal of the center heel seat allows for a better fit, it occasionally results in an infracalcaneal bursitis.) **(I)** The gait plate, which has an extension of the lateral shell, encourages subtalar joint pronation during the propulsive period and is often used to treat mild toe-in deformities in children (although its efficacy has never been demonstrated).**(J-L)**UC-BL, modified Whitman and modified Roberts, respectively. (UC-BL is an acronym for University of California Biomechanics Laboratory.) These orthotic shells are modern versions of the Whitman and Roberts forms that were originally developed the 1920s and 1930s when the perceived goal of orthotic treatment was to change the shape of the foot, not necessarily to control motion. (These shells are typically not posted.) Because the bulk of these orthotics make for difficulties with shoe fit and because their restrictive nature may impair proprioception, these shells are rarely used, except in children with hypermobile flat feet and individuals with flaccid paralysis. **(M)** Heel stabilizer. This shell shape is used to control rearfoot motion in children by maintaining the calcaneus perpendicular to the supporting surface. Heel stabilizers may be fabricated with a variety of options, including deep heel cups, lateral clips, medial flanges, etc.

Figure 6.6. The compressible post to sulcus. Besides providing continued control of subtalar motion during the propulsive period, this addition lessens the risk of iatrogenic injury by supporting the metatarsal heads *(A)*, thereby distributing pressure away from the distal edge of the forefoot post *(star)*.

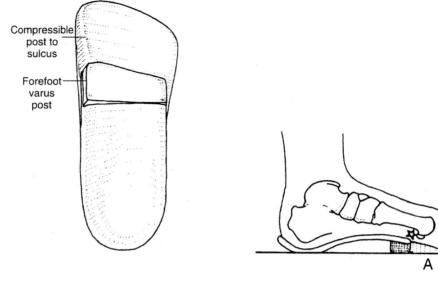

the most commonly used material. The post is then ground in such a way that it brings the rearfoot to vertical (C). Critics of this technique claim that the extrinsic material often cracks off the shell and the added bulk makes for difficulty with shoe fit.

In situations requiring large forefoot posts, a common practice is to partially correct the forefoot deformity with an intrinsic post and then add the remaining number of degrees necessary to bring the heel to vertical with an extrinsic post. For example, a 12° forefoot varus deformity may have 6° built intrinsically into the shell via a posting platform, while the remaining 6° of varus posting is added extrinsically. As a rule, limitations associated with shoe fit prevent use of a forefoot varus post greater than 9°, while forefoot valgus posts should not exceed 6°. Also, if a large forefoot post is indicated, it is suggested that a compressible post to sulcus be added so that the distal orthotic shell does not dig into the metatarsal shafts (Fig. 6.6).

INTRINSIC REARFOOT POSTING

With the forefoot posting completed, it is now possible to post the rearfoot. As with forefoot posts, the rearfoot posts may be applied either extrinsically or intrinsically. As described by Lundeen (3), a true intrinsic rearfoot post requires sectioning the positive model to the axis of the subtalar joint and rotating the rearfoot section into the desired degree of valgus or varus (Fig. 6.7). The crease in the positive model is then blended smoothly with additional plaster to prevent the formation of an annoying edge that would otherwise be molded into the shell. This technique allows fairly large deformities to be posted without affecting how the device fits into the shoe.

An easier, albeit less effective method of posting is the modified intrinsic technique. This method of posting requires placing the heel of the molded plastic shell onto a

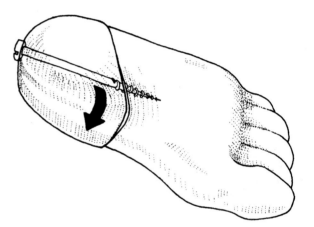

Figure 6.7 The biaxial intrinsic post. Prior to molding the shell to the positive, the cast is sectioned and rotated so as to capture the desired of rearfoot posting intrinsically. (Modified from Lundeen RO. Polysectional triaxial posting. A new process for incorporating correction in foot orthoses. J Am Podiatr Med Assoc 1988; 78(2): 55.)

horizontal sander and grinding the desired angulation into the shell (Fig. 6.8). While the modified intrinsic post allows for a nice shoe fit, it is relatively ineffective at controlling motion because the base of support provided by the intrinsic post is too narrow: whenever pressure is centered distal or medial to the plantar grind, the orthotic will rock medially, thereby nullifying the effectiveness of the post.

This is not to say that the modified intrinsic post is not useful. When placed in a shoe with a firm, flat inner sole, this post serves as a proprioceptive tool that allows the patient to feel the transition from the controlling lateral portion of the device to the unangled medial portion of the device. (Note that even though it is unangled, the medial portion of the orthotic still prevents the subtalar joint from pronating beyond heel vertical.)

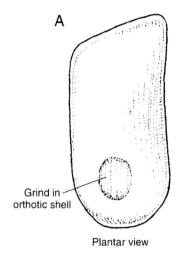

A

Grind in
orthotic shell

Plantar view

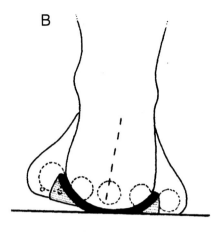

B

Figure 6.8. The modified intrinsic rearfoot post. The plantar heel of the orthotic shell is ground flat **(A)**, thereby maintaining the rearfoot in the desired angle **(B)**. Unfortunately, the degree of posting is limited by the thickness of the shell.

EXTRINSIC REARFOOT POSTING

While true intrinsic and modified intrinsic posts are occasionally used for controlling subtalar joint motion, by far the most popular method of posting is the extrinsic rearfoot post. This post is fabricated using the same grinding method used for the modified intrinsic post, only now the plantar aspect of the heel is reinforced with extrinsic posting material (Fig. 6.9).

One of the most important characteristics of the extrinsic rearfoot post with regards to its ability to control motion during stance phase relates to how far the posting material is extended distally beneath the shell. Normally, the extrinsic rearfoot post extends approximately one-half inch distal to the center of the heel seat, which maintains the entire orthotic in its posted angle until the progression of forces passes distal to the rock line (see Fig. 3.92). Once these forces pass distal to this line, the entire orthotic will evert onto its distal medial edge (or forefoot post, if present), making the rearfoot post nonfunctional.

As demonstrated in Figure 3.93, the standard extrinsic rearfoot post is effective only until the early midstance period. If desired, it is possible to request either a short rearfoot post (which typically ends at the center of the heel seat or slightly proximal to that point) or a long rearfoot post (which extends approximately 3/4 inch distal to the center of the heel seat). Because the short rearfoot post basically moves the rock line proximally, an orthotic made with this post will control motion only during the contact period, with the orthotic everting onto its distal edge during late contact. This may be helpful when treating an individual with a compensated rearfoot varus deformity who has a history of recurrent inversion ankle sprains (which would make maintaining the rearfoot in an inverted position during midstance period a contraindication).

Conversely, a long rearfoot post displaces the rock line distally, thereby allowing for improved control during the latter half of stance phase. Of course, it is also possible

to control motion during the propulsive period by placing the desired rearfoot post beneath the distal medial edge of the orthotic shell or by adding a compressible post to the sulcus.

The decision as to the exact number of degrees that an orthotic shell should be posted is a matter of controversy. It has been suggested that the rearfoot post angle should equal the total degrees of rearfoot varus deformity and that the range of subtalar pronation necessary for shock absorption should be supplied by adding a 4° or 6° biplanar grind to the plantar surface of the rearfoot post (6). The theory behind the biplanar grind is that the unaltered aspect of the rearfoot post maintains ideal osseous alignment while the biplanar grind enables the orthotic (and therefore the subtalar joint) to evert through the exact range necessary for ideal function (Fig. 6.10).

Unfortunately, this logic is incorrect, even dangerous, as the biplanar grind basically behaves as a short extrinsic rearfoot post that maintains the heel in an inverted position during early contact, delaying pronation until the early midstance period. This is particularly dangerous when you consider that the majority of pronation occurs during the first 50% of the contact period (7). A fully posted orthotic with its biplanar grind essentially blocks subtalar joint pronation at a time when it is needed the most: during the early contact period. This risks iatrogenic injury from decreased shock absorption and predisposes to knee injury, as it prevents the range of talar adduction necessary to accommodate the internally rotating lower extremity, i.e., inertial forces drive the internally rotating femur into the immobilized tibia which, together with the talus, is held stationary by the rearfoot post. This may eventually produce laxity of the ligaments responsible for limiting tibiofemoral rotation.

The industry-wide use of biplanar grinds with extrinsic rearfoot posts most likely explains anecdotal reports relating rigid orthotics (rohadur) to knee injuries. Note that it is not the firmness of the shell that produces such injury, it is the inappropriate use of an oversized and rigid post that

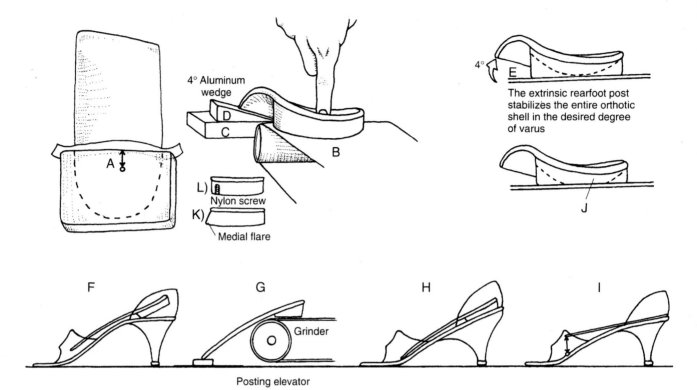

Posting elevator

Figure 6.9. Method for fabricating an extrinsic rearfoot varus post. The plantar proximal orthotic shell is scuffed, and an extrinsic post is glued so that its distal edge rests approximately 1/2 inch distal to the center of the heel seat (**A**). The edges of the post are then filed down, and the heel is placed on a horizontal sander (**B**). The distal orthotic is positioned on a supporting platform (**C**), and the edge of the orthotic shell is angled a specific number of degrees with an aluminum wedge (**D**). The heel of the orthotic is then firmly pressed into the sander, which allows the plantar rearfoot post to stabilize the entire orthotic shell in the desired of varus (**E**). If the orthotic is to be worn in dress shoes, it is frequently necessary to use a posting elevator to ensure that the post will rest flat against the heel seat of the shoe. For example, if the extrinsic rearfoot post was ground on a level surface and then placed in a high heel shoe, the plantar surface of the post would be unable to adequately contact the heel, thereby negating the post's ability to control rearfoot motions (**F**). This problem can be avoided by placing the orthotic on a posting elevator when grinding the rearfoot post (**G**). By duplicating the relationship between the plantar heel seat and forefoot of the shoe, the posting elevator allows the entire rearfoot post to sit flush against the heel seat (The finished post in **G** would fit perfectly into shoe F). As a general rule, shoes with 1/2- , 1-, and 1 1/2-inch heels are accommodated by using 4-, 8-, and 12-

mm posting elevators, respectively. However, as demonstrated by Ross and Gurnick (5), it is not so much the height of the heel that determines the size of the posting elevator as it is the angulation of the heel slope in the shoe. An example of this is illustrated in **H**. Despite the height of its heel, an orthotic for this shoe should be ground flat because of the acute angulation of the heel seat. Because of this, the height of the posting elevator should be selected by placing a *flat bar* (a tongue depressor works well) flush against the heel seat and noting the distance between the bar and the point where the orthotic will end (**I**). This distance represents the ideal height of the posting elevator. In addition to using a posting elevator, it is also possible to allow for improved shoe fit by requesting the rearfoot post be ground into the shell (**J**). This modification significantly reduces the bulk of the extrinsic post by decreasing the height that the orthotic will raise the heel. The stability and resiliency of the rearfoot post may be improved by adding a medial or lateral flare to the post (**K**) (to control excessive pronation or supination, respectively) and by reinforcing the post material with nylon screws (**L**). Because the most common posting material is a compressible crepe, the plantar surface of the post is usually covered with a thin, high-density plastic in order to prevent excessive wear. (This is referred to as a "post-protector".)

blocks the necessary range of subtalar and midtarsal pronation necessary for shock absorption during the early contact period. The major problem associated with incorporating a biplanar grind is that although it does allow for subtalar pronation, the range it allows is too little (a 4° grind allows only 4° of rearfoot motion, which is not enough to ade-

quately absorb shock), and it allows this motion to occur too late in the gait cycle. (By midstance all pronatory motions should have ended.)

The problems associated with biplanar grinds are further complicated by the fact that the ability of the orthotic to rock medially is dependent upon the firmness of the sole. In

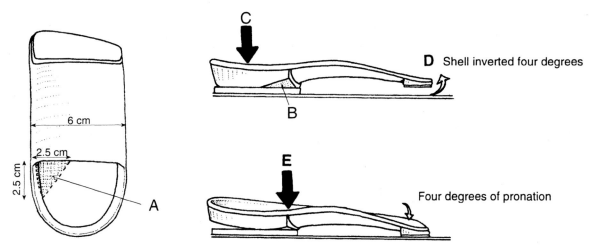

Figure 6.10. The biplanar grind. The distal medial portion of the extrinsic rearfoot post corresponding to the shaded area (**A**) is ground to a depth of approximately 4 mm (this is a gradual grind that peaks at the distal medial corner of the post **B**). According to Weed et al. (6), the biplanar grind allows the rearfoot post to maintain perfect osseus alignment during the contact period; i.e., when weight is centered posterior to the axis of the grind (C), the rearfoot post maintains the subtalar joint in an inverted position (D) while allowing the subtalar joint to pronate the four degrees necessary for shock absorption once the progression of forces are centered distal to the axis of the biplanar grind (E). (Adapted from Weed JH, Ratliff FD, Ross SA. Biplanar grind for rearfoot posts on functional orthoses. J Am Podiatr Assoc 1978;69 (1): 35.)

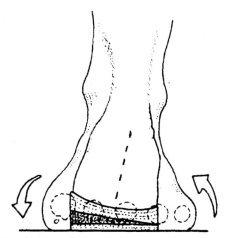

Figure 6.11. By excessively inverting the rearfoot during static stance, a large rearfoot varus post may allow for the development of a functional forefoot valgus deformity (arrows). Another important consideration is that the rearfoot post should never be so high that the knee, when flexed during static stance, rotates external to the sagittal plane.

softer slip-lasted sneakers or shoes with soft heel seats, the lateral portion of the extrinsic rearfoot post actually sinks into the shoe, negating the ability of the biplanar grind to allow for the additional range of subtalar pronation.

A safer, more effective method of determining the size of the rearfoot varus post is to find the total of the rearfoot varus deformity (i.e., add subtalar varum, lower tibial varum, and any varum associated with a cross-over gait pattern) and subtract either 6 or 8° from this number in order to allow for an adequate range of subtalar pronation. For example, an individual with a 4° subtalar joint varum, an 8° lower tibial varum, and a normal base of gait would require a 4° rearfoot varus post (4 plus 8 minus 8) in order to allow the subtalar joint to pronate through an 8° range of motion during the contact period. By using this method, the subtalar joint would have already pronated through its ideal range before the medial calcaneus strikes the shell. At that time, the orthotic would act to block only the excessive motion, allowing for the ideal range necessary for shock absorption.

There is some concern that maintaining the rearfoot in a constantly inverted position during static stance will result in the development of a functional plantarflexed first ray and/or functional forefoot valgus (Fig. 6.11). However, this is not a consideration since, as long as the subtalar joint is allowed to pronate 8°, the forefoot is able to evert 6° beyond neutral secondary to the increased range of midtarsal joint motion associated with the pronated position of the subtalar joint. This means that the rearfoot varus post may be as high as 6° (although it is seldom necessary to post the rearfoot at anything more than 4°) without fear of creating a functional forefoot valgus deformity. If a large rearfoot varus post is deemed necessary (Blake [8] claims the rearfoot varus post may be as high as 10°), a compressible post to sulcus should be added to support the medial metatarsal heads.

In situations in which the total rearfoot varus deformity is less than 8°, but exaggerated pronation is still a concern (e.g., individuals with a vertical oblique midtarsal joint axis, single articulated subtalar joint, or hypermobile first

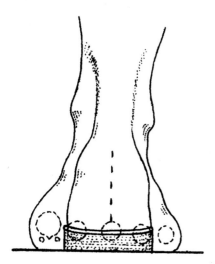

Figure 6.12. The 0° rearfoot post stabilizes the heel in a vertical position.

ray), the rearfoot should be posted at 0° (Fig. 6.12), and the range of excessive pronation would now be controlled by the orthotic shell, not the post angle, i.e., support of the medial longitudinal arch in these individuals is helpful in controlling the overall range of motion.

ORTHOTIC ADDITIONS

With the orthotic shell posting the desired number of degrees, it is occasionally necessary to reinforce beneath the medial longitudinal arch with a filler material to protect against shell breakage. Although the strength of a thermoplastic shell usually obviates the need for reinforcement, certain situations dictate that additional support be added, e.g., if the orthoses were to be worn by obese patients or patients involved in high-impact sporting activities. Also, if an accommodative shell had been chosen (such as leather or low-density polyethylene), it is necessary to attach a filler material to the plantar surface in order to reinforce the arch. The shell and attached filler material are completed by grinding the borders down to the desired shape and width.

Besides choosing from different shell and filler materials, an orthotic can be further modified by adding any of a variety of top covers and/or additions. These modifications are outlined as follows.

Top covers. The most commonly used top covers, which may be extended to the proximal metatarsal heads (covering only the orthotic), to the sulcus (ending at the base of the toes), or to the distal toes (full length), are typically made from glove leather, Spenco (a neoprene foam with a thin layer of nylon on its upper surface), vinyl, nylon, or any of a variety of synthetic suedes. With the exception of Spenco, top cover materials are most often layered with either a 1/8- or 1/16-inch piece of PPT (a very resilient open-cell foam available from the Langer Biome-

chanics Group, Inc., Deer Park, NY) or Plastazote (a more compressible closed-cell foam). The layered material may be added from the distal edge of the orthotic shell to the distal edge of the cover (referred to as an extension) or, it may run beneath the entire length of the top cover.

For example, a vinyl top cover may be requested with a 1/8-inch PPT extension to the sulcus (in which case only the vinyl will cover the orthotic while a combination of vinyl and PPT are extended from the distal edge of the orthotic to the base of the toes). Or, a vinyl/PPT top cover to the sulcus may be requested, which would consist of a layered vinyl/PPT combination being extended from the heel of the orthotic to the base of the toes. Note that it is also possible to request that a bottom cover be added beneath the entire orthotic. Bottom covers are usually used with accommodative orthotics where filler materials would otherwise be susceptible to wear.

Heel lifts. Heel lifts may be invaluable in the treatment of a multitude of conditions. In the treatment of leg length discrepancy, a heel lift will level the pelvis and decrease lateral shear forces on the side of the short leg (9). Heel lifts may also be used bilaterally to treat injuries associated with compensation for a decreased range of ankle dorsiflexion. While usually made from rubber or cork, heel lifts can also be made from more shock-absorbing materials, such as PPT or sorbothane, in order to more effectively treat a high-impact foot (e.g., an uncompensated rearfoot varus or a rigid forefoot valgus deformity).

The ability of PPT to lessen impact forces was demonstrated by Millgrom et al. (10), as they noted that a generic flexible orthotic with a 3° rearfoot varus post and a 1/8-inch PPT heel lift decreased the incidence of femoral stress fractures in military recruits by 8.1%. This is consistent with the findings by Voloshin (11), who noted that viscoelastic heel lifts decreased the amplitude of bone oscillations during walking.

Furthermore, because some people adapt to added cushioning by decreasing the velocity of knee flexion at heel-strike (12), shock-absorbing heel lifts may also be of benefit in treating retropatella arthralgias. (Although as demonstrated by Nigg et al. [13], it is not necessary to replace the standard EVA insole found in running shoes with the more expensive sorbothane insoles, as the stock insoles are just as effective at reducing vertical forces at heel-strike.) With regards to treating injuries of the achilles tendon, Lee et al. (14) concluded that heel lifts can be an effective form of treatment, as progressively larger heel lifts produce linear decreases in EMG activity of the medial gastrocnemius muscle.

Regardless of the potential benefits, heel lifts should always be prescribed with caution, as they produce an increase in vertical forces bilaterally (9) and may initially increase the range of subtalar pronation during the contact period (15). (Note that there is much conflicting information regarding the effects of heel lifts on contact period subtalar motions [16-18].) Also, because they displace the body's center of mass anteriorly, heel lifts may produce a facet syndrome (the lumbar spine hyperextends to accommodate the displaced center of mass) and/or precipitate a painful forefoot condition, as a greater percentage of weight is now borne by the metatarsal heads. (Because of this, heel lifts may actually aggravate a plantar fascia problem.)

Bar posts.   A bar post is a flat forefoot post that may effectively decrease pressure on the metatarsal heads by supporting the metatarsal necks. It is common to request a 2–5 bar post when treating a plantarflexed first ray. Note that when treating a large deformity, a compressible 2–5 bar post may be extended to the sulcus.

Balance for Lesion.   This is an invaluable addition providing customized cushioning for painful bony or soft tissue prominences. The practitioner marks the lesion on either the patient's foot (the ink will transpose onto the cast) or on a diagram located on the laboratory order form. A custom doughnut-, U-, or J-shaped pad is then contoured around the lesion and attached beneath the top cover. The finished balance allows for a redistribution of pressure away from the involved prominence. The most commonly used balances, which are usually made from cork or PPT, are illustrated in Figure 6.13.

In situations in which a painful lesion is located directly over the orthotic shell (such as a prominent calcaneal condyle), it is possible to build the balance for lesion directly into the orthotic shell. This addition, referred to as

pocket accommodation, requires adding a small amount of plaster directly over the corresponding location on the positive model (Fig. 6.14A). The shell that is molded over this modified positive model will have an indentation or pocket that distributes pressure away from the painful lesion (Fig. 6.14B).

Morton's extension.   An 1/8-inch platform is shaped from cork or crepe and placed beneath the top cover in order to support a short first metatarsal (refer back to Fig. 3.104). Please note that this addition should not be used to treat a long second metatarsal, which is more appropriately treated with metatarsal pads, toe crests, and/or a sub 2 balance for lesion.

Kinetic wedge.   Developed by Howard Dananberg, DPM, this addition requires adding a dense crepe extension beneath the second through fifth metatarsal heads, while a softer triangularly shaped piece of PPT is placed beneath the first metatarsal head. According to Dananberg (20), the softer material placed beneath the medial forefoot allows the first metatarsal to "plantarflex and evert during peroneus longus activity," thereby allowing for the dorsal-posterior shift of the first metatarsophalangeal joint's transverse axis that is necessary for the hallux to reach its full range of dorsiflexion.

Unfortunately, the logic for this addition is questionable since the most common cause for impaired first ray plantarflexion during propulsion is excessive subtalar pronation. Because the soft material placed beneath the me-

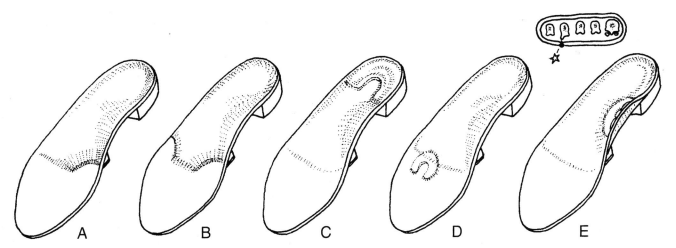

Figure 6.13.   The various balances for lesions. (A) The sub 1 balance for lesion (aka "dancer's pad") is used to accommodate a plantarflexed first ray while the sub 1,5 balance **(B)** (aka "double dancer's pad") is used to accommodate the plantarflexed first and fifth rays often associated with cavus foot types. **(C and D)** The horseshoe pad accommodation may be used to accommodate a calcaneal spur, a plantarflexed lesser metatarsal, a prominent plantar condyle *(inset)* or a plantar wart, i.e., because pressure stimulates growth of the virus (19), any addition that decreases pressure beneath the

wart (such as a bar post, metatarsal pad, toe crest or sub-metatarsal balance) is clinically indicated. **(E)** An accessory navicular, which may be attached to the parent navicular via a synchondrosis, often requires protection from tensile, shear, and compressive forces. This may be accomplished by adding a U-shaped balance to a large medial flange. This balance is usually used in conjunction with the appropriate rearfoot and/or forefoot varus posts in order to minimize excessive subtalar pronation that would otherwise irritate this osseous anomaly.

Figure 6.14.   (**A** and **B**) The pocket accommodation.

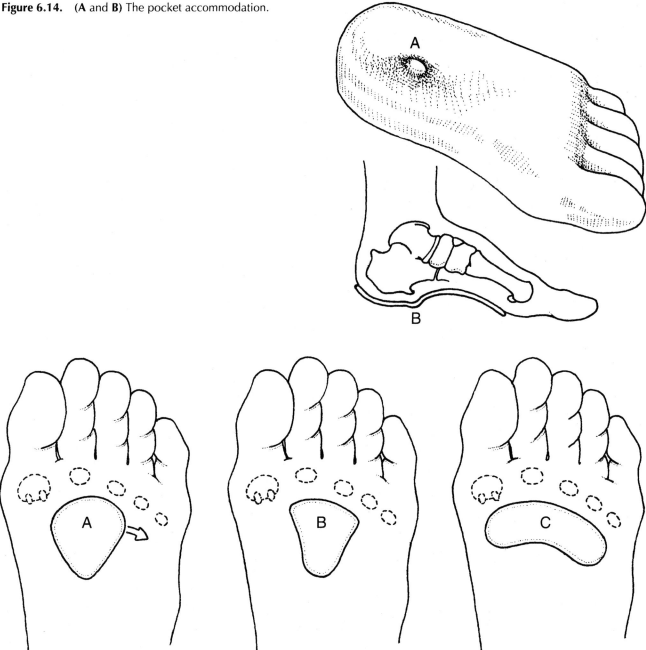

Figure 6.15.   (A) Heart-, (B) stomach-, and (C) kidney-shaped metatarsal pads.

dial forefoot may actually encourage subtalar pronation, the kinetic wedge has the potential to create the exact condition it was designed to prevent: functional hallux limitus.

This is not to say the kinetic wedge should never be used. In situations in which deformity of the first metatarsophalangeal joint is secondary to a long first metatarsal, the kinetic wedge may allow for the improved range of first ray plantarflexion necessary to prevent continued deformity. (As long as it is used in conjunction with a long rearfoot varus post in order to prevent excessive subtalar pronation.)

Metatarsal pads.   These pads, which are typically made from either sponge rubber, felt, or PPT, allow for a redistribution of pressure away from the metatarsal heads by supporting the distal metatarsal shafts (21). As a result, metatarsal pads may be an effective form of treatment for elongated second metatarsals, plantar keratoses, interdigital neuromas, intermetatarsophalangeal bursitis, plantar warts, and/or plantarflexed lesser metatarsals. To be effective, the metatarsal pad, which comes in a variety of shapes and sizes (Fig. 6.15), should be positioned just proximal to the metatarsal heads.

Because each person responds to pad placement differently, it is often necessary to have the metatarsal pad shifted proximally, distally, medially, or laterally in order to find the exact location that provides the best results. In some situations, it is necessary to use a temporary metatarsal pad and allow the patient to experiment with size and location. When the ideal position is located, a permanent metatarsal pad may be attached beneath the top cover of the orthotic.

It should be stressed that when the goal of treatment is to reduce pressure beneath the first metatarsal head (as with sesamoiditis), it is necessary that a large metatarsal pad be used since small metatarsal pads have no effect on reducing pressure patterns beneath the hallux or first metatarsal head (21). If it is necessary to incorporate a large metatarsal pad, the practitioner is cautioned against using the hard rubber materials since they may irritate the central band of the plantar fascia and may even produce heel pain secondary to a bowstring effect on the plantar fascia.

Toe crests. This addition is used in the treatment of hammer and claw toe deformities. By supporting the central portions of the second through fifth digits, toe crests function to reduce pressure beneath the metatarsal heads and distal toes by distributing pressure over a larger surface area (Fig. 6.16). Also, because toe crests effectively stabilize the distal phalanges, their addition helps improve the propulsive period function of flexor digitorum longus, which is severely compromised by digital contractures.

Please note that individual variation in the angulation of the second through fifth metatarsals makes ideal placement of toe crests difficult. A helpful method for ensuring proper positioning is to initially prescribe a vinyl top cover with a Plastazote extension to the toes. After 2 weeks of wear, the lesser metatarsal heads will form a groove in the Plastazote that allows for exact placement.

Interdigital plugs. Used to treat a painful inter-metatarsophalangeal bursitis, this teardrop-shaped addition, which is placed directly between the involved metatarsal heads, actively opens the interspace theoretically allowing for a reduction of shear forces on the bursa (Fig. 6.17).

Because this addition may potentially increase compressive forces at the neighboring interspaces, and may even result in entrapment of the interdigital nerve between the plug's dorsal surface and the transverse metatarsal ligament, it is suggested that the interdigital plug be used only as a last resort in the treatment of a painful interspace.

Cuboid pad. This small pad, which is placed directly beneath the cuboid, is typically used only with prefabricated orthotics as a way to accommodate plantarflexed fourth and fifth rays. (The shell of a custom-molded orthotic will naturally contour the plantar lateral foot, thereby negating the need for this addition.) Care must be taken when prescribing a cuboid pad as inappropriate use may result in a premature locking of the calcaneocuboid joint, which may potentially sprain the midtarsal restraining ligaments, contuse the quadratus plantae muscle, and may even produce a neuropraxia of the lateral plantar nerve (which is chronically sheared between the pronating cuboid and the pad).

It is worth mentioning that some orthotic laboratories put this addition on all of their orthotics, claiming it supports the "lateral arch." For obvious reasons, this approach is discouraged.

SPORT-SPECIFIC VARIATIONS

Besides choosing from the previously listed additions, it is often necessary to further modify an orthotic so that it may accommodate the biomechanical demands associated with a specific sport. For example, a tennis player with a rearfoot varus deformity would be posted differently than a long distance runner with the same varus angulation. Basically, unidirectional sporting activities (such as walk-

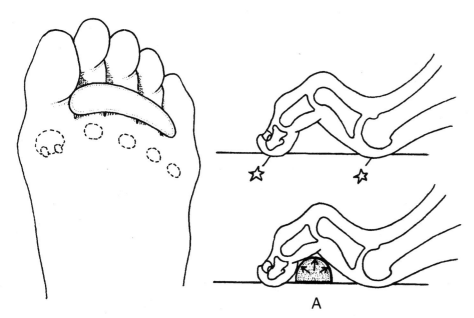

Figure 6.16. By supporting the entire digit (A), toe crests effectively reduce pressure beneath the metatarsal heads and distal digits *(stars).*

A

Figure 6.17.   The interdigital plug.

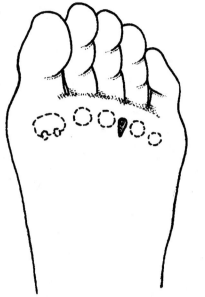
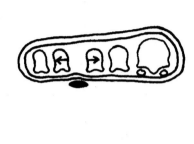

ing and running) are typically treated with semirigid shells with maximum amounts of rearfoot and if necessary, forefoot posting. If the running athlete strikes the ground in a toe-heel sequence, the rearfoot post should be placed beneath the forefoot and a compressible post to sulcus added. Also, in order to meet the training requirements of a long-distance runner, it is suggested that the medial longitudinal arch in these individuals be reinforced with either PPT or cork and that a compressible post to sulcus be used to protect against propulsive period injury.

Because weight of the orthotic is a legitimate concern to the running athlete (because of the length of the lever arm to the hip, each 100 g added to the foot increases the aerobic demands of running by 1% [22]), many distance runners prefer to train in the heavier thermoplastic orthoses and race in the lighter Plastazote or graphite laminates. Sprinting athletes also have specific needs in that they require control of the excessive rearfoot motions associated with speed work (contrary to previous reports, speed work is associated with an increase in rearfoot motion [2] that is worsened by the fact that racing flats are less able to control subtalar pronation [23]), while also requiring the ideal rearfoot/leg alignment necessary for the achilles tendon to maximally participate in an explosive propulsive period.

Because of these concerns, it is suggested that orthoses for these athletes incorporate large rearfoot posts with compressible posts extended beneath the metatarsal heads in order to more effectively control motion during early and late stance phase. In fact, to control the propulsive period motions for the longest possible time, Sisney (24) suggested extending the compressible posts all the way to the toes. Because of the limited space and extreme lasts frequently seen in racing flats, it is recommended that flats be sent to the laboratory for custom fitting of the orthotic.

Another unidirectional sport that requires accommo-

dation is race walking. Because of their extended length of stride, these athletes maintain their heels on the ground for such long periods that it is not uncommon for these individuals to require as much as 35° of ankle dorsiflexion to allow for noncompensated function. Since this range greatly exceeds the norm, the use of bilateral heel lifts has become the rule rather than the exception. As with other unidirectional sports, these individuals respond best to fully posted orthotics made from non-weight-bearing neutral position plaster casts.

When dealing with athletes involved in multidirectional sports, however, the exact opposite situation occurs. In order to allow for the various cuts, pivots and lateral movements necessary for these athletes to "feel" the playing surface, it is customary to use semi-weight-bearing impression techniques with minimal rearfoot posting (0° is the most common request) in conjunction with the soft Plastazote or leather shells (although graphite is an excellent alternative because of its ability to flex in the frontal plane). If necessary, the forefoot deformity may be fully or partially posted (i.e., while a forefoot valgus post may be essential for stability with lateral motions, a large forefoot varus post may irritate the distal first metatarsal shaft and possibly produce an inversion ankle sprain during the propulsive period). With multidirectional sports that include much jumping (e.g. basketball, volleyball, aerobics), full length top covers are used and additional shock absorbing materials are typically placed beneath the metatarsal heads and heel.

Golf is a multidirectional sport that provides an interesting biomechanical dilemma because of its asymmetrical requirements: the right foot of the right-handed player must be able to pronate through a large range during the end stage of the swing, while the left foot requires firm digital stabilization with protection against lateral instability (Fig. 6.18).

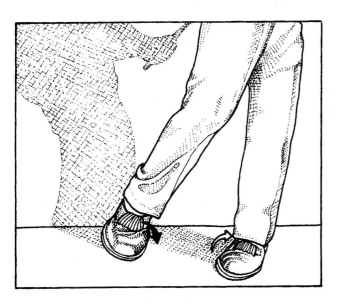

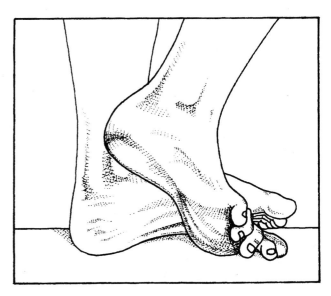

Figure 6.18. Foot motions during the end-stage of a golf stroke. Notice how the right foot is maximally pronated while the left foot is inverted with its digits clawing or grasp- ing in an attempt to gain a "toe hold." (Modified from photographs in Segesser B, Pforringer W (eds). The Shoe in Sport. Chicago: Yearbook Medical Publishers, 1989: 125.)

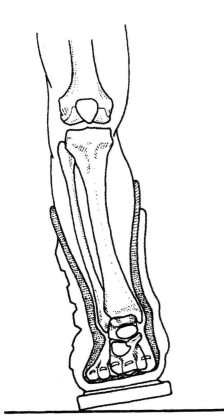

Figure 6.19. A tibial varum deformity will force the skier to stand on the outside of the ski. Witherel (28) noted that 80% of the ski community has this problem. (Adapted from Matheson GO, Macintyre JG. Lower leg varum alignment in skiing: relationship to foot pain and suboptimal performance. Phys Sports Med 1987; 15(9): 163.)

One method to accomplish this is to use a thermoplastic shell posted at 0° rearfoot bilaterally, with a kinetic wedge placed on the right orthoses (which allows for continued subtalar pronation during the drive) and toe crests added bilaterally to improve proprioception and stabilize the digits. If forefoot posts are indicated, a compressible post to sulcus should be used to distribute pressure onto the metatarsal heads. It should be mentioned that Williams and Cavanagh (25) believe that orthotics for golfers should be posted with the rearfoot in valgus in order to provide greater stability and reduce shear force during the swing. They suggested that the right-handed golfer have a lateral flare on the left shoe and a medial flare on the right shoe "to facilitate and support the rolling movements of the feet." While the concept of adding flares to improve stability has merit, the routine incorporation of rearfoot valgus posts cannot be recommended as it would most likely produce symptoms associated with excessive pronation.

Athletes involved in edge sports (such as skiing, hockey, and ice skating) typically require orthotic therapy to accommodate even mild varus deformity of the leg and foot. In a beautifully written article describing the biomechanical demands associated with skiing, Matheson and Macintyre (27) stated that the ski boot serves as a rigid mechanical extension of the lower leg that forces the individual with a tibial varum to ride on the lateral edge of the ski (Fig. 6.19). This predisposes to injury and/or poor performance in that the skier is more likely to fall by catching the outside edge. It also requires that turns be initiated with a hopping motion that serves to unlock the lateral edge.

The first step in accommodating the tibial varum is to make the appropriate correction in the cuff of the ski boot

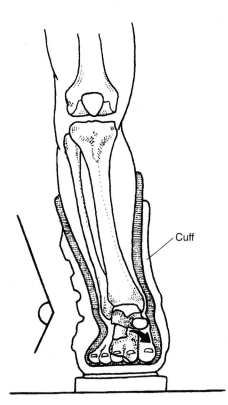

Figure 6.20.   The cuff of the ski boot may be angled laterally to accommodate a tibial varum. (Adapted from Matheson GO, Macintyre JG. Lower leg varum alignment in skiing: relationship to foot pain and suboptimal performance. Phys Sports Med 1987; 15(9): 163.)

(Fig. 6.20). Unfortunately, while this adjustment accommodates the bowed tibia, it also allows the subtalar joint to shift into its pronated position (arrow in Fig. 6.20). This is deleterious in that when standing in a functional ski position (knees flexed, ankles dorsiflexed), the body's center of gravity rests directly over the metatarsal heads and the tips and tails of the skis are controlled evenly throughout a turn via a continual shift of pressure between the heel and the metatarsal heads. In order to control the distal ends of the skis, the foot must function as a rigid beam with the subtalar joint being maintained in a neutral position with the midtarsal joint locked and stable.

If the subtalar joint is pronated, the midfoot will buckle as pressure is shifted from the heels to the metatarsal heads and the distal ends of the skis can only be controlled via great muscular effort (27). Furthermore, when the subtalar joint is maintained in a pronated position (which is amplified by tight-fitting ski boots which flatten the medial arch), it is often impossible to gain access to the inner edge of the ski without internally rotating the lower extremity and creating a valgus thrust at the knee (Fig. 6.21). This may result in faulty upper body rotation (the torso turns into the hill making counterrotation difficult), side slipping (the tail end of the ski often washes out due to unequal tip to tail pressure), excessive muscular effort and an increased po-

tential for retropatella arthralgia (which is extremely common in the ski community).

These problems may be avoided by prescribing an orthotic with full forefoot and rearfoot posting and minimal lowering of the medial longitudinal arch. Note that because there is no heel-strike in skiing, it is not necessary to allow the 6–8° of pronation necessary for normal shock absorption as the goal of orthotic therapy is to align the lower extremity so that a vertical line drawn from the midpoint of the patella falls directly over the second toe while the skier stands in a functional ski position. The fully posted orthotic, which should incorporate a compressible post to sulcus and a top cover to the toes, enables the skier to evenly pressure the tips and tails of the skis while also allowing for easier access to the inner edges of the skis (thereby lessening the potential for knee injury). To ensure the orthotic does not rock in the boot, the plantar surfaces of the forefoot and rearfoot posts should always rest on the same transverse plane.

This may be accomplished by placing the desired forefoot and rearfoot posts beneath the distal orthotic and then posting the rearfoot flat to stabilize the heel. Matheson and Macintyre (27) stated that the adequacy of the post angles may be tested by placing an additional varus wedge beneath the medial forefoot while the skier stands in a functional position. If the original post angles were insufficient, the skier would feel more stable with the added wedges.

Conversely, if the skier complains of discomfort or an outward rolling of the knees, the built-up orthotic is overposted. The authors claim that advanced skiers are remarkably sensitive to even subtle changes in post angulation. It is noteworthy that because they lack the angulation necessary to accommodate various forefoot/rearfoot deformities, the custom-molded orthotics sold in ski shops are of little value to the more advanced skier and/or individuals with significant varus deformity (27).

The biomechanical requirements associated with bike riding are similar to skiing in that because there is no heel-strike or toe off, the goal of treatment is to improve functional alignment of the patella and allow the foot to function as a rigid lever. The cyclist presenting with excessive subtalar pronation often demonstrates exaggerated medial deviation of the knee during the power stroke and chronic muscle fatigue in the arch secondary to an inability to effectively transfer forces through an unstable midtarsal joint. Treatment with an appropriately sized post will both improve functional alignment of the knee and allow for the locking of the midtarsal joint necessary for the foot to effectively transfer forces during the power stroke.

The improved biomechanical efficiency associated with properly posted orthotics was clearly demonstrated by Hice et al. (29), as they noted that the same five cyclists were able to consume less oxygen and maintain a lower heart rate as they performed at a given submaximal work

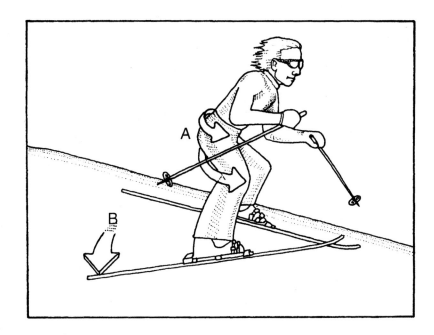

Figure 6.21. Excessive pronation results in an exaggerated internal rotation of the entire lower extremity and pelvis (A). While this may allow the medial edge of the ski to carve a turn, it is associated with a "washing-out" of the tail **(B)**, wider turns, and an increased sense of muscular effort, as the upper torso must counterrotate for the next turn. (Adapted from Matheson GO, Macintyre JG. Lower leg varum alignment in skiing: relationship to foot pain and suboptimal performance. Phys Sports Med 1987; 15(9): 163.)

rate while wearing orthotics. Because toe-clips maintain the forefoot in a fixed position with the center of pressure located directly beneath the metatarsal heads, it is important the desired rearfoot and forefoot posting be combined and placed beneath the forefoot with a compressible post to sulcus added to support the metatarsal heads. Note that because some cycling shoes have contoured bottoms, it may be necessary to have the cyclist switch to a different shoe. If this is a concern, it is possible to completely avoid using an in-shoe orthotic by adding a specifically designed replacement pedal.

Without doubt, the athletic activity that presents the most difficulties for orthotic management is ballet dancing. Because of the limited confines of the ballet slipper, it is necessary to fabricate an orthotic in which only the forefoot is posted. Allied OSI Laboratories (Indianapolis, IN) suggests using a semiflexible thermoplastic shell with an extrinsic forefoot post and suede top cover that is held in place with an elastic band and a thong. This orthotic, which may include metatarsal pads, bar posts, and/or balances for lesions (dancers frequently require balances beneath the first and fifth metatarsal heads), may be invaluable when treating metatarsal stress fractures, capsulitis, interdigital neuromas, and/or plantar fasciitis.

Of particular interest with regard to treating ballet dancers, Miller et al. (30) recently demonstrated that modifying a standard technique ballet shoe with 1/8-inch PPT extended from the heel to the metatarsals, 1/16-inch PPT extended under the toes, and a high PPT arch support was able to successfully redistribute pressure away from the overworked and often injured first and second metatarsal heads without compromising the dancer's subjective comfort and feel for the floor.

IN-OFFICE FABRICATION TECHNIQUES

So far, the discussion of orthotic fabrication has been limited primarily to the role of the commercial laboratory. However, it is also possible to use various in-office techniques to manufacture effective, inexpensive orthotics.

The most popular technique for manufacturing in-office orthoses is the direct mold method. This method requires heating a layered strip of Plastazote in a convection oven for approximately 7 minutes (the edges lift up and drop when the material is ready). The heated Plastazote is then placed on a block of high-density foam and directly molded to the patient's foot. (The patient is wearing a sock to prevent burns.) The formed Plastazote is then cut and ground into the desired shell shape and if indicated, various top covers, additions, balance for lesions and/or posts may then be added. It is important to note that the inherent compressibility of Plastazote dictates that forefoot and/or rearfoot posts be evaluated after 2 weeks of regular wear to determine the need for possible reinforcement. Because of the accommodative nature of the Plastazote, the direct mold orthoses are particularly effective when treating individuals with inflammatory arthritis or diabetes mellitus.

In fact, because of their tendency for plantar ulcerations, Mueller et al. (31) suggest that diabetics who are insensitive to a 5.07 Sems Weinstein monofilament, possess less than 5° ankle dorsiflexion or have less than 30° subtalar range of motion, should begin treatment with accommodative footwear designed to lessen plantar pressure points coupled with mobility exercises and education in foot protection methods.

In addition to treating arthritic and diabetic individuals, the direct mold Plastazote orthoses may also be helpful

Figure 6.22. The Biopedal (Biosports, Mill Valley, CA), which is used to replace the existing pedal, may provide up to 12° of forefoot varus or valgus angulation (A), 6° of in or out-toe positioning (B), and structural leg length discrepancies of up to 1 inch.

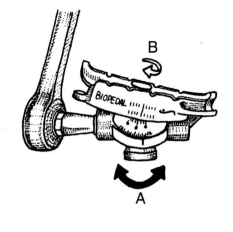

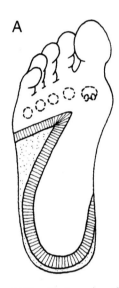 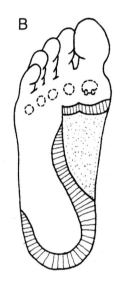 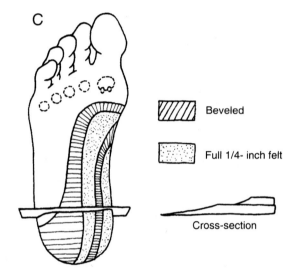

Figure 6.23. By tapering the edges of felt strips or Plasta-zote, paste-in orthotics may be used to treat forefoot valgus deformities (A), forefoot varus (B), and rearfoot varus defor- mities **(C).** (Modified from McPoil TC. The cobra pad–an or-thotic alternative for the physical therapist. J Orthop Sports Phys Ther 1983; 5(1): 30.)

in treating athletes involved in cutting sports (particularly basketball and soccer) where a more functional orthotic might not be tolerated. The only drawbacks to the direct mold methods are that they are time-consuming (they take anywhere from 25 minutes to 2 hours to fabricate, depending upon the individual's experience) and the process requires the use of noisy, fairly expensive machinery. Also, because the choice of materials is limited to the closed cell polyethylene foams (these are the only shells that will readily mold to the patient), the finished orthotics are not very durable and must be reevaluated every 6 months for possible reinforcement or replacement.

A simple alternative to the direct mold method is the paste-in technique. This technique involves shaping various accommodative materials (usually felt, Plastazote or PPT) into different posts and/or balances and then gluing these forms onto the bottom of an innersole (either the patient's present innersole or a generic Spenco or PPT innersole may be used). Figure 6.23 illustrates the more commonly used modifications.

Despite their relatively simple design, paste-in orthotics are able to effectively reduce both the range and speed of subtalar pronation (32, 33). As with direct mold techniques, these orthotics should be evaluated biannually for possible reinforcement or replacement.

References

1. McPoil TG, Adrian M, Pidcoe P. Effects of foot orthoses on center of pressure pattern in women. Phys Ther 1989; 69(2): 149.
2. Smith LS, Clarke TE, Hamill CL, Santopietro F. The effects of soft and semi-rigid orthoses upon rearfoot movement in running. J Am Podiatr Med Assoc 1986; 76(4): 227.
3. Lundeen RO. Polysectional triaxial posting. A new process for incorporating correction in foot orthoses. J Am Podiatr Med Assoc 1988; 78(2): 55.
4. Jorgensen U, Bojsen-Moller F. Shock absorbency of factors in the shoe/heel interaction--with special focus on role of the heel pad. Foot Ankle 1989; 9(11): 294.
5. Ross AS, Gurnick KL. Elevator selection in rearfoot posted orthoses. J Am Podiatr Assoc 1982; 72(12): 621.

6. Weed JH, Ratliff FD, Ross SA. Biplanar grind for rearfoot posts on functional orthoses. J Am Podiatr Assoc 1978; 69(1): 35.

7. Cavanagh PR. The shoe-ground interface in running. In: Mack RP (ed). Symposium on the Foot and Leg in Running Sports. St. Louis: CV Mosby, 1982: 30–44.

8. Blake RL, Common sports injuries and their treatment. In: Foot and Leg Function. Deer Park, NY: Langer Biomechanics Group, 1989; 1(3): 7.

9. Schuit D, Adrian M, Pidcoe P. Effects of heel lifts on ground reactive force patterns in subjects with structural leg length discrepancies. Phys Ther 1989; 69: 41–48.

10. Milgrom C, Giladi M, Kashton H, et al. A prospective study of the effect of a shock-absorbing orthotic device on the incidence of stress fractures in military recruits. Foot Ankle 1985; 6(2): 101.

11. Voloshin WJ. Low back pain: conservative treatment with artificial shock absorbers. Arch Phys Med Rehabil 1985; 66: 145.

12. McMahon TA, et al. Groucho running. J Appl Physiol 1987; 62: 326–337.

13. Nigg BM. Effect of viscoelastic shoe insoles on vertical impact forces in heel-toe running. Am J Sports Med 1988; 16(1): 70–76.

14. Lee KH, Shieh JC, Matteliano A, Smiehorowski T. Electromyographic changes of leg muscles in women: therapeutic implications. Arch Phys Med Rehabil 1990; 71: 31–33.

15. Nike Sport Research Review. Rearfoot stability. Beaverton, OR: Nike, Nov/Dec. 1989.

16. Bates BT, Osternig LR, Mason B, James SL. Lower extremity function during the support phase of running. In: Asmussen E, Jorgensen K (eds). Biomechanics VI. Baltimore: University Park Press, 1978.

17. Clark TE, Frederick EC, Hamill CL. The effect of shoe design on rearfoot control in running. Med Sci Sports Exerc 1983; 15: 376–381.

18. Stacoff A, Kaelin X. Pronation and sport shoe design. In: Nigg BM, Kerr BA (eds). Biomechanical Aspects of Sports Shoes and Playing Surfaces. Canada: University of Calgary:143–151.

19. Glover MG. Plantar warts. Foot Ankle 1990; 11(3): 172.

20. Dananberg HG. Letter to the editor. The kinetic wedge. J Am Podiatr Med Assoc 1988; 78(2).

21. Holmes GB, Jr, Timmerman L. A quantitative assessment of the effect of metatarsal pads on plantar pressures. Foot Ankle 1990; 11:141–145.

22. Frederick EC. The energy cost of load carriage on the feet during running. In: Winter DA, et al. (eds). Biomechanics IX. Champaign, IL. Hum Kinet 1985: 295–300.

23. Hamill J, Freedson PS, Boda W, Reichsman F. Effects of shoe type on cardiorespiratory responses and rearfoot motion during treadmill running. Med Sci Sports Exerc 1988; 20(5): 515.

24. Sisney P. Triathlons and associated injuries. In: Subotnick S (ed). Sports Medicine of the Lower Extremity. New York: Churchill Livingstone, 1989: 637.

25. Williams KR, Cavanagh PR. The mechanics of foot action during the golf swing and implications for shoe design. Med Sci Sports Exerc 1983; 15(3): 247.

26. Segesser B, Pforringer W (eds). The Shoe in Sport. Chicago: Yearbook Medical Publishers, 1989: 125.

27. Matheson GO, Macintyre JG. Lower leg varum alignment in skiing: relationship to foot pain and suboptimal performance. Phys Sports Med 1987; 15(9): 163.

28. Witherel W. If you can't ski parallel, cant. Skiing, January 1977.

29. Hice GA, Kendrick Z, Weeber K, Bray J. The effect of foot orthoses on oxygen consumption while cycling. J Podiatr Med Assoc 1985; 75(10): 513.

30. Miller CD, Paulos LE, Parker RD, Fishell M. The ballet technique shoe: a preliminary study of eleven differently modified ballet technique shoes using force and pressure plates. Foot Ankle 1990; 11(2): 97.

31. Mueller MJ, Diamond JE, Delitto A, Sinacore DR. Insensitivity, joint mobility and plantar ulcers in patients with diabetes mellitus. Phys Ther 1989; 69: 453–458.

32. Nigg BM, Luthis, Segesser A, et al. Sportschuhkorrekturen. Ein biomechanicsher Vergleich von drei verschiedenen. Sportschuhkorrekturen Z Orthop 1982; 120: 34–39.

33. Clarke TE, Frederick EC, Hlavac HF. Effects of a soft orthotic device on rearfoot movement in running. Podiatr Sports Med 1983; 1(1): 20.

34. McPoil TC. The cobra pad–an orthotic alternative for the physical therapist. J Orthop Sports Phys Ther 1983; 5(1): 30.

Chapter Seven

Orthotic Dispensing, Shoe Gear, and Clinical Problem-Solving

ORTHOTIC DISPENSING

On receiving the orthotics from the laboratory, the practitioner should evaluate the finished posts to make sure that they match the requested angles. Although this is difficult with an extrinsic forefoot post, and impossible with an intrinsic forefoot post, the accuracy of the rearfoot post may be determined by pressing a finger into the center of the heel cup and noting how far the distal medial edge of the orthotic raises from the table: a 4° rearfoot post will raise the edge approximately 7 mm. If the orthotics are to be worn in dress shoes with curved shanks, the accuracy of the laboratory's posting elevator can be determined by placing the heel of the orthotic on a variable height platform (a deck of cards works well) and noting the amount of heel lift necessary for the extrinsic post to rest flat while the distal orthotic shell just barely contacts the supporting surface. Of course, the orthotic should also be evaluated in the shoe to ensure proper anterior-posterior stability.

The next step is to place the orthotic against the patient's foot and evaluate all contours. If the orthotic shell extends more than 1 cm proximal to the first metatarsal head, it will most likely be a source of future irritation and should accordingly be shaved down. The patient is then asked to stand on the orthotic and gently move through a full range of inversion and eversion. Painful contact points around the heel cup or medial edge may have to be filed down. (Every practitioner should own a small dremel.)

With the patient still standing on the orthotic, talonavicular congruency should be evaluated, and the head of the talus should project just medially to the navicular acetabulum. Note that it is not uncommon for the patient to state that he or she still "feels pronated." In these cases, it is necessary to explain how the orthotic must allow enough pronation for shock absorption and how an orthotic is actually more effective at controlling motion during dynamic function than during static stance (1).

Regardless of whether the prescribed orthotic is functional, accommodative, direct mold, or paste-in, the finished device will alter functional interactions along the entire kinetic chain and/or produce a redistribution of plantar foot pressures. Because of this, the patient should be told to expect minor aches and pains during the first few weeks of wear and that the orthotic should be broken-in gradually, i.e., the orthotic should be worn for 1 hour the first day, 2 hours the second day, 3 hours the third day, etc., until it can be worn for 8 consecutive hours without discomfort. After that, the orthotic may be worn constantly.

Depending on the type of orthotic and the degree of posting used, it is possible to anticipate the location of potential problem spots and to caution the patient accordingly. For example, a rigid orthotic with a large rearfoot varus post is more likely to produce lateral knee and ankle discomfort, while an orthotic with a large forefoot valgus post is more likely to produce soleus strain. If these or other symptoms do develop despite the gradual break-in, the patient should be told to decrease wearing time to a point at which there is no discomfort and then to increase wearing time again gradually by approximately 1/2 hr/day.

As might be expected, rigid orthotics with large posts are more difficult to break-in than the softer, unposted accommodative orthotics. In fact, it is often possible to completely bypass the break-in process when prescribing accommodative orthotics. It is of clinical interest that individuals who proceed through the break-in period without incident are more likely to have a favorable prognosis (2).

In order for the patient to fully tolerate the orthotic, it may be necessary to begin a treatment program that incorporates various manipulative and physiological therapeutics. Although this approach may be essential for treating functional foot deformities and equinus conditions, the routine use of ultrasound, electric muscle stimulation, and foot exercises are of questionable value, as Donatelli et al. (2) demonstrated that individuals treated with these therapies plus orthotics had the same success rate as individuals treated with orthotics alone.

A similar observation was noted by Awbrey et al. (3), as they discovered that ice, stretches, and shin curl exercises were ineffective in the treatment of plantar fasciitis (7 of 7 patients treated showed no change in symptoms after 3 months) while individuals treated with off-the-shelf stock orthoses presented with a 50% reduction in pain after 1 month, a 90–95% reduction after 3 months, and no pain at 6 months. This study was particularly interesting in that it demonstrated that lidocaine/cortisone injections were not as effective as stock orthotics (2 of 7 treatment failures with injections alone) and that the combined use of injections and orthotics showed no significant improvement over the use of orthoses alone.

SHOE GEAR

Possibly the most important factor to consider when fabricating an orthotic is that the orthotics are only as functional as the shoes in which they are worn. As demonstrated by McPoil et al. (4), a well- designed shoe, even without an orthotic, has the ability to favorably alter the center of pressure recordings in individuals with forefoot varus deformities. Unfortunately, the reverse of this is also true, in that a poorly designed shoe may serve as an extrinsic source of pronation. Because of this, the patient should be educated as to the proper choice of shoe gear.

The more important qualities to look for in a shoe include a firm, deep heel counter that closely contours the patient's calcaneus (this may require adding felt to the inner aspects of the heel counter), a strong shank that does not flex upon weight-bearing (the shank is the section of the shoe that corresponds to the medial longitudinal arch), and a spacious toe box that does not compress the metatarsal heads (Fig. 7.1).

When being fit for a shoe, the patient's larger foot should be measured (oddly enough, a study of 125 individuals indicated that the foot opposite the dominant hand is the larger of the two in almost 80% of those evaluated [5]), and the length of the shoe should be determined by the position of the metatarsal heads: the widest portion of the shoe should parallel the bisection of the metatarsal heads. If the patient has an Egyptian foot-type with its long first toe (note that this refers to the length of the big toe, not to the length of the first metatarsal), then the distal toe box should be evaluated to make sure that it is not compressing the hallux, which if it happens might precipitate a hallux abductovalgus deformity. Also, to allow for adequate frontal plane stability, the plantar surface of the heel should be fairly wide (unlike most women's dress shoes) and should be replaced when excessive signs of wear are present. The patient should always be informed that the orthotic may not significantly change wear patterns (which are secondary to abrasion and not vertical forces) and may actually increase varus wear when a large rearfoot varus post is used (1).

In addition to choosing from the various stock changes in shoe design, certain cases require that a given shoe be modified by a cobbler in order to better accommodate a specific foot type. The more common modifications are detailed in Figure 7.2.

Whenever possible, the patient should be encouraged

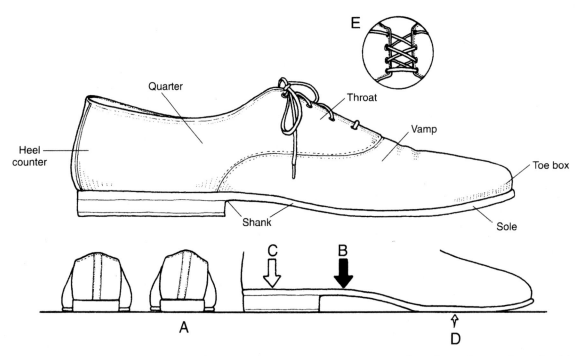

Figure 7.1. Components of a well-made shoe. The heel counter should fit securely (it may be necessary to balance Haglund's deformity with felt), and its bisection should be vertical to the supporting surface. (Poor quality control often allows for an asymmetrical heel counter that is either inverted or everted relative to the table top; see **A**). Also, the shank should be able to resist forceful compression without deforming **(B)**, and it should be angled in such a way that when the heel seat is compressed **(C)**, the plantar forefoot lifts no more than a few millimeters **(D)**. (A-P instability is present if the forefoot lifts more than this.) The toe box should provide ample space so as not to compress a dorsomedial or lateral bunion. Because it allows for greater separation of the upper, Blucher lacing may be necessary to accommodate the bulkier orthoses **(E)**. If the patient complains that his or her foot is sliding forward on the orthotic (which often occurs when heel lifts are used), a strip of adhesive felt may be placed along the undersurface of the tongue that gently presses the foot posteriorly onto the orthotic, thereby preventing slippage and improving control.

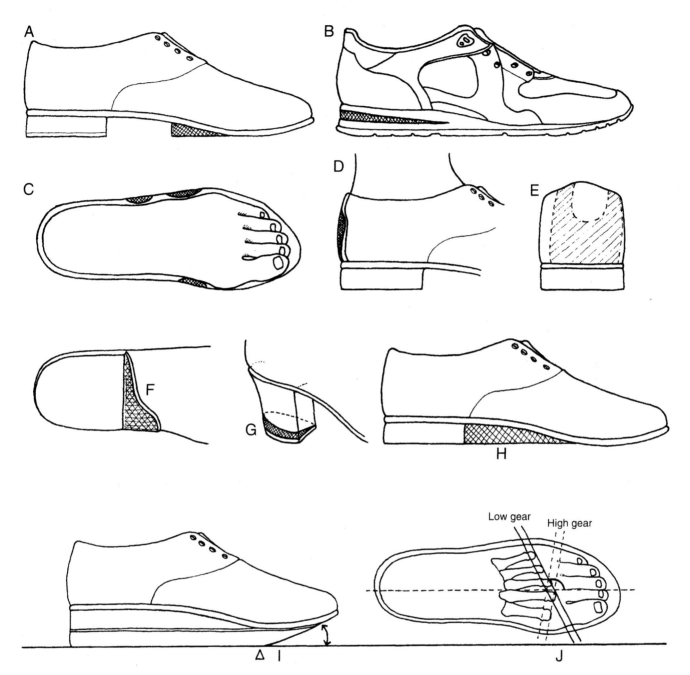

Figure 7.2. Shoe modification. (A) By supporting the metatarsal necks, a Thomas bar may decrease pressure beneath the metatarsal heads. **(B)** A Schuster heel wedge is useful when heel lifts greater than 7 mm are required. **(C–E)** Decompression pads may be used to distribute pressure away from a variety of bony prominences (including dorsomedial and lateral bunions and Haglund's deformity). **(F)** A wing-heel may be added to reinforce the medial heel while a varus wedge may also be incorporated into the heel itself **(G).** (Note that external modifications of shoes are not as effective at controlling motion as in-shoe orthoses [6].) **(H)** An overly flexible shank may be reinforced with a filler material while the addition of a rocker-bottom **(I)** allows the patient to proceed through the propulsive period without bending the metatarsophalangeal joints. (This modification is often essential when treating hallux rigidus deformities.) The final modification requires making cuts in the sole of the shoe in order to encourage a high or low gear push-off **(J):** A high gear push-off should be encouraged in an individual with a rigid forefoot valgus and recalcitrant interdigital neuritis while a low gear push-off should be encouraged in an individual with a hallux abductovalgus deformity associated with excessive propulsive period pronation.

to wear running shoes, as advances in materials technology coupled with large variation in shoe design allows for accommodation of a wider variety of foot types. For example, the practitioner may recommend either curved or straight-lasted sneakers in order to accommodate a metatarsus adductus or metatarsus rectus (Fig. 7.3). The practitioner should also make recommendations for either slip-, combination-, or board-lasted sneakers (Fig. 7.4).

The use of sneakers is also preferable to shoes because it is possible to modify subtalar motion at heel strike by choosing from different density midsoles, e.g., Frederick

(8) notes a direct correlation between midsole durometer (density) and the range of subtalar pronation (Fig. 7.5).

Because softer midsoles improve shock absorption while the firmer midsoles more effectively control motion, it has become standard practice for manufacturers to combine a softer lateral midsole with a firmer medial midsole. Referred to as a duodensity midsole, the softer material on the lateral side softens impact forces and decreases the initial velocity of pronation while the firmer material on the medial side provides protection against excessive pronation. The duodensity midsole essentially creates a functional

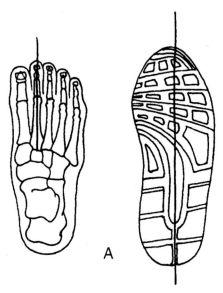
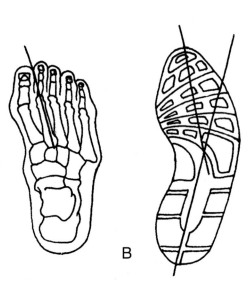

Figure 7.3. The last refers to the foot-shaped high-density polyethylene mold that a shoe is constructed around. At present, shoes are either straight or curve-lasted. A straight-lasted shoe is well-aligned in the forefoot and rearfoot and should be recommended for individuals with rectus foot types **(A).** On the contrary, curve-lasted shoes are angled medially at the forefoot and should be recommended only for individuals with metatarsus adductus **(B).** (The inadvertent use of a curve-lasted shoe by an individual with a metatarsus rectus most often results in a painful adventitious bursa forming over the dorsolateral fifth metatarsal head.)

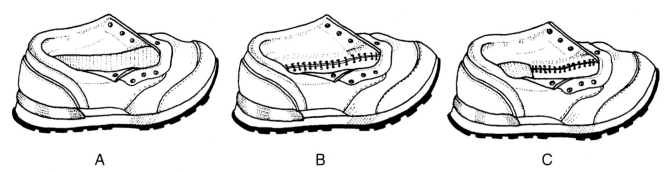

Figure 7.4. A board-lasted shoe (A) has a hard fibrous board on its inner surface that provides stability and is more appropriate for individuals who overpronate (7). Unfortunately, the board-lasted shoe is stiffer and may precipitate an achilles tendon injury. In a slip-lasted shoe **(B),** the upper is stitched into a one-piece moccasin and then glued to the sole. These shoes provide less stability but are lighter, more flexi-ble, and roomier in the toe box (making them an excellent choice for individuals with cavus foot types). The combination last shoe **(C)** provides the best of both worlds by providing rearfoot stability with a board-lasted heel while maintaining flexibility with a slip-lasted forefoot. This is a nice combination when treating individuals with rearfoot varus deformities.

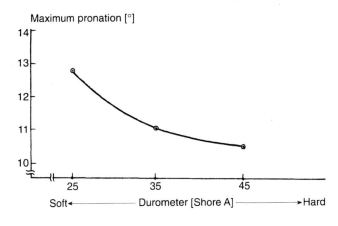

Figure 7.5. Relationship between midsole density and maximum pronation. (Adapted from Frederick EC. The Running Shoe: Dilemmas and Dichotomies in Design. In: Segesser B, Pforringer W (eds). The Shoe in Sport. Chicago: Yearbook Medical Publishers, 1989: 31.)

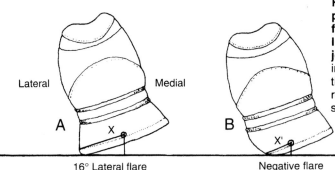

16° Lateral flare   Negative flare

Figure 7.6 Although the overall range of pronation will remain unchanged, a large lateral flare (A) provides ground-reactive forces with a longer lever arm (X) for pronating the subtalar joint at heel strike. This feature produces significant increases in the initial range and velocity of pronation. Note that a midsole with a negative flare (B) provides ground-reactive forces with a shorter lever arm (X') for pronating the subtalar joint.

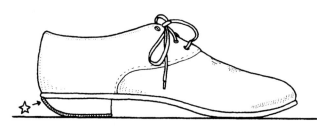

Figure 7.7. The negative posterior heel flare.

rearfoot varus post that has been proven to be effective in controlling rearfoot motion at heel-strike (9).

In addition to choosing from different density midsoles, the amount of subtalar pronation present during the contact period may also be modified by varying the amount of lateral heel flare. As demonstrated by Nigg and Morlock (10), a large lateral flare increases the length of the lever arm between the subtalar joint axis and the ground, which produces a concomitant increase in both the range and speed of initial subtalar joint pronation (Fig. 7.6A). The authors also demonstrated that a negative flare effectively lessens the length of the lever arm (X' in Fig. 7.6B), which produces a concomitant decrease in the range and speed of initial pronation .

The same biomechanical principle applies to the negative posterior flare (Fig. 7.7), in that it shortens the lever arm between the ankle joint axis and the ground, thereby lessening the velocity and range of initial ankle

plantarflexion during heel-strike. (This modification should be considered in all recreational and competitive walkers as a method of reducing strain on the anterior compartment musculature.) It is also important to note that while a large lateral flare may initially increase velocity of pronation, a large medial flare effectively reduces the range of pronation by acting as a physical barrier that blocks excessive motion (8). This is also true of sneakers that have extra midsole material placed directly beneath the medial longitudinal arch (11).

One of the most important qualities of a sneaker is that the heel counter securely stabilize the rearfoot. In addition to maintaining the fat pad (which protects the plantar calcaneus from injury), a well-formed heel counter has the ability to lessen musculoskeletal transients, decrease activity in the quadriceps and triceps surae musculature, and reduce VO_2 (12). In addition, the deeper heel counters present in most running shoes allow for a better fit with the orthotic. (Note that the stock insole present when the sneaker is purchased should be removed, as it may adversely tilt or angle the orthotic.)

The final stock modification that makes running shoes preferable to a standard shoe is the upward curve of the distal midsole (Fig. 7.8). Referred to as a toe-spring, the superior angulation of the midsole basically represents a modified rocker bottom that serves to shorten the functional length of the shoe while also allowing the metatarsophalangeal joint to move through a lessened range of motion

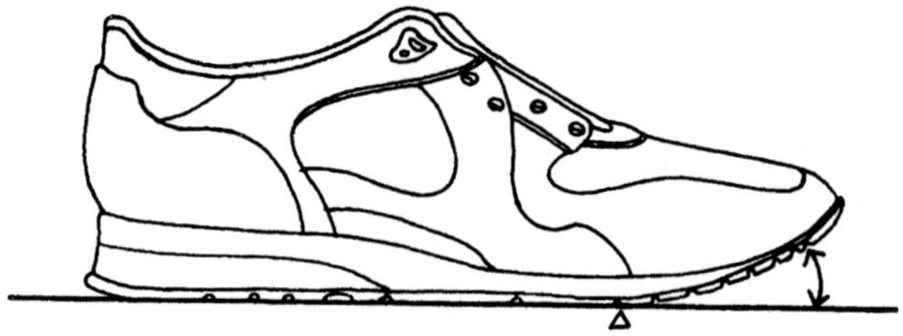

Figure 7.8. Many running shoes have a superior angulation of the distal midsole that allows for a more efficient propulsive period.

during propulsion. Because of these improvements, this modification is invaluable in the treatment of achilles tendinitis, plantar fasciitis, metatarsal stress syndrome, and/or hallux limitus/rigidus.

In all cases, the practitioner should try to match the patient's foot type to a specific shoe. For example, patients with rigid foot types typically respond best to slip-lasted sneakers with the softest possible midsoles. Because of their ability to decrease both the range and velocity of subtalar pronation at heel strike, individuals with a rearfoot varus deformity respond best to a combination last sneaker with a duodensity midsole, a 30° medial flare, and a negative lateral flare. (Because they are not yet commercially available, it is necessary that the lateral flare be modified either in-office or by sending the sneakers to an orthotic laboratory.)

For patients presenting with extreme ranges of calcaneal eversion (e.g., individuals with large forefoot varus deformities or obese patients with hypermobile flatfeet), additional support may be afforded by a midsole that is reinforced beneath the medial longitudinal arch, coupled with a plastic external heel stabilizer. Although Nigg et al. (13) demonstrated that an external heel stabilizer may actually increase the initial velocity of pronation, this fact does not

outweigh the beneficial effect of a stable, vertical heel counter.

CLINICAL PROBLEM-SOLVING

Regardless of how thorough your evaluation is, there will always be cases in which a patient's response to treatment is less than wonderful. Fortunately, it is frequently possible to determine in advance which patients will respond poorly to treatment, as the majority of these individuals will have large rearfoot and/or forefoot deformities, rigid cavus foot types (which are notoriously difficult to treat), congenitally limited amounts of ankle dorsiflexion (equinus conditions often defy orthotic management), and/or advanced stages of soft tissue damage (which is often difficult to resolve even with the most thorough rehabilitative procedures). Patients with these problems should always be informed in advance that the orthotic may not produce a substantial reduction in symptomatology and that it is in no way a cure-all. (However, there is always the pleasant exception to these rules in which a patient with large structural deformity and seemingly untreatable amounts of soft tissue degeneration will have a complete resolution of all symptoms.)

Unfortunately, there are also other instances in which patients with seemingly manageable deformities are unable to wear their orthotics for more than a few hours without discomfort. Although the list of possible causes for treatment failure is long (and would include faulty measurements during evaluation, poor casting techniques, laboratory error, incorrect selection of materials, and/or unanticipated proprioceptive deficits that are not responding to the rehabilitative program), it is often possible to determine the source of the problem by relating the location of the discomfort to the specifics of the patient's foot type and the type of orthotic fabricated.

Table 7.1 (adapted from ref. 14) relates specific prob-

Table 7.1 [a]
SPECIFIC PROBLEMS: PROBABLE CAUSES AND CORRECTIVE ACTIONS

Location of Discomfort	Possible Causes and Rationale	Corrective Action
Bunion pain increases with use of orthotic.	a. Large rearfoot/forefoot varus post lifting the medial forefoot (and bunion) into shoe gear.	a. Reevaluate need for posting. If the post angles are correct, have laboratory grind the posts to the shell. This lowers the overall height of the orthotic without affecting function. Another method of treatment is to have a cobbler stretch the leather over the bunion or switch to shoe with wider toe box.

Location of Discomfort	Possible Causes and Rationale	Corrective Action
Sesamoid pain continues despite use of orthotic.	a. Not enough rearfoot control; the patient continues to pronate excessively, thereby compressing the sesamoids.	a. Consider increasing post angles and/or using a more controlling orthotic. To control propulsive period pronation, the rearfoot posts may be placed beneath the distal edge of the orthotic, and the soles of the shoes may be cut to allow for low gear push-off.
Sesamoid pain develops with orthotic.	a. Orthotic too long. b. Large forefoot valgus post causing forefoot to slide medially.	a. Return to laboratory for adjustment or simply taper the distal edge in office. b. Reevaluate need for post. If the post is correct, use Spenco top to prevent slippage.
Distal end of orthotic extension (particulary those that end at sulcus).	a. Overly sensitive soft tissues.	a. Have patient wear thick socks until the soft tissues can accommodate the extension or simply taper the plantar surface of the extension. Another consideration is to have the patient rest a flat Spenco insert over the orthotic. (This also serves to cushion the toes.)
Dorsal 5th metatarsal head.	a. Large forefoot valgus post lifting lateral forefoot into shoe gear. b. A large forefoot varus post causing the patient to slide laterally off the orthotic, jamming the 5th metatarsal head into the shoe. c. Incorrect use of a curve-lasted shoe in patient with rectus foot type.	a. Have cobbler stretch shoe gear over 5th metatarsal head (especially if a tailor's bunion is present). b. Reevaluate post angles: if correct, consider adding Spenco top cover to prevent slippage or have patient insert felt strip under tongue of shoe. c. Switch to straight-lasted shoe.
Dorsal first metatarsophalangeal joint pain and/or first interphalangeal joint pain develops with orthotic.	a. Incorrect use of a forefoot varus post. The posting material prevents the normal plantarflectory motions of the first metatarsal necessary for a full range of hallux dorsiflexion. The interphalangeal joint may be injured as it hyperextends to compensate for the limited metatarsophalangeal joint motion.	a. Reevaluate need for forefoot varus post.

Table 7.1 —*continued*

Location of Discomfort	Possible Causes and Rationale	Corrective Action
	b. Incorrect use of Morton's extension, which also limits the plantarflectory movements of the first metatarsal.	b. Reevaluate need for Morton's extension.
	c. Cast was taken with forefoot supinated.	c. Recast patient.
Interdigital neuritis continues despite use of orthotic.	a. Suspect double-crush syndrome from entrapment in tarsal tunnel or spine (particularly if the interdigital pain is bilateral).	a. Order appropriate diagnostic tests.
	b. Patient continues to wear tight-fitting shoes or overly flexible shoes that allow for a range of digital dorsiflexion that tractions the interdigital nerve against the transverse ligament.	b. Switch to shoes with a more spacious toe box and stiffer soles that lessen the range of digital dorsiflexion. Also, subtle changes in the position of metatarsal pad may have a dramatic effect on reducing interdigital pain.
Medial arch pain develops with orthotic.	a. Rearfoot varus posting is too high.	a. Reevaluate need for posting. Consider softer posting material.
	b. Inadequate strength, flexibility, and/or proprioception.	b. Increase frequency of treatments and/or home rehab procedures.
	c. Incorrect choice of material (particularly if rigid shell is used for rigid foot type).	c. Consider changing materials or add soft top cover to present orthotic.
	d. Full arch height used with equinus foot type: as the midtarsals attempt to compensate for limited ankle dorsiflexion, the plantar medial arch is compressed into the orthotic.	d. Add temporary bilateral heel lifts, have laboratory lower the medial longitudinal arch, and/or use softer materials.
	e. Negative impression is taken with the subtalar joint supinated.	e. Have laboratory lower arch. Consider recasting patient.
Medial border of orthotic digging into soft tissues.	a. Laboratory error: failure to lower arch for equinus foot type.	a. Have laboratory lower arch, add bilateral heel lifts, and/or use softer orthotics.
	b. Inadequate shoe gear: patient rolling over orthotic.	b. Change shoe gear and/or remake orthotic with medial flange.
	c. Inadequate levels of proprioception and/or muscle strength.	c. Address with appropriate rehabilitation techniques.
	d. Overweight patient with a large genu valgum.	d. Remake orthotic with medial flange, reinforce shoe gear, strengthen intrinsic musculature.

Location of Discomfort	Possible Causes and Rationale	Corrective Action
Plantar fascial/medial arch discomfort continues despite use of orthotic.	a. Too little control or tissues too inflamed to tolerate a functional orthotic. b. Inadequate strength/ flexibility and/or proprioception. c. Incorrect diagnosis of mechanical foot pain. The seronegative spondylo-arthropathies often produce symptoms at the medial tuberosity of the calcaneus.	a. Consider using more functional orthotic and/or use low-dye taping procedures with orthotic. b. Increase frequency of treatment and/or home rehabilitation procedures. **Consider night brace.** c. Request appropriate labora-tory tests.
Plantar first metatarsal shaft pain at distal end of orthotic.	a. Large rearfoot/forefoot varus post lifting medial orthotic into first metatarsal. b. Laboratory error, the medial distal edge of device too long.	a. Reevaluate need for post-ing: if correct, have patient wear thick pair of socks until soft tissues accommodate new stress or send to laboratory and add a compressible post to sulcus. (This distributes weight off the metatarsal necks onto the metatarsal heads.) b. Return to laboratory for adjustment (or just grind edge down in office).
Tissues over metatarsal pad become uncomfortable.	a. Normal part of break-in as tissues accommodate new stresses. b. Metatarsal pads too large or poorly positioned, creating bowstring effect on central band of plantar fascia.	a. Proceed more slowly with break-in and/or wear thick pair of socks. b. Return to laboratory for smaller and/or softer pads, or for repositioning.
Tarsometatarsal pain after using balance for lesion beneath a painful metatarsal head.	a. Normal part of break-in. b. Balance too deep, allowing for excessive plantarflexion of involved metatarsal head (thereby straining the proximal tarsometatarsal articulation).	a. Proceed more slowly with break-in. b. Have laboratory partially fill balance, remove if necessary.
Medial, posterior, and/or lateral heel pain at edge of heel cup.	a. If the laboratory does not allow for sufficient displacement of calcaneal fat pad when modifying the positive model of an off-weight-bearing impression, the edge of the orthotic heel seat will become a source of chronic irritation as it digs into the displacing soft tissues. Also, shoes with	a. Initially, make sure the shoe's heel counter is firm and snug (consider adding felt to the inside of heel counter) and feather the edge of heel seat at point of irritation. If necessary, return to laboratory for modifi-cation (always pinpoint the painful area by marking the edge) and consider

Table 7.1 —*continued*

Location of Discomfort	Possible Causes and Rationale	Corrective Action
	inadequate heel counters may allow for excessive displacement of the fat pad and may therefore be a source of chronic discomfort at the edge of the orthotic.	requesting a deeper heel seat to allow for improved containment of the fat pad.
Plantar-lateral surface of calcaneus.	a. This is frequently a normal part of the break-in process, as a rearfoot varus post will redistribute a greater percentage of **vertical** forces toward the lateral heel.	a. Proceed more slowly through break-in. If discomfort continues, reevaluate need for rearfoot posting or use softer material for shell or post.
Plantar-medial surface of calcaneus.	a. Too little control. (The patient continues to pronate excessively, jamming the medial condyle into orthotic.)	a. Increase post angle, check shoe gear, strengthen gastrocnemius/soleus and **tibialis posterior**.
	b. Too much control (Overposting with rearfoot varus wedge will compress and irritate the medial plantar heel.)	b. Reevaluate post angle; consider softer posting material.
	c. Heel height of orthotic is shifting weight to the forefoot, thereby stressing plantar fascia and, in turn, its origin on the medial tuberosity.	c. Test by having patient walk on toes for 30 sec: if heel symptoms increase, remove heel lifts and grind the rearfoot posts into the shells.
Lateral heel pain at edge of heel cup.	a. Patient slides off orthotic secondary to large varus post.	a. Reevaluate need for post. Consider adding Spenco cover to prevent slippage. Also, check fit of heel counter.
Achilles tendinitis develops or continues, despite use of the orthotic.	a. Orthotic under- or over-posted with resultant misalignment of rearfoot and leg.	a. Reevaluate post angles.
	b. Failure to lower medial arch for equinus foot type; this increases work load on the achilles tendon as midtarsal compensation is disallowed.	b. Lower medial arch of orthotic, add bilateral heel lifts, and/or use softer orthotics.
	c. contracture of triceps surae	c. increase stretching, consider night brace
Soleus strain develops with orthotic.	a. Incorrect use of forefoot valgus post: the faulty post is prematurely locking the midtarsal joint prior to heel lift, thereby preventing the rearfoot from inverting to	a. Remove post and stretch soleus.

Location of Discomfort	Possible Causes and Rationale	Corrective Action
	its vertical position. The soleus muscle is constantly strained as it attempts to bring the rearfoot to vertical by lifting the entire medial foot up and over the oversized forefoot valgus post.	
Medial tibial stress reaction continues despite use of orthotic.	a. Too little control.	a. Reevaluate post angles, orthotic selection (consider more controlling orthotic), shoe gear, and casting technique. (Consider neutral position technique.)
	b. Inadequate amounts of strength, flexibility, and/or proprioception.	b. Reevaluate treatment program.
	c. Problem not mechanical, rule out vascular disorder. (Note: If thrombophlebitis is present, a blood pressure cuff wrapped around the calf will produce pain when inflated to 40–80 mm Hg. Myositis will not produce pain even when the cuff is inflated to 120 mm Hg.)	c. Reevaluate patient; consider referral if necessary.
Peroneus longus and/or brevis discomfort develops with orthotic.	a. Normal part of break-in as peroneals attempt to accommodate rearfoot varus post.	a. Slow down break-in and incorporate peroneal stretches.
	b. Excessive rearfoot varus post straining peroneus brevis as it attempts to bring the subtalar joint back to its neutral position	b. Reevaluate post angles.
	c. Incorrect use of forefoot varus post: the faulty post inverts forefoot during late midstance, thereby unlocking the midtarsal joint. Peroneus longus, by virtue of its insertion into the base of the first metatarsal, attempts to stabilize the midtarsals by forcefully plantarflexing the first metatarsal (which would evert the forefoot and lock the midtarsal joint). However, resistance from the post prevents this action and is thereby responsible for chronically straining this muscle.	c. Remove post.

Table 7.1 —*continued*

Location of Discomfort	Possible Causes and Rationale	Corrective Action
Medial knee (typically a pes anserine bursitis) and/or retropatella discomfort continue despite use of orthotic.	a. Too little control; the subtalar joint continues to pronate excessively. This most frequently results from use of an overly flexible shell with a hypermobile foot type and/or inadequate shoe gear.	a. Reevaluate post angles. Consider a more controlling orthotic and check shoe gear (especially the fit of the heel counter).
High-impact symptoms continue, despite use of orthotic.	a. Inadequate posting of rigid forefoot valgus/plantar-flexed first ray, allowing for continued supinatory compensation by the subtalar joint.	a. Increase post angles as needed and consider adding shock-absorbing material beneath the heel.
High-impact symptoms develop with orthotic: typically, lateral knee pain (a diffuse bony ache) and/or chronic sacroiliac instability.	a. Normal part of break-in as tissues attempt to accommodate new stresses b. Too much control: the orthotic is disallowing the amount of subtalar pronation necessary to absorb shock. This may result from excessive rearfoot/forefoot varus posting, faulty casting technique (especially if subtalar joint was supinated), and/or incorrect choice of materials, e.g., a rigid orthotic was used to treat a rigid foot type.	a. Proceed more slowly with break-in. b. Reevaluate post angles, consider having lab lower the medial arch (or recast), and/or switch to a softer orthotic.

*a*Langer S. Orthotic adjustments ready-reference guide. Langer Biomechanics Newsletter. Deer Park, NY: Langer Biomechanics Group, 1987; 14(2): 4.

lems to probable causes and corrective actions. While the list may seem intimidating in size, remember that break-in problems requiring more than changes in shoe gear are relatively uncommon and are readily avoided as the practitioner becomes proficient with the principles of biomechanics and orthotic fabrication.

References

1. Novick A, Kelley DL. Position and movement changes of the foot with orthotic intervention during the loading response of gait. J Orthop Sports Phys Ther 1990; 11(7): 301–312.
2. Donatelli R, Hulbert C, Conaway D, St. Pierre R. Biomechanical foot orthoses: a retrospective study. J Orthop Sports Phys Ther 1988; 10(6): 211.
3. Awbrey BJ, Bernardone JJ, Connolly TJ. The prospective evaluation of invasive and non-invasive treatment protocols for plantar fasciitis. Rehabil Res Dev Prog Rep 1989; 50.
4. McPoil TG, Adrian M, Pidcoe P. Effects of foot orthoses on center of pressure patterns in women. Phys Ther 1989; 69(2): 149.
5. Baum I, Spencer A. Limb dominance: its relationship to foot length. J Am Podiatr Assoc 1980; 70(10): 505–507.
6. Rose GK. Correction of the pronated foot. J Bone Joint Surg (Br) 1962; 44: 642.
7. McKenzie DC, Clement DB, Taunton JE. Running shoes, orthotics and injuries. Sports Med 1985; 2: 334–347.
8. Frederick EC. The running shoe: dilemmas and dichotomies in design. In: Segesser B, Pforringer W (eds). The Shoe in Sport. Chicago: Yearbook Medical Publishers, 1989: 31.
9. Nigg BM, Bahlsen HA. The influence of running velocity and

midsole hardness on external impact forces in heel-toe running. Int J Sports Biomech 1988; 4: 205–219.

10. Nigg BM, Morlock M. The influence of lateral heel flare of running shoes on pronation and impact forces. Med Sci Sports Exerc 1987; 19(3): 294.

11. Hamill J, Freedson PS, Boda W. Reichsman F. Effects of shoe type on cardiorespiratory responses and rearfoot motion during treadmill running. Med Sci Sports Exerc 1988; 20(5): 515.

12. Jorgenson J. Body in heel-strike running: the effect of a firm heel counter. Am J Sports Med 1990; 18:177–181.

13. Nigg BM, et al. Effect of viscoelastic shoe insoles on vertical forces in heel-toe running. Am J Sports Med 1988; 16(1): 70–76.

14. Langer S. Orthotic adjustments ready-reference guide. Langer Biomechanics Newsletter. Deer Park, NY: Langer Biomechanics Group, 1987; 14(2): 4.

Index

Page numbers in italics denote figures; those followed by "t" denote tables.